Bodies and Barriers

Literature and Medicine
MARTIN KOHN AND CAROL DONLEY, EDITORS

1. *Literature and Aging: An Anthology*
   EDITED BY MARTIN KOHN, CAROL DONLEY, AND DELESE WEAR

2. *The Tyranny of the Normal: An Anthology*
   EDITED BY CAROL DONLEY AND SHERYL BUCKLEY

3. *What's Normal? Narratives of Mental and Emotional Disorders*
   EDITED BY CAROL DONLEY AND SHERYL BUCKLEY

4. *Recognitions: Doctors and Their Stories*
   EDITED BY CAROL DONLEY AND MARTIN KOHN

5. *Chekhov's Doctors: A Collection of Chekhov's Medical Tales*
   EDITED BY JACK COULEHAN

6. *Tenderly Lift Me: Nurses Honored, Celebrated, and Remembered*
   BY JEANNE BRYNER

7. *The Poetry of Nursing: Poems and Commentaries of Leading Nurse-Poets*
   EDITED BY JUDY SCHAEFER

8. *Our Human Hearts: A Medical and Cultural Journey*
   BY ALBERT HOWARD CARTER III

9. *Fourteen Stories: Doctors, Patients, and Other Strangers*
   BY JAY BARUCH

10. *Stories of Illness and Healing: Women Write Their Bodies*
    EDITED BY SAYANTANI DASGUPTA AND MARSHA HURST

11. *Wider than the Sky: Essays and Meditations on the Healing Power of Emily Dickinson*
    EDITED BY CINDY MACKENZIE AND BARBARA DANA

12. *Lisa's Story: The Other Shoe*
    BY TOM BATIUK

13. *Bodies and Barriers: Dramas of Dis-Ease*
    EDITED BY ANGELA BELLI

Bodies and Barriers

❦

Dramas of Dis-Ease

❦

Edited by Angela Belli

❦

The Kent State

University Press

KENT, OHIO

℘

© 2008 by The Kent State University Press, Kent, Ohio 44242
All rights reserved
Library of Congress Catalog Card Number 2007021838

ISBN 978-0-87338-922-8

Manufactured in the United States of America

Library of Congress Cataloging-in-Publication Data
Bodies and barriers : dramas of dis-ease / edited by Angela Belli.
p. cm. — (Literature and medicine ; 13)
Includes bibliographical references.
ISBN-13: 978-0-87338-922-8 (pbk. : alk. paper) ∞
1. Medical drama. 2. American drama—20th century. 3. English drama—
20th century. I. Belli, Angela.
PS627.M42B63 2007
822'.9140803561—DC22   2007021838

British Library Cataloging-in-Publication data are available.

12 11 10 09 08   5 4 3 2 1

In Memoriam

James Walter Smith, M.D.
1926–2006

Contents

ℒ

Introduction ix

Whose Life Is It Anyway?
  BRIAN CLARK 1

The Elephant Man
  BERNARD POMERANCE 58

W;t
  MARGARET EDSON 96

Wings
  ARTHUR KOPIT 142

The Sandbox
  EDWARD ALBEE 183

The Shadow Box
  MICHAEL CRISTOFER 193

Before It Hits Home
  CHERYL L. WEST 251

Introduction

ℰ

At the age of eighty-seven, being of sound mind, Sophocles created one of the wonders of the classical theater, the *Philoctetes*. The drama was unparalleled for its clear and puissant representation of a moral dilemma that posits a man in conflict with himself. The tale of the titular hero, bitten on the foot by a sacred serpent for treading on holy ground, has its origin in Greek mythology, which served, for one, to validate the religious life of a people. In creating the artistic form in which Philoctetes reappears in 409 B.C., Sophocles constructed him anew amidst a recognizable landscape traced by divine intervention. The "spin" that the dramatist places on the known account is its reflection of his own view of life. Sophocles acknowledged the continuance of powerful supernatural laws guiding the universe but viewed existence as a fundamentally human affair with man determining his own destiny.

En route to battle in Troy, Philoctetes and his fellow warriors follow divine directives. Along the way they make mortal choices. When his companions fail to heal Philoctetes' wound, finding human medicine no match for divinely inflicted injury, they turn from him, repulsed by the foul stench issuing from the festering sore and intolerant of his shrieks of anguish for pain they cannot feel. No longer able to bear his presence, the Greeks abandon Philoctetes on the uninhabited island of Lemnos and sail on to their destination. No divine agency guides the action. Following some ten years of futile warfare, an oracle reveals that the Greeks can overcome the Trojans only with the aid of the discarded man.

Sophocles opens his drama in medias res when emissaries of the Greeks arrive on Lemnos to retrieve Philoctetes, no small task considering the outcast's hatred of his former comrades. Still suffering from the unhealed wound,[1] added to which is the trauma of abandonment and betrayal, the diminished hero makes an initial entrance expressing intense, overwhelming pain. The audience first hears his howls from a distance; then the cries grow louder as the figure draws closer. The action takes up a good bit of stage time, bearing in mind that the entrance to the orchestra in the Athenian theater was approximately thirty yards long (Kitto 115). The aural impact is swelled by the visual image of a tattered figure slowly limping across the stage. Barely a trace remains of the noble presence that once defined the young man. What the audience feels as it gazes at the stumbling figure is open to question. Physical pain cannot be shared. In instances of intense pain, such as that experienced by Philoctetes, communication is shattered as language is displaced by primitive vocal sounds. Intense pain disintegrates the self and splinters its connection to the surrounding world as the universe compresses to the space containing the body. While such experience is private, there are occasions when it is of value to share one's distress with another, however limited the perception of the beholder.

A sensitive observer can interpret, if not feel, the pain of the sufferer. Such is often the case in medicine when the physician who trusts the patient as a reliable narrator of his own sentient needs can interpret such expression as an aid in restoring health (Scarry 4–11).

Outside the medical context, one area in which pain may be interpreted is in literature. Frequently physicians and writers share sensibilities and skills in defining somatic disorder. While the physician interacts with living beings, the literary artist constructs a reality wherein the experience of his fictional characters must be realized imaginatively. The writer is most advantaged in the theater, where a variety of stimuli combine to engage the senses of the spectator while opening the imagination to a world brought to life by actors, objects, and lights, as well as language—all of which enable the interaction between narrative and performance. Besides its sensory appeal, drama speaks to the intellect as well. All great dramas have been dramas of ideas. Nowhere is this more evident than in the *Philoctetes*. The moral dilemma at the core of Sophocles' play tests the fiber of leaders in whose hands rests the fate of a civilization. But it falls to a teenager to resolve the issue. Neoptolemus, the young son of the slain Achilles, is the first of the returning party of Greeks to encounter Philoctetes on coming ashore at Lemnos. Struck by the joy with which the abandoned warrior greets the sight of another living being—and one who speaks his native tongue—Neoptolemus grasps instantly and completely the inhumanity wrought by his fellow Greeks upon the injured man. Having been advised in advance by his elders that deception is the sole means by which the embittered Philoctetes can be enlisted in their cause, Neoptolemus experiences a crisis of conscience. He must weigh his loyalty to his nation and the promise of personal gain against his fundamental honesty and his noble breeding that demand that he refrain from trickery. When he decides on action, his choice is not based on reason but on emotion. He feels compassion for the wretched man. Not revolted by deteriorating flesh, Neoptolemus offers him the comfort of his touch: "Thou art oppressed with ills on every side. / Give me thy hand. Come, wilt thou lean upon me?" (ll. 764–65). Emerging as the true hero, Neoptolemus makes the crucial decision of the drama: to withdraw from the conspiracy. Instead of betrayal he offers friendship and courage to bolster the targeted man's spirit as he predicts a cure for his ailing body. As if to sanction the young man's personal integrity, the god Heracles appears deus ex machina to uphold Neoptolemus and to ensure the restoration of health to the wounded man. He promises the mortal patient "My Aesculapius will I send e'en now / To heal thy wounds" (ll. 1438–39).

Sophocles' work is most remarkable from our perspective for its treatment of issues that remain viable in our culture some thousands of years later. The depiction of the human form under assault from within has become dominant in the modern theater as evidenced by the many contemporary plays with a similar dramatic focus. Both the classical play and current works reveal a similar concern for cultural attitudes vis-à-vis the impaired. Given the individual suffering a health crisis, the Greek playwright dramatized societal attitudes toward the afflicted, particularly those that cast such people aside and prevent their full participation in community life. In the United States at present the same discrimination has met with federal legislation as a mode of address. Sophocles' resolution is of another kind. He teaches the power of love and compassion as a healing and conciliatory force. And he acknowledges the rare gift of one who can share the pain of another. Within the theological framework of the *Philoctetes,* Neoptolemus' act of self-sacrifice is upheld by a god. The drama's resolution points to the existence of a beneficent order to guide man's destiny in defiance of moral depravity. A question remains: How can the Greek dramatist transmit truth to a culture where science has replaced religion as a guiding force? Sophocles answers with linguistics. The play's language is closer to conversational Greek than that of any other Greek drama (Lind 158). Deus ex machina aside, the dramatic conflict and its resolution are addressed in the language of the common man. The values that guide Neoptolemus are communicated as recognizable markers of our shared humanity. They transcend cultural differences and can cure our world as well as his. The play, more tangible than the myth that inspired it, presents contemporary dramatists with a blueprint for transmitting essential truths of human behavior as well as providing a model of tolerance.

In the spring of 409 B.C. the *Philoctetes* received the first prize in tragedy at the Greater Dionysia, the yearly festival held to honor the work of poets.

In the centuries following the appearance of Sophocles' play, the human body under stress continued in various degrees to be a source of fascination for dramatists and audiences. Interest has been particularly keen in our time where the stage illusion has been shaped by two intersecting currents—one scientific and one artistic. By the early twentieth century, the mortal heirs of Aesculapeus were practicing medicine as defined by research and specialization. A rapid succession of technological advances allowed for the body to be penetrated and its mysteries revealed as objective data was collected to diagnose disease. Antiseptic surgery and other technologies were employed to effect healing. The phenomenon of psychic functioning became a subject of much interest and theorizing and led to increased awareness of psychological motivation in daily life. A scientific, rational view of the world came to be centered on the human subject. Simultaneously, beginning with the naturalists, playwrights brought a scientific view into the theater. Emile Zola, most notably, maintained that drama could explore social realities by applying the scientific method to the study of human nature. The convergence of theater and medicine at this time has been well noted (Gardner, "Physiologies of the Modern" 529–42). Zola failed to create any memorable works for the stage himself. Much of his theory can be found in the Preface to his drama *Thérèse Raquin,* with the theory outliving the play. It remained to such seminal playwrights as August Strindberg, Luigi Pirandello, and Anton Chekhov to probe the extent to which scientific observation could shape drama. In each instance, biographical events served to catalyze the developing form.

Strindberg's history of marital strife and his own mental turmoil led him to delve into areas that would later be fully explored in twentieth-century psychopathology. The dramatic focal point in his work is the body under psychic duress. Similarly, Pirandello's reflections on life were shaped by his troubled marriage to a neurotic woman, prompting him to add the discourse of medicine to the drama of ideas. In the case of Chekhov, the biographical interactions are particularly notable since the Russian author was both a practicing physician and a celebrated writer, equally devoted to both crafts. In discussing his art, Chekhov firmly maintained that knowledge of medicine and a commitment to the scientific method enabled him to bring a fundamental truth to his creations that was essential to the engagement of an audience:

> My work in medical sciences has undoubtedly had a serious influence on my literary development; it significantly extended the area of my observations, enriched my knowledge, and only one who is himself a physician could understand the true value of all this for me as a writer; this training has also been a guide, and probably because of my closeness to medicine, I have managed to avoid many mistakes. Familiarity with the natural sciences and scientific method has always kept me on my guard, and I have tried, whenever possible, to take scientific data into consideration, and where that was impossible, I've preferred not to write at all. (qtd. in Simmons 479)

Chekhov's descriptions of certain pathologies, a rarity in fiction, provide data accurate enough for current practitioners to diagnose disease in a character and analyze a medical situation in a tale. In terms of his dramatic art, he added innovations in form, dispensing with linear plot and foregrounding the interior lives of his fictional beings to provide a paradigm for the future theater of the absurd (Corrigan 139–67).

Despite the acceptance by audiences of the above dramatists, public interest has not been absorbed with the medicalized body. Beginning in the late nineteenth century, a physical culture movement that aimed at corporeal perfection gained support among health enthusiasts. Disciplined, communal training of the body gave rise to gymnastic organizations and revised curricula in the schools to accommodate physical education. An emphasis on sports unequaled in history became another means of worshipping the perfect body. Recognition of the homage paid to physical achievement in the ancient world resulted in the revival of the Olympic Games, broader in scope and less brutal than the original. The female body as well was viewed as capable of perfection as physical training was not gender restricted and women came to distinguish themselves in athletic competition (Segel 3–5). To create a cult of the body cognizant of its classical and aesthetic perfectibility, however, has a dark side when the supporting social structure concurrently marginalizes the impaired body. Developing means by which the impaired body could be transformed and pathologies reversed became the goal of medical technology and experimentation. Despite its rejection of the impaired individual, the public has maintained a curiosity regarding all aspects of health care that has kept pace with scientific advances.

The nonprofessional confronts the institution of medicine primarily through its practitioners, though other contact occurs by means of publications geared to the lay public and other mass media resources. An enormously popular venue, easily within reach of millions, is television, where medicine and creativity frequently meet. The viewer, in such instances, is likely to encounter a fictional world where similarities to real life are purely coincidental. The brilliant, devoted, benevolent individuals in white coats whose practices are limited to the tube battle all manner of disease, often of the exotic variety, as they attain the status of hero, at least according to television standards. As more public health issues become matters of wide concern, as with HIV/AIDS, they are introduced as regular television fare (Jones 12–19). A satiric view of the doctor, never far from the popular imagination, is that of the malevolent experimenter in the occult or the erstwhile dabbler in the supernatural. Such figures are found commonly in popular fiction where they assume a mythic identity.[2] One is included by reference in Brian Clark's play *Whose Life Is It Anyway?* when the frustrated paraplegic hero, given to black humor, instructs a social worker to report to his physician: "Go and convince Dr. Frankenstein that he has successfully made his monster and he can now let it go" (51).

In addition to the audience that responds to television drama and popular fiction, there is another, more sophisticated and discriminating group of spectators that are spellbound before images of less than perfect beings and their caregivers as represented in the theater. The contemporary plays are situated in a line of descent, however indirect, from Sophocles. What is new about the modern works is their centrality in a wider discursive field where the body and its pathologies are referenced within the framework of medical science. Current theatrical representations of medical discourse take their authority, language, images, and characters—a roster of professionals—all from medicine. Contemporary medicine is a rich source of material for playwrights taken with the conflict between human values and a rapidly changing technology that has come to prevail in the delivery of health care, as indeed in other vital areas of human experience. Frequently the conflict of the drama has its origin in an issue that is the focus of debate among bioethicists. In such instances the theater becomes the domain where the debate is acted out before a live audience for whom the questions are part of everyday reality. Represented on stage in graphic terms are crises involving end-of-life issues, including the termination of treatment, the "Do Not Resuscitate" order, the use of human subjects for research, the option of hospice care, and the need to recognize human freedom and dignity in deciding a dispute—these among other matters of increasing concern.

The plays included in this collection tell of the experience of men and women who suffer a dis-ease of the body, an absence of ease or a disturbance likely to cause a loss of physical and/or emotional well-being. The condition could be morbid, as with cancer or AIDS; it could define a progressive physical decline, as with aging; or it could indicate a disability that is lasting, though not life threatening. In all instances, the most damaging assault on the afflicted is that which is socially directed, as the impaired protagonist is cast out of the company of those who would ignore his imperfection as they would the finite nature of life. In bringing their novel discourse before the public, playwrights most often use nontraditional constructs to project their vision with maximum effect.

Clark's *Whose Life Is It Anyway?* foregrounds the body as a receptor of manipulative machinery. The striking visual image perceived by the spectator is that of a hopelessly paralyzed young man, Ken Harrison, whose spinal cord was severed in an automobile accident. The hero is seen for the duration of the play as a sentient being entrapped by confining apparatus—bed, wheelchair, tubes. Further, he is found in a hospital setting, totally dependent and transformed into an object. Kept alive by mechanical means, the hero has lost his personal freedom and, more grievously, he has lost his artistic freedom as well since he can no longer exercise his craft as a sculptor. Having lived through his art, his loss brings him to the edge of annihilation. The character's situation is particularly poignant since the disability he must deal with is an acquired one. Having lived a normal adult life prior to the accident, he recalls in pain his previous physical capacity. The play is far from humorless, but it is a dark humor that directs our attention frequently to his inability to function sexually. In this regard the audience is challenged to consider the popular myth that for those who are incapacitated in the manner of quadriplegics, the loss of sexual function equates with a loss of sexuality, including emotional and sensual components. As such, the disabled person is not considered a sexual being. The misconception reinforces the observation that disability does not reside solely in the impaired but is, in large measure, a creation of social attitudes.

Ken Harrison's position remains consistent throughout the drama. The situation in which he finds himself is not of his choosing. But he remains capable of personal choices, the most crucial of which is whether to live or die. The greatest cruelty he suffers is in having the choice removed from him. The dramatic conflict comes about when the hero chooses to be free of the sustaining apparatus that has replaced his human will and elects to die with dignity. He is opposed by a physician who believes that to acquiesce to his patient's will is to betray his oath as a doctor to sustain life. Opposed to the hero on ethical grounds, he assumes the moral as well as the technical agency for his patient. His action is consistent with the traditional paternalistic interaction between physician and patient that has long characterized medical practice.

A similar relationship exists between the hero of Bernard Pomerance's *The Elephant Man*, John Merrick, and his physician, Frederick Treves. Merrick suffers from a medical condition popularly regarded as neurofibromatosis. During the course of the drama, his genetic disorder is revealed in vivid detail; his markedly distorted body dominates the stage. The facts are true enough since the patient in Pomerance's work is modeled on a man who actually lived in England a century ago and whose history can be reconstructed.

The historical truth of the dramatized tale invites a comparison: Merrick's dilemma has been witnessed numerous times in current experience by scores of patients. The fundamental difference between the hero of the drama and the live patients who have followed is in the advantage that the latter enjoy as beneficiaries of the work of research teams that strive to control the symptoms that cause suffering. While treatment at present is predominantly surgical, including plastic and reconstructive surgery, studies in molecular genetics points a direction to nonsurgical and/or pharmacological treatment. Psychological assessment is also available, as is genetic counseling. In treating his patient, the physician in *The Elephant Man* cannot avail himself of medical advances that mark progress in our time nor can he reach beyond scientific inquiry to access certain social constructs, such as support groups, that respond to patients' needs. His imagination cannot encompass the use of a computer as a means of communication between patients who rely on online bulletin boards and discussion forums to reach others. Such bonding in the face of social marginalization is an immeasurable emotional benefit, frequently a factor in enabling individuals to lead productive lives. In the end, one is led to question whether it is not the social factor that is of greatest significance in helping the afflicted to endure.

Despite the fact that Treves cannot rely on recent scientific data in treating Merrick, he is sufficiently attuned to people's wants to comprehend the import of human interaction, whether it occurs via a computer or, more satisfactorily, in a nineteenth-century drawing room. To carry out the only experiment he can control, Treves shapes an exclusive society for his patient. His action validates the principles of acceptance and tolerance at the same time that it repudiates the social structure that casts aside those who fail to meet its standards. The tragedy of the drama is in the failure of the experiment. Its triumph is in the celebration of human values.

Physical incapacity restricts a character once privileged to enjoy the most luxurious of freedoms—the freedom to pursue knowledge—in Margaret Edson's drama *W;t*. The play charts the ordeal of Vivian Bearing, a prominent professor of English literature, who is confined to a hospital as she undergoes treatment for cancer. While the female body has been traditionally exploited on "the wicked stage" as an erotic object of male sexual desire, current dramatists, a significant number of whom are women, offer another view of female corporeal experience (Garner, *Bodied Spaces* 198–99). The female body is revealed as a physiological site, with the attention of the audience directed to the distress of women whose bodies come under physical and emotional attack. The heroine of *W;t* suffers from advanced metastatic ovarian cancer. Her harrowing decline occurs in a medical setting where she is the object of the most advanced and aggressive experimentation attempted. The theatrical context is marked by performance elements that reinforce her presence on stage as the dramatic focal point. Throughout the play she appears in a hospital gown, in bed, or attached to an IV pole that visually extends her corporeal dimensions. By far the most striking theatrical effect is the character's monologues in direct address to the audience. These are interchanged frequently with passages of dialogue, the heroine moving freely from one to the other as she remains ever present within the audience's sight. As with the Chorus in classical drama, the heroine of the contemporary play often acts as narrative voice, interrupting the action of the plot. The technique allows her to contrast her previous life with her present one for the benefit of the audience. *W;t* explores questions of identity, particularly those likely to occur when a person becomes the subject of an experiment. Vivian Bearing undergoes a reversal of fortune likely to occur on the Greek stage. The professor becomes an object of study, with both her body and her ego undergoing deconstruction.

The heroine's point of view prevails as she meets the challenges to her sense of self. Cut off from the university that has been her sole life, she now seeks the companionship of the spectators who, however compassionate, must remain forever separated from her by the distance separating life from art. Only in the final act of her life does she turn her back on the audience as she begins a solitary journey toward redemption.

The disintegration of self is a consequence of massive physical impairment in Arthur Kopit's *Wings*. Grounded in actual experience, the work has its impetus in the major stroke suffered by the playwright's father. Rendered incapable of speech, the afflicted man suffered a number of complications related to aphasia. Kopit maintains that his work is essentially about language disorder and its implications. In observing his father, he was most aware of the utter isolation the older man endured with the loss of comprehension and communication skills.

The catastrophic event occurred some months before the playwright was commissioned to write an original radio play for Earplay, the drama project of National Public Radio. No stipulation was made regarding subject; a limitation of one hour was set on playing time. Kopit availed himself of the opportunity to transform a personal disaster into a universal statement on human frailty and human courage. He found himself both terrified and fascinated in beholding the effects of brain damage. His fear was overpowered by curiosity. As he struggled to reach his father, to penetrate the prison his body had become, he questioned the extent to which the man was aware of what had happened to him. Was he essentially the same man as before? Kopit was convinced that he was. The playwright recognized the advantage that radio presented as an appropriate medium to explore the questions. For one, it imposed the necessity of a contoured script to exclude a myriad of peripheral issues in relation to aphasia. In exploring the matter of identity, the author could very well have been diverted to any number of related issues. And, in fact, had the piece been conceived originally for the stage, such would, no likely, have been the case. The stage presents an extended range for investigating a subject in broad terms. Kopit was grateful for the rigor of radio that kept him focused on his central character's condition. His task as an artist was a daunting one. He needed to convey what the spectator could never feel—the inner turmoil, the terror of another (Kopit 179–80).

When the work was eventually adapted for the stage, some expansion was necessary to accommodate various visual components of the character's external world. But the dramatist's vision remains fixed. Finding it necessary to work by analogy, he created another character with another history, Emily Stilson, to relive his father's experience. Each scene is constructed to expose reality as it is received through her senses. All sounds and images are filtered through her mind. Seen in the company of assorted medical staff, she remains distant due to her inability to decode the information they send; facts become scrambled as she receives them. Her frustration and isolation is total. Only in the company of her extraordinary therapist, Amy, is she able to form any comforting relationship. And only in her final moments of life, in Amy's company, is she able to suit her words to the action. Free of terror at last, smiling faintly, she offers a soft "Thank you."

Another elderly woman to take center stage and confront the audience appears in Edward Albee's *The Sandbox*. In this brief, one-act drama the main character, Grandma, suffers no violent trauma, no terminal illness. She is rendered powerless and marginalized by a pervasive canker in the social fabric that targets older individuals, ageism. Like racism and sexism, ageism is a prejudice that is engrained in the culture, with de facto discrimination omnipresent in the workplace, in education, within the medical community, and in the media. Albee locates the bias in American society and spotlights the family structure as another likely site. He reveals the cruelest form of rejection, the abuse of relatives on whom a person depends for protection and sustenance. The abuse frequently involves ignoring the physical and emotional needs of the subject. The prejudice has its origin in the minds of those younger adults who, like Grandma's family, repress the truth of their own vulnerability and mortality.

The myth that ageing and cognitive decline are one has led to the erroneous conclusion that older citizens are incapable of significant contributions to communal life, including aesthetic creations that add beauty to our lives. Indeed, the elderly are frequently regarded with pity, sometimes revulsion, for the loss of their own youthful beauty, beauty as culturally determined. The perception leads to further stereotyping that links physical attractiveness with sexuality. Individuals over a certain age who are considered physically unattractive are also looked on as sexually undesirable. A suspect morality condemns sex among older people as downright shameful and even perverse. In sum, the achievements of seniors are regarded as being of little value and deserving of little in return. The conclusion translates commonly into contempt and disregard.

In *The Sandbox* Albee draws attention to a continual issue in daily life; he calls on the spectator to ponder a disturbing reality it would otherwise ignore. Making supreme use of theatrical form with its reliance on riveting images and distilled language, the dramatist rapidly destroys the stereotype, breaking the mold and freeing a vital, loving being to be our animated companion for some brief moments.

The confrontation with mortality is sudden for characters of varying ages in Michael Cristofer's *The Shadow Box*, where we meet no less than three terminally ill patients. Appearing in the late 1970s, the play provided an artistic perspective from which to ponder the emerging hospice movement on the American scene. Many in the audience were unfamiliar with the hospice philosophy that offered dying patients an alternative to traditional, impersonal care provided by the established medical system. Dying patients were often isolated in hospitals where their pain and discomfort received inadequate relief. Committed to social change, hospice provided a refuge for individuals in the last stages of incurable disease. Its goal was to provide palliative and supportive care that enabled patients to live as fully as possible in the days that remained to them. The quality of life rather than its length was of paramount import. Offering a humanistic and holistic approach, hospice was devoted to treating the person rather than the disease by taking into account both the psychosocial and physical needs of the dying. The care is distinguished for being family-centered, with loved ones sharing feelings and making decisions together.

Often the most difficult decision faced by patients and physicians alike is when to initiate hospice care. The decision requires a wrenching admission that the illness has advanced beyond curing. In truth, a condition may improve and hospice care may itself be terminated. But hope does not induce pity and fear in an audience at a play. Cristofer's intention was to reveal the conflicting emotions that hamper individuals who would come to terms with a grim diagnosis. Providing a glimpse of the hospice structure as it exists in an inpatient facility, the playwright suggests the presence of caregivers by aural rather than by visual effect, contributing to the ethos he would transmit. His foremost intention is to represent the response of people who, like those in attendance, are new to the concept. The drama concentrates on the value in affirming life as the sole means of embracing the quality of the time that remains. Questions about relationships, feelings, regrets, and accomplishments—questions about how to live—compose the dialogue. On stage the dramatist presents an assortment of patients, friends, and family who are torn between accepting a life that has been altered irrevocably in some manner for each or disallowing the reality they cannot escape. As spectators we share in their fears and despair. We are led to consider the tragic view of life as inevitable doom that prevailed in ancient Greece. We witness the passing of those involved from ignorance to awareness, from denial to acceptance in the manner of the Sophoclean hero. Finally, we share in the reconciliation of Cristofer's characters as they live each day in the company of one another.

Appearing frequently in current works for the theater is the body of the gay male, which has become a subject of recurrent interest, particularly since the 1980s when HIV/AIDS was identified as a health crisis of global proportions to affect a significant number of homosexual men.

Homosexuality is, of itself, an isolative experience. The gay man is further marginalized when viewed as a toxic body likely to spread a fatal disease. The objective of playwrights who deal with the issue and make heroes of the infected is to gain the attention of mainstream audiences who have long remained aloof and unsympathetic as the contagion has grown. In American experience, encounters with epidemics have been recorded largely in the non-imaginative literature of medicine. Such encounters have been recorded more often than not as success stories with the medical community vanquishing the disease while creating a new type of hero, the medical researcher. The dimensions and cultural ramifications of HIV/AIDS have galvanized discourses within medical, political, and artistic spheres. The theater provides its own sanctuary within which the public may consider the effects of a baffling disease that has shaken its security and confidence in biomedical advances. While constructing an admittedly illusory world, drama locates the dialogue in public space, providing a unique opportunity within a communal setting for raising awareness as it promulgates the facts and spurs socio/political action.

In *Before It Hits Home* Cheryl L. West recounts the dissolution of an African American family as they react to the unexpected crisis of an infected son, Wendal Bailey, in their midst.

Presented in the 1990s, the play reached a public for whom the medical disaster and its depiction in art were common fare. Where the disease was denied was within the African American community, on stage and off. West's task was a daunting one in that she had to battle the toxicity of ignorance and intolerance among a population with which she, as a black writer, was identified. She succeeds admirably, largely because she shifts the focus of the drama away from the disease itself and on to all who suffer its consequences, including those who, disease-free, remain to bear witness. She invites both homosexuals and heterosexuals alike to view the perils that assault the human heart. Projecting the universal meaning of tragedy, the plot moves from conflict to reconciliation.

The plays to follow are disturbing for arousing their audiences to a reality they would ignore but must perforce comprehend and deal with. In the despair of the protagonists echo the distant cries of Philoctetes in testimony to man's brutality to man. One further similarity links Sophocles' work to that of the modern dramas: each play has gained critical acclaim and has been among those awarded the highest honors in the dramatic contests in which they have competed.

Notes

1. In the absence of a medical explanation for the unchanging character of Philoctetes' wound over the preceding ten years, including any hint of pernicious effects on the hero, we grant Sophocles poetic license.

2. For an overview of images of doctor figures in literature, see Leslie Fiedler, "Images of the Doctor in Literature and the Popular Arts," in *Tyranny of the Normal: Essays in Bioethics, Theology and Myth* (Boston: D.R. Godine, 1996), 107–20.

Works Cited

Clark, Brian. *Whose Life Is It Anyway?* New York: Dodd, 1979.

Corrigan, Robert W. "The Plays of Chekhov." In *The Context and Craft of Drama*. Ed. Robert W. Corrigan and James L. Rosenberg. Scranton, Pa.: Chandler, 1964. 139–67.

Fiedler, Leslie. "Images of the Doctor in Literature and the Popular Arts." In *Tyranny of the Normal: Essays on Bioethics, Theology and Myth*. Boston: D.R. Godine, 1996. 107–20.

Garner, Stanton B., Jr. *Bodied Spaces: Phenomenology and Performance in Contemporary Drama*. Ithaca, N.Y.: Cornell Univ. Press, 1994.

———. "Physiologies of the Modern: Zola, Experimental Medicine, and the Naturalist Stage." *Modern Drama* 48 (Winter 2000): 529–42.

Jones, Therese. "As the World Turns on the Sick and the Restless, So Go the Days of Our Lives: Family and Illness in Daytime Drama." *Journal of Medical Humanities* 18.1 (1997): 5–20.

Kitto, H. D. F. *Form and Meaning in Drama*. London: Methuen, 1956.

Kopit, Arthur. *Wings: Three Plays*. New York: Hill and Wang, 1997. 179–270.

Lind, L. R. *Ten Greek Plays in Contemporary Translations*. Boston: Houghton Mifflin, 1957.

Russo, Ann. "Exploring AIDS in the Black Community." *Sojourner: The Women's Forum* 15.1 (1989): 37–38.

Scarry, Elaine. *The Body in Pain*. New York: Oxford Univ. Press, 1985.

Segel, Harold. *The Body Ascendant*. Baltimore: Johns Hopkins Univ. Press, 1998.

Simmons, Ernest J. *Chekhov*. Boston: Little, Brown, 1962.

Sophocles. *Philoctetes*. Trans. Thomas Francklin. *The Complete Greek Drama*. Ed. Whitney J. Oates and Eugene O'Neill Jr. Vol. 1. New York: Random House, 1938.

West, Cheryl L. *New Traditions Compendium Forums and Commentaries: 1992–96*. 1994. http://www.ntcp.org/compendium/artists/CHERYL.html. Accessed May 31, 2005.

Whose Life Is It Anyway?

ℒ

Brian Clark

INTRODUCTION

The title of Brian Clark's *Whose Life Is It Anyway?* poses the question to the audience. During the course of the drama, the issue is examined from three perspectives: medical, philosophical, and legal. The protagonist, Ken Harrison, is a hopelessly paralyzed young sculptor who sustained his injury in a road accident. His physical condition has been stabilized, but he remains confined to the hospital with only the prospect of a long-term care facility as a change of address. Effectively removed from society by reason of his injuries, it is Ken himself who willfully determines to make the separation permanent by choosing to end his life rather than endure an existence where he has no control over his body and where his brain is kept alive with no prospect of carrying out the directives of his spirit. He believes that to continue him in such a state is to deny that which distinguishes him as a person. While there exists an argument to counter his, namely the view that locates the tragedy of disability within an unaccommodating society rather than within the disabled, for Ken a life worth living must include the capacity to express himself as a sculptor. To the social worker who argues that unimagined mechanical devices can help restore him, he questions, "How about an electronically operated hammer and chisel?" (55). In short, technology has taken over his human will, and he no longer has the ability to make free and rational choices.

In truth, Ken seeks a privilege beyond that of the right to remove or refuse life-sustaining therapy. He fights to repossess his liberty. When he makes his stand, it is on the firmest ground—the entire tradition of Western social and political philosophy that rests on individual liberty as its moral basis. In terms of clinical practice, where the autonomy of the patient is acknowledged as a value, it is a contractual relationship that characterizes the physician-patient transaction. The hero's actions in the play are an assertion of those contractual rights viewed in terms of current philosophical arguments which hold that

1

the dual principles of autonomy and contract keeping, conceptually linked, provide the sole moral foundation for clinical practice consistent with the social context in which the practice occurs (Smith and Newton 43–60).

In *Whose Life Is It Anyway?* the hero's antagonist is Dr. Michael Emerson, the consultant physician. Dr. Emerson opposes Ken on two grounds: he maintains that his patient lacks the necessary knowledge to challenge any medical decisions; and he believes that Ken is caught in the effects of a medical syndrome—that is, his decision results from clinically depressed thinking occasioned by his massive physical injuries. Emerson argues that "a doctor cannot accept the choice for death; he's committed to life" (91). He firmly believes that if he allows Ken to die, he will be aiding him in an act of suicide. Consequently, he assumes the moral as well as the technical agency for his patient. If his position is erroneous, it is due to his failure to recognize that the functions of an individual extend beyond the physical and the psychological. That which makes us human is our cognitional-volitional or social function, which enables us to integrate all other powers to fulfill our human destiny. Once that power is destroyed, Ken can no longer strive to fulfill his purpose in life. If a goal of medical ethics is the restoration of health, and if therapy is inadequate to restore those functions that enable us to pursue our spiritual goals, then medicine need not assume an aggressive role. Ethically, as well as legally, Ken Harrison has the right to the conscious decision he makes.

Reaching to the larger society beyond the hospital walls, Ken turns to the law to settle the dispute. The legal resolution in the play is inevitable, for the courts have little choice but to reaffirm the patient's contractual rights. Any moral guidelines set by the medical profession or any other subculture must, of necessity, harmonize with the philosophical preconceptions of the larger society. The dramatic resolution does not solve the dilemma in medical practice that the work explores, however. The paternalistic tradition continues to dominate the physician-patient interaction. Contrary to the egalitarian spirit of the contractual relationship, inequality is intrinsic when illness renders the patient's capacity to make rational choices open to question and shifts the balance of power to the physician who possesses both the knowledge and the obligation to restore health. Emerson affirms, "My power isn't arbitrary; I've earned it with knowledge and skill" (127). The fact remains that the initial decision regarding the patient's competence to act autonomously rests with the physician. Moreover, even for the skilled professional, the determination may be difficult, depending on the clinical situation. An added complication is the fact that while a patient is limited by his illness, so, too, is the physician constrained by forces beyond his control, those that invade his domain from the areas of government and the law. Bemoaning the fact that patients are becoming so litigious that doctors will soon fear to offer any opinion or take any action at all, Emerson must acknowledge that such failure in itself is grounds for a malpractice suit. His reluctance to participate in what he considers an act of suicide is based partly on his moral outlook and partly on the traditional view of the criminality of the act.

While the challenges to his power frustrate Emerson, they have a similar effect on the various health professionals who support him. The nurses, social worker, psychiatrist, and junior physician are all unsettled by their contact with the hero, who obliges them to confront their own limitations. They are, however, restricted only partially by such challenges as patients' rights and the legal system; by far the greater restraint is their human fallibility, which renders them powerless to cure their patient. Ken is keen to their vulnerability in this regard. In one scene he turns tables on the examining psychiatrist by pointing out his "tidiness compulsion" and drawing from him the defensive statement that he was an only child. The humor inherent in the reversal of patient-physician roles is consistent in aim with Ken's rapid black humor gags that center on his sexual incapacity. His goal is to embarrass and disarm his antagonists so that they will drop their professional veneer. Along with the discarded veneer, it is to be hoped that scientific objectivity will be abandoned as well, for it is detachment that impairs clinical empathy.

Although no satisfactory solution to the paternalism/autonomy conflict is found in the drama, there are moments that suggest that the clinical relationship can evolve to a point where the personhood and self-determination of the patient can be respected without giving ground to the professional competence and moral agency of the physician. Such an instance occurs when Ken manages to convince Dr. Clare Scott, the junior registrar, not to give him the tranquilizer she had prescribed earlier for him. On reflection she sympathizes with his need to keep his consciousness clear. Taken to task by Dr. Emerson for ignoring her initial, objective decision, she argues the case for the greater validity of subjectivity at such a time. However, Emerson's response—forcibly to inject the protesting hero with the undesired tranquilizer—precipitates the climax of the play, with Ken having recourse to the law. Having won the battle to be discharged and free at last to die away from his constrainers, the hero accepts his doctor's promise to stop treatment, and he expresses what amounts to a final choice—a desire to spend his last days in their company.

Certainly the issues explored in *Whose Life Is It Anyway?* are of major concern to physicians, patients, medical ethicists, and whoever may ponder matters of life and death. But it remains to the audience to answer the question of the title. The spectator is presented with no resolution yet witnesses a rare reconciliation of the conflicting parties. It is to the playwright's credit that he can balance both sides and depict ordinary individuals—no villains or faultless heroes—acting with the best of intentions. In terms of audience empathy, the balance shifts towards the maimed hero, whose immobile form is the dominant stage image in virtually every scene. And while the facts of a patient's physical state may be the total of technological data, added to which is the physician's assessment, the playwright can offer his audience something more, something that cannot be seen or measured but is essential in helping it to determine whose life is in question. He can provide a glimpse of his hero's spirit.

WORKS CITED

Clark, Brian. *Whose Life Is It Anyway?* New York: Dodd, 1979.
Smith, D. G., and L. H. Newton. "Physician and Patient: Respect for Mutuality." *Theoretical Medicine* 5 (1984): 43–60.

WHOSE LIFE IS IT ANYWAY?
By Brian Clark

For Maggie

CHARACTERS

KEN HARRISON	*The Patient*
SISTER ANDERSON	*Ward Sister (Supervisor)*
NURSE KAY SADLER	*A Probationer Nurse*
JOHN	*A West Indian Ward Orderly*
DR. CLARE SCOTT	*Junior Registrar*
DR. MICHAEL EMERSON	*Consultant Physician*
MRS. GILLIAN BOYLE	*A Medical Social Worker*
PHILIP HILL	*Ken's Solicitor*
DR. PAUL TRAVERS	*Consultant Psychiatrist*
PETER KERSHAW	*Ken's Barrister*
DR. BARR	*Consultant Psychiatrist (from Norwood Park Hospital)*
ANDREW EDEN	*Hospital's Barrister*
MR. JUSTICE MILLHOUSE	*Judge*

The action is continuous and takes place in a side ward, offices, corridors and a road outside a general hospital.

ACT ONE

(SISTER ANDERSON *and* NURSE KAY SADLER *enter with trolley*)

SISTER: Good morning, Mr. Harrison. A new face for you today.

KEN: That's nice.

NURSE: Hello.

KEN: Hello. I'm afraid I can't offer you my hand. You'll just have to make do
    with my backside like all the other nurses.

(*They lower the bed*)

Going down–Obstetrics, Gynecology, Lingerie, Rubber wear.

(*They roll* KEN *over and start to massage his back and heels with spirit and talc*)

It's funny, you know. I used to dream of situations like this.

SISTER: Being injured?

KEN: No! Lying on a bed being massaged by two beautiful women.

SISTER:

(*Mock serious*)

If you go on like this, Mr. Harrison, I shan't be able to send my young
    nurses in here.

KEN: They're perfectly safe with me, Sister.

(*The phone rings outside*)

SISTER: Can you manage for a moment, Nurse?

NURSE: Oh, yes, Sister.

SISTER: Wipe your hands and put the pillows behind Mr. Harrison; we
    don't want to have him on the floor.

KEN: Have me on the floor, Sister, please. Have me on the floor.

(SISTER *goes out*)

What's your name?

NURSE: Kay.

KEN: That's nice, but don't let Sister hear you say that.

NURSE: What?

KEN: What's your second name?

NURSE: Sadler.

KEN: Then you must answer "Nurse Sadler" with a smile that is full of
    warmth, but with no hint of sex.

NURSE: I'm sorry.

KEN: I'm not. I'm glad you're called Kay. I shall call you Kay when we're
    alone, just you and me, having my backside caressed . . .

NURSE: I'm rubbing your heels.

KEN: Well, don't spoil it. After all, it doesn't matter. I can't feel anything wherever you are. Is this your first ward?

NURSE: Yes. I'm still at P.T.S.

KEN: What's that? Primary Training School?

NURSE: Yes. I finish next week

KEN: And you can't wait to get here full time.

NURSE: I'll be glad to finish the school.

KEN: All students are the same.

NURSE: Were you a teacher?

KEN: Tut tut; second lesson. You mustn't use the past tense.

NURSE: What do you mean?

KEN: You said: "Were you a teacher?" You should have said: "Are you a teacher?" I mean, you are now part of the optimism industry. Everyone who deals with me acts as though, for the first time in the history of medical science, a ruptured spinal column will heal itself–it's just a bit of a bore waiting for it to happen.

NURSE: I'm sorry

KEN: Don't be. Kay, you're a breath of fresh air.

(SISTER *comes back*)

SISTER: Finished, Nurse?

KEN: What do you mean? Have I finished Nurse. I haven't started her yet!

NURSE: Yes, Sister.

(*They roll him back and remake the bed*)

KEN: I must congratulate you, Sister, on your new recruit. A credit to the monstrous regiment.

SISTER: I'm glad you got on.

KEN: Well, I didn't get quite that far. Not that I didn't try, Sister. But all I could get out of her was that her name was . . . Nurse Sadler . . . and that she's looking forward to coming here.

SISTER: If she still feels like that after being five minutes with you, we'll make a nurse of her yet.

KEN: I don't know quite how to take that Sister—lying down I suppose.

SISTER: Night Sister said you slept well.

KEN: Ah-thew. I fooled her . . . After her last round, a mate of mine came in and smuggled me out . . . We went midnight skateboarding.

SISTER: Oh yes . . . I hope it was fun . . .

KEN: It was all right . . . The only problem was that I was the skateboard.

SISTER: There, that's better. Comfortable?

KEN: Sister, it's so beautifully made, I can't feel a thing.

SISTER: Cheerio, Mr. Harrison

(*They leave*)

NURSE: Won't he ever get better, Sister?

SISTER: No.

NURSE: What will happen to him?

SISTER: When we have him fully stabilized, he'll be transferred to a long-stay hospital.

NURSE: For the rest of his life?

SISTER: Yes.

(JOHN, *an orderly, comes along the corridor carrying shaving tackle on a tray*)

JOHN: Morning, Sister.

SISTER: Morning, John. Are you going to Mr. Harrison?

JOHN: That's right.

SISTER: He's all ready.

JOHN: Right.

(JOHN *goes into the sluice room to collect an electric razor*)

NURSE: How long has he been here?

SISTER: Four months.

NURSE: How much longer will he be here?

SISTER: Not much longer now, I should think. Take the trolley into the ward, Nurse. I should start on Mr. Phillips.

(SISTER *goes into her office.* JOHN *goes into* KEN's *room. He plugs in the razor and shaves* KEN)

JOHN: Good morning, Mr. Harrison . . .

KEN: Come to trim the lawn?

JOHN: That's right.

KEN: Good . . . Must make sure that all the beds and borders are neat and tidy.

JOHN: That's my job.

KEN: Well, my gardening friend, isn't it about time you got some fertilizer to sprinkle on me and get some movement going in this plant?

JOHN: Ah, now there you have me. You see, I'm only a laborer in this here vineyard. Fertilizers and pruning and bedding out is up to the head gardener.

KEN: Still, you must be in charge of the compost heap. That's where I should be.

(SISTER *puts her head around the door*)

SISTER: John.

JOHN: Yes?

SISTER: Don't be long, will you. Dr. Scott will probably be early today; there's a consultant's round this morning.

JOHN: Right, Sister.

(SISTER *goes back to her office*)

KEN: The visitation of the Gods.

JOHN: Eh?

KEN: The Gods are walking on earth again.

JOHN: Oh yes–they think they're a bit of all right.

KEN: What happened to the other chap–Terence, he was called . . . I think?

JOHN: They come and they go . . . I think he left to get married up north somewhere.

KEN: Terence, getting married? Who to? A lorry driver?

JOHN: Catty!

KEN: No. Bloody jealous. From where I'm lying, if you can make it at all–even with your right hand–it would be heaven . . . I'm sorry . . . feeling sorry for myself this morning . . . I can't even say I got out of the wrong side of the bed. Are you down to the bone yet? . . . Anyway, how long will you be staying?

JOHN: Just till we go professional, man.

KEN: Doing what?

JOHN: Music. We got a steel band–with some comedy numbers and we're getting around a bit . . . We're auditioning for Opportunity Knocks in four months.

KEN: That's great . . . Really great . . . I like steel bands . . . There's something fascinating about using oil drums–making something out of scrap . . . Why not try knocking a tune out of me?

JOHN: Why not, man!

(*He puts down his razor and, striking* KEN *very lightly up and down his body like a xylophone, sings a typical steel band tune, moving rhythmically to the music.* KEN *is delighted.* DR. CLARE SCOTT *comes in.* JOHN *stops*)

DR. SCOTT: Don't stop . . .

JOHN: It's all right . . . I've nearly finished.

(*He makes one more pass with the razor*)

KEN: I was just making myself beautiful for you, Doctor.

JOHN: There . . . Finished.

(*He goes to the door*)

KEN: Work out some new tunes . . . Hey, if Doctor Scott could drill some holes in my head, you could blow in my ear and play me like an ocarina.

JOHN: I'll see you later.

(*He grins and goes out*)

DR. SCOTT: You're bright and chirpy this morning.

KEN:

(*Ironically*)

It's marvelous, you know. The courage of the human spirit.

DR. SCOTT:

(*Dryly*)

Nice to hear the human spirit's OK. How's the lungs?

(*She takes her stethoscope from her pocket. She puts the stethoscope to* KEN'S
   chest)

KEN:

(*Sings*)

Boom boom.

DR. SCOTT: Be quiet. You'll deafen me.

KEN: Sorry.

(*She continues to listen*)

And what does it say?

DR. SCOTT:

(*Gives up*)

What does what say?

KEN: My heart, of course. What secrets does it tell?

DR. SCOTT: It was just telling me that it's better off than it was six months
   ago.

KEN: It's a brave heart. It keeps its secrets.

DR. SCOTT: And what are they?

KEN: Did you hear it going boom boom, like that? Two beats.

DR. SCOTT: Of course.

KEN: Well, I'll tell you. That's because it's broken, broken in two. But each
   part carries on bravely, yearning for a woman in a white coat.

DR. SCOTT: And I thought it was the first and second heart sounds.

KEN: Ah! Is there a consultant's round this morning?

DR. SCOTT: That's right.

KEN: I suppose he will sweep in here like Zeus from Olympus, with his
   attendant nymphs and swains.

DR. SCOTT: I don't think that's fair.

KEN: Why not?

DR. SCOTT: He cares; he cares a lot.

KEN: But what about?

DR. SCOTT: His patients.

KEN: I suppose so.

DR. SCOTT: He does. When you first came in he worked his guts out to keep you going; he cares.

KEN: I was a bit flip, wasn't I . . .

DR. SCOTT: It's understandable.

KEN: But soon we shall have to ask the question why.

DR. SCOTT: Why?

KEN: Why bother. You remember the mountain labored and brought forth not a man but a mouse. It was a big joke. On the mouse. If you're as insignificant as that, who needs a mountain for a mummy?

DR. SCOTT: I'll see you later . . . with Dr. Emerson.

KEN: And Cupbearers Limited.

DR. SCOTT: Oh no . . . I assure you . . . We're not at all limited.

(*She goes out. She opens the door of* SISTER*'s room. The* SISTER *is writing at the desk*)

Sister. It's Mr. Harrison. He seems a little agitated this morning.

SISTER: Yes, he's beginning to realize what he's up against.

DR. SCOTT: I'm changing the prescription and putting him on a small dose of Valium. I'll have a word with Dr. Emerson. Thank you, Sister.

(*She closes the door and looks up the corridor toward* KEN*'s room.* NURSE SADLER *is just going in with a feeding cup*)

KEN: An acolyte, bearing a cup.

NURSE: I beg your pardon?

KEN: Nothing. I was joking. It's nothing.

NURSE: It's coffee.

KEN: You're joking now.

NURSE: I'm not.

KEN: What you have there is a coffee-flavored milk drink.

NURSE: Don't you like it?

KEN: It's all right, but I would like some real coffee, hot and black and bitter so that I could chew it.

NURSE: I'll ask the Sister.

KEN: I shouldn't.

NURSE: Why not?

KEN: Because in an hour's time, you'll be bringing round a little white pill that is designed to insert rose-colored filters behind my eyes. It will calm me and soothe me and make me forget for a while that you have a lovely body.

NURSE: Mr. Harrison . . . I'm . . .

KEN:

(*Genuinely concerned*)

I'm sorry. Really, I *am* sorry. I don't want to take it out on you–it's not your fault. You're only the vestal virgin . . . Sorry I said virgin.

NURSE: You'd better drink your coffee before it gets cold.

(*She feeds him a little, sip by sip*)

KEN: I was right; it's milky . . . What made you become a nurse?

NURSE: I'm not a nurse yet.

KEN: Oh yes you are.

(NURSE SADLER *smiles*)

Nurse Sadler.

NURSE: You must have thought me a real twit.

KEN: Of course not!

NURSE: The Sister-Tutor told us we would say it.

KEN: Well then . . .

NURSE: But I was so sure I wouldn't.

KEN: You haven't told me what made you become a nurse.

NURSE: I've always wanted to. What made you become a sculptor?

KEN: Hey there! You're learning too fast!

NURSE: What do you mean?

KEN: When you get a personal question, just ignore it–change the subject, or better still, ask another question back.

(NURSE SADLER *smiles*)

Did Sister-Tutor tell you that too?

NURSE: Something like it.

KEN: It's called being professional, isn't it?

NURSE: I suppose so.

KEN: I don't want any more of that, it's horrid. Patients are requested not to ask for credit for their intelligence, as refusal often offends.

NURSE: You sound angry. I hope I . . .

KEN: Not with you, Kay. Not at all. With myself I expect. Don't say it. That's futile isn't it?

NURSE: Yes.

(SISTER *opens the door*)

SISTER: Have you finished, Nurse? Dr. Emerson is here.

NURSE: Yes, Sister. I'm just coming.

SISTER: Straighten that sheet.

(*She goes, leaving the door open*)

KEN: Hospitals are weird places. Broken necks are acceptable, but a wrinkled sheet! . . .

(NURSE SADLER *smooths the bed. She goes out as* DR. EMERSON *comes in with* SISTER *and* DR. SCOTT)

DR. EMERSON: Morning.

KEN: Good morning.

DR. EMERSON: How are you this morning?

KEN: As you see, racing around all over the place.

(DR. EMERSON *picks up the chart and notes from the bottom of the bed*)

DR. EMERSON:

(*To* DR. SCOTT)

You've prescribed Valium, I see.

DR. SCOTT: Yes.

DR. EMERSON: His renal function looks much improved.

DR. SCOTT: Yes, the blood urea is back to normal and the cultures are sterile.

DR. EMERSON: Good . . . Good. Well, we had better go on keeping an eye on it, just in case.

DR. SCOTT: Yes, of course, sir.

DR. EMERSON: Good . . . Well, Mr. Harrison, we seem to be out of the woods now . . .

KEN: So when are you going to discharge me?

DR. EMERSON: Difficult to say.

KEN: Really? Are you ever going to discharge me?

DR. EMERSON: Well, you'll certainly be leaving *us* soon, I should think.

KEN: Discharged or transferred?

DR. EMERSON: This unit is for critical patients; when we have reached a position of stability, then you can be looked after in a much more comfortable, quiet hospital.

KEN: You mean you only grow the vegetables here–the vegetable store is somewhere else.

DR. EMERSON: I don't think I understand you.

KEN: I think you do. Spell it out for me, please. What chance have I of only being partly dependent on nursing?

DR. EMERSON: It's impossible to say with certainty what the prognosis of any case is.

KEN: I'm not asking for a guarantee on oath. I am simply asking for your professional opinion. Do you believe I will ever walk again?

DR. EMERSON: No.

KEN: Or recover the use of my arms?

DR. EMERSON: No.

KEN: Thank you.

DR. EMERSON: What for?

KEN: Your honesty.

DR. EMERSON: Yes, well . . . I should try not to brood on it if I were you. It's surprising how we can come to accept things. Dr. Scott has prescribed something which will help.

(*To* DR. SCOTT)

You might also get Mrs. Boyle along . . .

DR. SCOTT: Yes, of course.

DR. EMERSON: You'll be surprised how many things you will be able to do. Good morning.

(*They go into the corridor area*)

DR. EMERSON: What dose was it you prescribed?

DR. SCOTT: Two milligrams T.I.D.

DR. EMERSON: That's very small. You might have to increase it to five milligrams.

DR. SCOTT: Yes, sir.

DR. EMERSON: We ought to aim to get him moved in a month at most. These beds are very precious.

DR. SCOTT: Yes.

DR. EMERSON: Well, thank you, Doctor. I must rush off. Damned committee meeting.

DR. SCOTT: I thought you hated those.

DR. EMERSON: I do, but there's a new heart monitoring unit I want . . . very much indeed.

DR. SCOTT: Good luck, then.

DR. EMERSON: Thank you, Clare.

(*He goes.* DR. SCOTT *looks in at* SISTER's *office.*)

DR. SCOTT: Did you get that Valium for Mr. Harrison, Sister?

SISTER: Yes, Doctor. I was going to give him the first at twelve o'clock.

DR. SCOTT: Give him one now, will you?

SISTER: Right.

DR. SCOTT: Thank you.

(*She begins to walk away, then turns*)

On second thoughts . . . give it to me. I'll take it. I want to talk with him.

SISTER: Here it is.

(*She hands a small tray with a tablet and a feeding cup of water*)

DR. SCOTT: Thank you.

(*She walks to* KEN's *room and goes in*)

I've brought something to help you.

KEN: My God, they've got some highly qualified nurses here.

DR. SCOTT: Only the best in this hospital.

KEN: You're spoiling me you know, Doctor. If this goes on I shall demand that my next enema is performed by no one less than the Matron.

DR. SCOTT: Well, it wouldn't be the first she'd done, or the thousandth either.

KEN: She worked up through the ranks, did she?

DR. SCOTT: They all do.

KEN: Yes, in training school they probably learn that at the bottom of every bed pan lies a potential Matron. Just now, for one or two glorious minutes, I felt like a human being again.

DR. SCOTT: Good.

KEN: And now you're going to spoil it.

DR. SCOTT: How?

KEN: By tranquilizing yourself.

DR. SCOTT: Me?

KEN: Oh, I shall get the tablet, but it's you that needs the tranquilizing; I don't.

DR. SCOTT: Dr. Emerson and I thought . . .

KEN: You both watched me disturbed, worried even perhaps, and you can't do anything for me—nothing that really matters. I'm paralyzed and you're impotent. This disturbs you because you're a sympathetic person and as someone dedicated to an active sympathy doing something—anything even—you find it hard to accept you're impotent. The only thing you can do is to stop me thinking about it—that is—stop me disturbing you. So I get the tablet and you get the tranquility.

DR. SCOTT: That's a tough diagnosis.

KEN: Is it so far from the truth?

DR. SCOTT: There may be an element of truth in it, but it's not the whole story.

KEN: I don't suppose it is.

DR. SCOTT: After all, there is no point in worrying unduly—you know the facts. It's no use banging your head against a wall.

KEN: If the only feeling I have is in my head, and I want to feel, I might choose to bang it against a wall.

DR. SCOTT: And if you damage your head?

KEN: You mean go bonkers?

DR. SCOTT: Yes.

KEN: Then that would be the final catastrophe, but I'm not bonkers—yet. My consciousness is the only thing I have and I must claim the right to use it and, as far as possible, act on conclusions I may come to.

DR. SCOTT: Of course.

KEN: Good. Then you eat that tablet if you want tranquility, because I'm not going to.

DR. SCOTT: It is prescribed.

KEN: Oh come off it, Doctor. I know everyone around here acts as though those little bits of paper have just been handed down from Sinai. But the writing on those tablets isn't in Hebrew . . .

DR. SCOTT: . . . Well, you aren't due for it till twelve o'clock. We'll see . . .

KEN: That's what I always say. If you don't know whether to take a tranquilizer or not–sleep on it. When you tell Dr. Emerson, impress on him I don't need it . . .

(DR. SCOTT *smiles. She leaves and goes to the* SISTER'S *room*)

DR. SCOTT: Sister, I haven't given it to him . . . Leave it for a while.

SISTER: Did you alter the notes?

DR. SCOTT: No . . . Not yet.

(*She picks up a pile of notes and begins writing*)

(*CROSS FADE on sluice room*)

(NURSE SADLER *is taking kidney dishes and instruments out of the sterilizer.* JOHN *creeps up behind her and seizes her round the waist.* NURSE SADLER *jumps, utters a muffled scream and drops a dish*)

NURSE: Oh, it's you . . . Don't do that . . .

JOHN: I couldn't help myself, honest, my Lord. There was this vision in white and blue, then I saw red in front of my eyes. It was like looking into a Union Jack.

(NURSE SADLER *has turned round to face* JOHN, *who has his arms either side of her against the table*)

NURSE: Let go . . .

JOHN: What's a nice girl like you doing in a place like this?

NURSE: Sterilizing the instruments . . .

(JOHN *gasps and holds his groin*)

JOHN: Don't say things like that! Just the thought . . .

(NURSE SADLER *is free and returns to her work*)

NURSE: I don't know what you're doing in a place like this . . . It's just a big joke to you.

JOHN: 'Course it is. You can't take a place like this seriously . . .

NURSE: Why ever not?

JOHN: It's just the ante-room of the morgue.

NURSE: That's terrible! They don't all die.

JOHN: Don't they?

NURSE: No! Old Mr. Trevellyan is going out tomorrow, for instance.

JOHN: After his third heart attack! I hope they give him a return ticket on the ambulance.

NURSE: Would you just let them die? People like Mr. Harrison?

JOHN: How much does it cost to keep him here? Hundreds of pounds a week.

NURSE: That's not the point.

JOHN: In Africa children die of measles. It would cost only a few pounds to keep them alive. There's something crazy somewhere.

NURSE: That's wrong too–but it wouldn't help just letting Mr. Harrison die.

JOHN: No . . .

(*He goes up to her again*)

Nurse Sadler, when your eyes flash, you send shivers up and down my spine . . .

NURSE: John, stop it . . .

(*She is backing away*)

JOHN: Why don't we go out tonight?

NURSE: I've got some work to do for my exam.

JOHN: Let me help . . . I'm an expert on anatomy. We could go dancing, down to the Barbados Club, a few drinks and then back to my pad for an anatomy lesson.

NURSE: Let me get on . . .

(JOHN *holds* NURSE SADLER*'s head and slides his hands down*)

JOHN:

(*Singing*)

Oh the head bone's connected to the neck bone, The neck bone's connected to the shoulder bone, The shoulder bone's connected to the . . . breast bone . . .

(NURSE SADLER *escapes just in time. She backs out of the room and into* SISTER, *who is coming to see what's causing the noise.*)

NURSE: Sorry, Sister.

SISTER: This hospital exists to cure accidents, not to cause them.

NURSE: No . . . Yes . . . Sister.

SISTER: Are you going to be all day with that sterilizer?

NURSE: No, Sister.

(*She hurries away*)

SISTER: Haven't you any work to do, John?

JOHN: Sister, my back is bowed down with the weight of all the work resting on it.

SISTER: Then I suggest you shift some.

JOHN: Right.

(*She goes.* JOHN *shrugs and goes*)

(*CROSS FADE on* DR. EMERSON*'s office*)

(DR. EMERSON *is on the phone*)

DR. EMERSON: Look, Jenkins, I know the capital cost is high, but it would save on nursing costs. I've got four cardiac cases in here at the moment. With that unit I could save at least on one nurse a day. They could all be monitored in the Sister's room . . . Yes I know . . .

(DR. SCOTT *knocks on the door. She goes in*)

Hello? . . . Yes, well, old chap, I've got to go now. Do impress on the board how much money we'd save in the long run . . . all right . . . Thank you.

(*He puts the phone down*)

DR. SCOTT: Still wheeling and dealing for that monitoring unit?

DR. EMERSON: Bloody administrators. In this job a degree in accountancy would be more valuable to me than my M.D. . . . Still, what can I do for you?

DR. SCOTT: It's Harrison.

DR. EMERSON: Some sort of relapse?

DR. SCOTT: On the contrary.

DR. EMERSON: Good.

DR. SCOTT: He doesn't want to take Valium.

DR. EMERSON: Doesn't want to take it? What do you mean?

DR. SCOTT: He guessed it was some sort of tranquilizer and said he preferred to keep his consciousness clear.

DR. EMERSON: That's the trouble with all this anti-drug propaganda; it's useful of course, but it does set up a negative reaction to even necessary drugs, in sensitive people.

DR. SCOTT: I'm not sure he's not right.

DR. EMERSON: Right? When you prescribed the drug, you thought he needed it.

DR. SCOTT: Yes.

DR. EMERSON: And when I saw him, I agreed with you.

DR. SCOTT: Yes.

DR. EMERSON: It's a very small dose–two milligrams T.I.D. wasn't it?

DR. SCOTT: That's right.

DR. EMERSON: The minimum that will have any effect at all. You remember I said you might have to go up to five milligrams. A psychiatric dose, you know, is ten or fifteen miligrams.

DR. SCOTT: I know, but Mr. Harrison isn't a psychiatric case, is he?

DR. EMERSON: So how did you persuade him to take it?

DR. SCOTT: I didn't.

DR. EMERSON: Now let's get this clear. This morning when you examined him, you came to a careful and responsible decision that your patient needed a certain drug.

DR. SCOTT: Yes.

DR. EMERSON: I saw the patient and I agreed with your prescription.

DR. SCOTT: Yes.

— DR. EMERSON: But in spite of two qualified opinions, you accept the decision of someone completely unqualified to take it.

DR. SCOTT: He may be unqualified, but he is the one affected.

DR. EMERSON: Ours was an objective, his a subjective decision.

DR. SCOTT: But isn't this a case where a subjective decision may be more valid? After all, you're both working on the same subject–his body. Only he knows more about how he feels.

DR. EMERSON: But he doesn't know about the drugs and their effects.

DR. SCOTT: He can feel their effects directly.

DR. EMERSON: Makes no difference. His knowledge isn't based on experience of a hundred such cases. He can't know enough to challenge our clinical decisions.

DR. SCOTT: That's what he's doing and he's protesting about the dulling of his consciousness with Valium.

DR. EMERSON: When he came in, shocked to hell, did he protest about the dextrose-saline? Or when he was gasping for breath, he didn't use some of it to protest about the aminophylline or the huge stat dose of cortisone . . .

DR. SCOTT: Those were inevitable and emergency decisions.

DR. EMERSON: And so is this one inevitable. Just because our patient is conscious, that does not absolve us from our complete responsibility. We have to maximize whatever powers he retains.

DR. SCOTT: And how does a depressant drug improve his consciousness?

DR. EMERSON: It will help him to use his consciousness, Clare. We must help him now to turn his mind to the real problem he has. We must help him to an acceptance of his condition. Only then will his full consciousness be any use to him at all . . . You say he refused to take the tablet?

(DR. SCOTT *nods.* DR. EMERSON *picks up the phone and dials. The phone rings in the* SISTER'*s office*)

SISTER: Sister Anderson speaking.

DR. EMERSON: Emerson here. Could you prepare a syringe with five milligrams of Valium for Mr. Harrison?

SISTER: Yes, sir.

DR. EMERSON: I'll be down myself immediately to give it to him.

SISTER: Yes, sir.

(*She replaces the phone and immediately prepares the syringe*)

DR. SCOTT: Do you want me to come?

DR. EMERSON: No . . . It won't be necessary.

DR. SCOTT: Thank you . . .

(*She moves to the door*)

DR. EMERSON: Harrison is an intelligent, sensitive and articulate man.

DR. SCOTT: Yes.

DR. EMERSON: But don't undervalue yourself. Clare, your first decision was right.

(DR. SCOTT *nods and leaves the room. She is unhappy.* DR. EMERSON *walks to the* SISTER'S *room*)

DR. EMERSON: Have you the Valium ready, Sister?

SISTER: Yes, sir.

(*She hands him the kidney dish.* DR. EMERSON *takes it.* SISTER *makes to follow him*)

DR. EMERSON: It's all right, Sister. You've plenty of work, I expect.

SISTER: There's always plenty of that.

(DR. EMERSON *goes into* KEN'S *room*)

KEN: Hello, hello, they've brought up the heavy brigade.

(DR. EMERSON *pulls back the bed clothes and reaches for* KEN'S *arm*)

Dr. Emerson, I am afraid I must insist that you do not stick that needle in me.

DR. EMERSON: It is important that I do.

KEN: Who for?

DR. EMERSON: You.

KEN: I'm the best judge of that.

DR. EMERSON: I think not. You don't even know what's in this syringe.

KEN: I take it that the injection is one of a series of measures to keep me alive.

DR. EMERSON: You could say that.

KEN: Then it is not important. I've decided not to stay alive.

DR. EMERSON: But you can't decide that.

KEN: Why not?

DR. EMERSON: You're very depressed.

KEN: Does that surprise you?

DR. EMERSON: Of course not; it's perfectly natural. Your body received massive injuries; it takes time to come to any acceptance of the new situation. Now I shan't be a minute . . .

KEN: Don't stick that fucking thing in me!

DR. EMERSON: There . . . It's over now.

KEN: Doctor, I didn't give you permission to stick that needle in me. Why did you do it?

DR. EMERSON: It was necessary. Now try to sleep . . . You will find that as you gain acceptance of the situation you will be able to find a new way of living.

KEN: Please let me make myself clear. I specifically refused permission to stick that needle in me and you didn't listen. You took no notice.

DR. EMERSON: You must rely on us, old chap. Of course you're depressed. I'll send someone along to have a chat with you. Now I really must go and get on with my rounds.

KEN: Doctor . . .

DR. EMERSON: I'll send someone along.

(*He places the dish on the side locker, throwing the needle in a waste bin. He goes out.* KEN *is frustrated and then his eyes close*)

(*CROSS FADE on* SISTER'S *office*)

(SISTER *and* DR. SCOTT *are sitting*)

SISTER: I'm always warning my nurses not to get involved.

DR. SCOTT: Of course . . . And you never do, do you?

SISTER:

(*Smiling*)

. . . Never.

DR. SCOTT: You're a liar, Sister.

SISTER: Dr. Scott!

DR. SCOTT: Come on, we all do. Dr. Emerson is as involved with Ken Harrison as if he were his father.

SISTER: But you don't feel like his mother!

DR. SCOTT: . . . No comment, Sister.

(NURSE SADLER *comes into* SISTER'S *office*)

NURSE: I've finished, Sister.

SISTER: All right . . . Off you go then, Nurse.

NURSE: Yes, Sister!

SISTER: Have you been running?

NURSE: No, Sister!

SISTER: Oh . . . You just looked . . . flushed.

NURSE: . . . Oh . . . Goodnight, Sister . . . Doctor.

SISTER:

DR. SCOTT:

Goodnight.

(*CROSS FADE to* KEN'S *room*)

(SISTER *and* NURSE SADLER *come in with the trolley*)

SISTER: Good morning, Mr. Harrison. How are you this morning?

KEN: Marvelous.

SISTER: Night Sister said you slept well.

KEN: I did. I had a lot of help, remember.

SISTER: Your eyes are bright this morning.

KEN: I've been thinking.

SISTER: You do too much of that.

KEN: What other activity would you suggest? . . . Football? I tell you what, Sister, just leave me alone with Nurse Sadler here. Let's see what the old Adam can do for me.

SISTER: I'm a Sister, not a Madame.

KEN: Sister–you dark horse you! All this time you've been kidding me. I've been wondering for months how on earth a woman could become a State Registered Nurse and a Sister and still think you found babies under a gooseberry bush–and you've known all along.

SISTER: Of course I've known. When I qualified as a midwife I learnt that when they pick up the babies from under the gooseberry bushes they wrap them up in women to keep them warm. I know because it was our job to unwrap them again.

KEN: The miracle of modern science! Anyway, Sister, as I said, I've been thinking, if I'm going to be around for a long time, money will help.

SISTER: It always does.

KEN: Do you remember that solicitor chap representing my insurance company a few months ago? Mr. Hill, I think he said his name was. He said he'd come back when I felt better. Do you think you could get him back as soon as possible? I'd feel more settled if we could get the compensation sorted out.

SISTER: Sounds a good idea.

KEN: You'll ring him up?

SISTER: Of course.

KEN: He left a card; it's in my drawer.

SISTER: Right.

(*She goes to the locker and takes out the card*)

Mr. Philip Hill, Solicitor. Right, I'll ring him.

KEN: Thanks.

SISTER: That's enough.

(*They cover him up again and straighten the bed*)

SISTER: Mrs. Boyle is waiting to see you, Mr. Harrison.

KEN: Mrs. Boyle? Who's she?

SISTER: A very nice woman.

KEN: Oh God, must I see her?

SISTER: Dr. Emerson asked her to come along.

KEN: Then I'd better see her. If I refuse, he'll probably dissolve her in water and inject her into me.

(SISTER *has to choke back a giggle*)

SISTER: Mr. Harrison! Come on, Nurse; this man will be the death of me.

KEN:

(*Cheerfully*)

Doubt it, Sister. I'm not even able to be the death of myself.

(SISTER *goes out with* NURSE SADLER. MRS. GILLIAN BOYLE *enters.*
She is thirty-five, attractive, and very professional in her manner. She is a
medical social worker)

MRS. BOYLE: Good morning.

KEN: Morning.

MRS. BOYLE: Mr. Harrison?

KEN: It used to be.

MRS. BOYLE: My name is Mrs. Boyle.

KEN: And you've come to cheer me up.

MRS. BOYLE: I wouldn't put it like that.

KEN: How would you put it?

MRS. BOYLE: I've come to see if I can help.

KEN: Good. You can.

MRS. BOYLE: How?

KEN: Go and convince Dr. Frankenstein that he has successfully made his
monster and he can now let it go.

MRS. BOYLE: Dr. Emerson is a first-rate physician. My goodness, they have
improved this room.

KEN: Have they?

MRS. BOYLE: It used to be really dismal. All dark green and cream. It's
surprising what pastel colors will do, isn't it? Really cheerful.

KEN: Yes; perhaps they should try painting me. I'd hate to be the thing that
ruins the décor.

MRS. BOYLE: What on earth makes you say that? You don't ruin anything.

KEN: I'm sorry. That was a bit . . . whining. Well, don't let me stop you.

MRS. BOYLE: Doing what?

KEN: What you came for, I suppose. What do you do? Conjuring tricks?
Funny stories? Or a belly dance? If I have any choice, I'd prefer the belly
dance.

MRS. BOYLE: I'm afraid I've left my bikini at home.

KEN: Who said anything about a bikini?

MRS. BOYLE: Dr. Emerson tells me that you don't want any more treatment.

KEN: Good.

MRS. BOYLE: Why good?

KEN: I didn't think he'd heard what I said.

MRS. BOYLE: Why not?

KEN: He didn't take any notice.

MRS. BOYLE: Well as you can see, he did.

KEN: He sent you?

MRS. BOYLE: Yes.

KEN: And you are my new treatment; get in.

MRS. BOYLE: Why don't you want any more treatment?

KEN: I'd rather not go on living like this.

MRS. BOYLE: Why not?

KEN: Isn't it obvious?

MRS. BOYLE: Not to me. I've seen many patients like you.

KEN: And they all want to live?

MRS. BOYLE: Usually.

KEN: Why?

MRS. BOYLE: They find a new way of life.

KEN: How?

MRS. BOYLE: You'll be surprised how many things you will be able to do with training and a little patience.

KEN: Such as?

MRS. BOYLE: We can't be sure yet. But I should think that you will be able to operate reading machines and perhaps an adapted typewriter.

KEN: Reading and writing. What about arithmetic?

MRS. BOYLE:

(*Smiling*)

I dare say we could fit you up with a comptometer if you really wanted one.

KEN: Mrs. Boyle, even educationalists have realized that the three r's do not make a full life.

MRS. BOYLE: What did you do before the accident?

KEN: I taught in an art school. I was a sculptor

MRS. BOYLE: I see.

KEN: Difficult, isn't it? How about an electrically operated hammer and chisel? No, well. Or a cybernetic lump of clay?

MRS. BOYLE: I wouldn't laugh if I were you. It's amazing what can be done. Our scientists are wonderful.

KEN: They are. But it's not good enough you see, Mrs. Boyle. I really have absolutely no desire at all to be the object of scientific virtuosity. I have thought things over very carefully. I do have plenty of time for thinking and I have decided that I do not want to go on living with so much effort for so little result.

MRS. BOYLE: Yes, well, we shall have to see about that.

KEN: What is there to see?

MRS. BOYLE: We can't just stop treatment, just like that.

KEN: Why not?

MRS. BOYLE: It's the job of the hospital to save life, not to lose it.

KEN: The hospital's done all it can, but it wasn't enough. It wasn't the hospital's fault; the original injury was too big.

MRS. BOYLE: We have to make the best of the situation.

KEN: No. "We" don't have to do anything. I have to do what is to be done and that is to cash in the chips.

MRS. BOYLE: It's not unusual, you know, for people injured as you have been, to suffer with this depression for a considerable time before they begin to see that a life is possible.

KEN: How long?

MRS. BOYLE: It varies.

KEN: Don't hedge.

MRS. BOYLE: It could be a year or so.

KEN: And it could last for the rest of my life.

MRS. BOYLE: That would be most unlikely.

KEN: I'm sorry, but I cannot settle for that.

MRS. BOYLE: Try not to dwell on it. I'll see what I can do to get you started on some occupational therapy. Perhaps we could make a start on the reading machines.

KEN: Do you have many books for those machines?

MRS. BOYLE: Quite a few.

KEN: Can I make a request for the first one?

MRS. BOYLE: If you like.

KEN: "How to be a sculptor with no hands."

MRS. BOYLE: I'll be back tomorrow with the machine.

KEN: It's marvelous, you know.

MRS. BOYLE: What is?

KEN: All you people have the same technique. When I say something really awkward you just pretend I haven't said anything at all. You're all the bloody same . . . Well there's another outburst. That should be your cue to comment on the light-shade or the color of the walls.

MRS. BOYLE: I'm sorry if I have upset you.

KEN: Of course you have upset me. You and the doctors with your appalling so-called professionalism, which is nothing more than a series of verbal tricks to prevent you relating to your patients as human beings.

MRS. BOYLE: You must understand; we have to remain relatively detached in order to help . . .

KEN: That's all right with me. Detach yourself. Tear yourself off on the dotted line that divides the woman from the social worker and post yourself off to another patient.

MRS. BOYLE: You're very upset . . .

KEN: Christ Almighty, you're doing it again. Listen to yourself, woman. I say something offensive about you and you turn your professional cheek. If you were human, if you were treating me as human, you'd tell me to bugger off. Can't you see that this is why I've decided that life isn't worth living? I am not human and I'm even more convinced of that by your visit than I was before, so how does that grab you? The very exercise of your so-called professionalism makes me want to die.

MRS. BOYLE: I'm . . . Please . . .

KEN: Go . . . For God's sake get out . . . Go on . . . Get out . . . Get out . . .

(*She goes into* SISTER's *room.* SISTER *hears* KEN's *shouts*)

SISTER: What's the matter, Mrs. Boyle?

MRS. BOYLE: It's Mr. Harrison . . . He seems very upset.

KEN:

(*Shouting*)

. . . I am upset.

(SISTER *closes the door*)

SISTER: I should leave him for now, Mrs. Boyle. We'll send for you again when he's better.

(SISTER *hurries in to* KEN. *He is very distressed, rocking his head from side to side, desperately short of breath*)

KEN: Sis . . . ter . . .

(SISTER *reaches for the oxygen mask*)

SISTER: Now, now, Mr. Harrison, calm down.

(*She applies the mask and turns on the oxygen.* KEN *gradually becomes calmer*)

SISTER: Now why do you go getting yourself so upset? . . . There's no point . . .

KEN:

(*Muffled*)

But . . .

SISTER: Stop talking, Mr. Harrison. Just relax.

(KEN *becomes calm.* SISTER *sees* NURSE SADLER *going past.* MRS. BOYLE *is still hovering*)

Nurse.

NURSE: Sister?

SISTER: Take over here, will you?

NURSE: Yes, Sister.

(NURSE SADLER *holds the mask.* SISTER *goes to the door*)

MRS. BOYLE: Is he all right?

SISTER: Yes, perfectly.

MRS. BOYLE: I'm sorry . . .

SISTER: Don't worry. It was not you . . . We'll let you know when he's better.

MRS. BOYLE: Right . . . Thank you.

(*She goes.* SISTER *stands at the open door*)

SISTER: Just give him another ten seconds, Nurse.

NURSE: Yes, Sister.

(SISTER *takes a pace back behind the door and listens. After ten seconds,*
    NURSE SADLER *removes the mask*)

KEN: Oh, she's a shrewd cookie, is our Sister.

(SISTER *smiles at this.* NURSE SADLER *glances backward.* KEN *catches on to*
    the reason)

It's all right, Sister. I'm still alive, bugger it. I don't want to give her too much
    satisfaction.

NURSE: She's gone.

(*She closes the door*)

KEN: Come on then, over here. I shan't bite you, Kay. Come and cool my
    fevered brow or something.

NURSE: What upset you?

KEN: Being patronized, I suppose.

NURSE: What did you mean about Sister?

KEN: She knew if she came in I'd shout at her, but if you were here I
    wouldn't shout.

NURSE: Why?

KEN: A good question. Because I suppose you're young and gentle and inno-
    cent and Sister knows that I am not the sort who would shout at you . . .

NURSE: You mean, you would rather patronize me.

KEN: Hey! Steady on there, Kay. If you show you're well able to take care of
    yourself I shall have to call you Nurse Sadler and shout at you too, and
    Sister and I will have lost a valuable asset.

NURSE: What were you? . . .

(*The door opens and* SISTER *and* DR. SCOTT *come in*)

KEN: What is this? Piccadilly Circus?

SISTER: All right, Nurse. Dr. Scott was just coming as it happened. Are you
    feeling better now, Mr. Harrison?

(NURSE SADLER *leaves*)

KEN: Lovely, thank you, Sister.

SISTER: I made your phone call to Mr. Hill. He said he'd try to get in tomorrow.

KEN: Thank you . . .

(SISTER *leaves*)

DR. SCOTT: And what was all the fuss about?

KEN: I'm sorry about that. The last thing I want is to bring down Emerson again with his pharmaceutical truncheon.

DR. SCOTT: I'm . . . sorry about that.

KEN: I don't suppose it was your fault.

DR. SCOTT: Can I give you some advice?

KEN: Please do; I may even take it.

DR. SCOTT: Take the tablets; the dose is very small–the minimum–and it won't really blunt your consciousness, not like the injection.

KEN: . . . You're on.

DR. SCOTT: Good . . . I was glad to hear about your decision to try and get your compensation settled.

KEN: How did you? . . . Oh, I suppose Sister checked with you.

DR. SCOTT: She did mention it . . .

KEN: You have lovely breasts.

DR. SCOTT: I beg your pardon?

KEN: I said you have lovely breasts.

DR. SCOTT: What an odd thing to say

KEN: Why? You're not only a doctor, are you? You can't tell me that you regard them only as mammary glands.

DR. SCOTT: No.

KEN: You're quite safe.

DR. SCOTT: Of course.

KEN: I'm not about to jump out of bed and rape you or anything.

DR. SCOTT: I know.

KEN: Did it embarrass you?

DR. SCOTT: Surprised me.

KEN: And embarrassed you.

DR. SCOTT: I suppose so.

KEN: But why exactly? You are an attractive woman. I admit that it's unusual for a man to compliment a woman on her breasts when only one of them is in bed, only one of the people that is, not one of the breasts, but that wasn't the reason, was it?

DR. SCOTT: I don't think it helps you to talk like this.

KEN: Because I can't do anything about it, you mean.

DR. SCOTT: I didn't mean that exactly.

KEN: I watch you walking in the room, bending over me, tucking in your sweater. It's surprising how relaxed a woman can become when she is not in the presence of a man.

DR. SCOTT: I am sorry if I provoked you . . . I can assure you . . .

KEN: You haven't "provoked" me, as you put it, but you are a woman and even though I've only a piece of knotted string between my legs, I still have a man's mind. One change that I have noticed is that I now engage in sexual banter with your nurses, searching for the double entendre in the most innocent remark. Like a sexually desperate middle-aged man. Then they leave the room and I go cold with embarrassment. It's fascinating, isn't it? Laughable. I still have tremendous sexual desire. Do you find that disgusting?

DR. SCOTT: No.

KEN: Pathetic?

DR. SCOTT: Sad.

KEN: I am serious you know . . . about deciding to die.

DR. SCOTT: You will get over that feeling.

KEN: How do you know?

DR. SCOTT: From experience.

KEN: That doesn't alter the validity of my decision now.

DR. SCOTT: But if we acted on your decision now, there wouldn't be an opportunity for you to accept it.

KEN: I grant you, I may become lethargic and quiescent. Happy when a nurse comes to put in a new catheter, or give me an enema, or to turn me over. These could become the high spots of my day. I might even learn to do wonderful things, like turn the pages of a book with some miracle of modern science, or to type letters with flicking my eyelids. And you would look at me and say: "Wasn't it worth waiting?" and I would say: "Yes" and be proud of my achievements. Really proud. I grant you all that, but it doesn't alter the validity of my present position.

DR. SCOTT: But if you became happy?

KEN: But I don't want to become happy by becoming the computer section of a complex machine. And morally, you must accept my decision.

DR. SCOTT: Not according to my morals.

KEN: And why are yours better than mine? They're better because you're more powerful. I am in your power. To hell with a morality that is based on the proposition that might is right.

DR. SCOTT: I must go now. I was halfway through Mr. Patel.

(*She walks to the door*)

KEN: I thought you were just passing. Oh, Doctor . . . one more thing . . .

DR. SCOTT: Yes?

KEN: You still have lovely breasts.

(*She smiles and goes out into the* SISTER'*s office. She is very upset.* SISTER *passes and looks at her*)

SISTER: Are you all right? Would you like a cup of tea?

DR. SCOTT: Yes, Sister, I would.

SISTER: . . . Nurse! Would you bring a cup of tea, please.

(NURSE SADLER *looks from the kitchen*)

NURSE: Yes, Sister.

(*They walk into the* SISTER'*s room and sit down*)

DR. SCOTT: I've never met anyone like Ken Harrison before.

SISTER: No.

DR. SCOTT: He's so . . . bright . . . intelligent . . . He says he wants to die.

SISTER: Many patients say that.

DR. SCOTT: I know that, Sister, but he means it. It's just a calm rational decision.

SISTER: I thought this morning, when he was talking about the compensation, he was beginning to plan for the future.

DR. SCOTT: Not really, you know. That was just to keep us happy. He probably thinks that if he pretends to be planning for the future we'll stop tranquilizing him, or something like that.

(*A knock on the door*)

SISTER: Come in.

NURSE: Here's the tea, Sister.

SISTER: Thank you, Nurse. For Doctor.

(NURSE SADLER *gives the cup to* DR. SCOTT *and goes out*)

DR. SCOTT: It's marvelous, you know. We bring him back to life using everything we've got. We give him back his consciousness, then he says: "But how do I use it?" So what do we do? We put him back to sleep.

(*CROSS FADE on* KEN'*s room*)

(JOHN *goes in to empty the rubbish. He taps* KEN *lightly as if to repeat the steel band game, but* KEN *is asleep*)

JOHN: Ping-Pong . . . You poor bastard.

(*He leaves*)

(*Curtain*)

ACT TWO

SISTER: A visitor for you, Mr. Harrison.

HILL: Good afternoon, Mr. Harrison.

KEN: Good afternoon.

HILL: You're looking very much better.

(SISTER *has placed a chair by the bed*)

KEN: It's the nursing, you know.

SISTER: I'm glad you realize it, Mr. Harrison.

KEN: Oh, I do, Sister, I do.

SISTER: I'll leave you gentlemen now.

HILL: Thank you, Sister.

(*She goes out*)

You really do look better.

KEN: Yes. I'm as well now as I shall ever be . . .

HILL:

(*Unzipping his briefcase*)

I've brought all the papers . . . Things are moving along very satisfactorily
now and . . .

KEN: I don't want to talk about the accident.

HILL: I understand it must be very distressing . . .

KEN: No, no. It's not that. I didn't get you along about the compensation.

HILL: Oh . . . Sister said on the phone . . .

KEN: Yes, I know. Could you come away from the door? Look, do you work
for yourself? I mean, you don't work for an insurance company or something, do you? . . .

HILL: No. I'm in practice as a solicitor, but I . . .

KEN: Then there's no reason why you couldn't represent me generally . . .
apart from this compensation thing . . .

HILL: Certainly, if there's anything I can do . . .

KEN: There is.

HILL: Yes?

KEN: . . . Get me out of here.

HILL: . . . I don't understand, Mr. Harrison.

KEN: It's quite simple. I can't exist outside the hospital, so they've got to
keep me here if they want to keep me alive and they seem intent on
doing that. I've decided that I don't want to stay in hospital any longer.

HILL: But surely they wouldn't keep you here longer than necessary?

KEN: I'm almost completely paralyzed and I always will be. I shall never
be discharged by the hospital. I have coolly and calmly thought it out

and I have decided that I would rather not go on. I therefore want to be discharged to die.

HILL: And you want me to represent you?

KEN: Yes. Tough.

HILL: . . . And what is the hospital's attitude?

KEN: They don't know about it yet. Even tougher.

HILL: This is an enormous step . .

KEN: Mr. Hill, with all respect, I know that our hospitals are wonderful. I know that many people have succeeded in making good lives with appalling handicaps. I'm happy for them and respect and admire them. But each man must make his own decision. And mine is to die quietly and with as much dignity as I can muster and I need your help.

HILL: Do you realize what you're asking me to do?

KEN: I realize. I'm not asking that you make any decision about my life and death, merely that you represent me and my views to the hospital.

HILL: . . . Yes, well, the first thing is to see the Doctor. What is his name?

KEN: Dr. Emerson

HILL: I'll try and see him now and come back to you.

KEN: Then you'll represent me? . . .

HILL: Mr. Harrison, I'll let you know my decision after I've seen Dr. Emerson.

KEN: All right, but you'll come back to tell me yourself, even if he convinces you he's right?

HILL: Yes, I'll come back.

(*CROSS FADE on the sluice room*)

(NURSE SADLER *and* JOHN *are talking*)

JOHN: So why not? . . .

NURSE: It's just that I'm so busy . . .

JOHN: All work and no play . . . makes for a boring day.

NURSE: Anyway, I hardly know you.

JOHN: Right . . . That's why I want to take you out . . . to find out what goes on behind those blue eyes . . .

NURSE: At present, there's just lists of bones and organs, all getting themselves jumbled up.

JOHN: Because you're working too hard . . .

NURSE: Ask me next week . . .

JOHN: OK. It's a deal . . .

NURSE: Right!

JOHN: And I'll ask you this afternoon as well.

(*CROSS FADE on* DR. EMERSON's *room*)

DR. EMERSON: Mr. Hill? Sister just rang through.

HILL: Dr. Emerson?

(*They shake hands*)

DR. EMERSON: You've been seeing Mr. Harrison?

HILL: Yes.

DR. EMERSON: Tough case . . . I hope you'll be able to get enough money for him to ease his mind.

HILL: Dr. Emerson. It's not about that I wanted to see you. I thought I was coming about that, but Mr. Harrison wishes to retain me to represent him on quite another matter.

DR. EMERSON: Oh?

HILL: Yes, he wants to be discharged.

DR. EMERSON: That's impossible.

HILL: Why?

DR. EMERSON: To put it bluntly, he would die if we did that.

HILL: He knows that. It's what he wants.

DR. EMERSON: And you are asking me to kill my patient?

HILL: I am representing Mr. Harrison's wishes to you and asking for your reaction.

DR. EMERSON: Well, you've had it. It's impossible. Now if that's really all you came about . . .

HILL: Dr. Emerson, you can, of course, dismiss me like that if you choose to, but I would hardly think it serves anyone's interests, least of all Mr. Harrison's.

DR. EMERSON: I am trying to save Mr. Harrison's life. There is no need to remind me of my duty to my patient, Mr. Hill.

HILL: Or mine to my client, Dr. Emerson.

DR. EMERSON: . . . Are you telling me that you have accepted the job of coming to me to urge a course of action that will lose your client his life?

HILL: I hadn't accepted it . . . no . . . I told Mr. Harrison I would talk to you first. Now I have and I begin to see why he thought it necessary to be represented.

DR. EMERSON: All right . . . Let's start again. Now tell me what you want to know.

HILL: Mr. Harrison wishes to be discharged from hospital. Will you please make the necessary arrangements?

DR. EMERSON: No.

HILL: May I ask why not?

DR. EMERSON: Because Mr. Harrison is incapable of living outside the hospital and it is my duty as a doctor to preserve life.

HILL: I take it that Mr. Harrison is a voluntary patient here.

DR. EMERSON: Of course.

HILL: Then I fail to see the legal basis for your refusal.

DR. EMERSON: Can't you understand that Mr. Harrison is suffering from depression? He is incapable of making a rational decision about his life and death.

HILL: Are you maintaining that Mr. Harrison is mentally unbalanced?

DR. EMERSON: Yes.

HILL: Would you have any objection to my bringing in a psychiatrist for a second opinion?

DR. EMERSON: Of course not, but why not ask the consultant psychiatrist here? I'm sure he will be able to convince you.

HILL: Has he examined Mr. Harrison?

DR. EMERSON: No, but that can be quickly arranged.

HILL: That's very kind of you Dr. Emerson, but I'm sure you'll understand if I ask for my own–whose opinion you are not sure of *before* he examines the patient.

DR. EMERSON: Good afternoon, Mr. Hill.

HILL: Good afternoon.

(MR. HILL *takes up his briefcase and leaves*)

DR. EMERSON:

(*Picks up the phone*)

Could you find out where Dr. Travers is, please? I want to see him urgently, and put me through to the hospital secretary, please. Well, put me through when he's free.

(*CROSS FADE on* KEN'*s room*)

(*The door opens and* MR. HILL *comes in*)

KEN: Well, how was it on Olympus?

HILL: Cloudy.

KEN: No joy then?

HILL: Dr. Emerson does not wish to discharge you.

KEN: Surprise, surprise. So what do we do now?

HILL: Mr. Harrison, I will be perfectly plain. Dr. Emerson claims that you are not in a sufficiently healthy mental state to make a rational decision, especially one of this seriousness and finality. Now, my position is, I am not competent to decide whether or not he is right.

KEN: So how will you decide?

HILL: I should like to have you examined by an independent psychiatrist and I will accept his view of the case and advise you accordingly.

KEN: Fair enough. Will Dr. Emerson agree?

HILL: He has already. I ought to warn you that Dr. Emerson is likely to take steps to have you admitted here as a person needing treatment under the Mental Health Act of 1959. This means that he can keep you here and give you what treatment he thinks fit.

KEN: Can he do that?

HILL: He probably can.

KEN: Haven't I any say in this?

HILL: Oh yes. He will need another signature and that doctor will have to be convinced that you ought compulsorily to be detained. Even if he agrees, we can appeal.

KEN: Let's get on with it then.

HILL: One thing at a time. First, you remember, our own psychiatrist.

KEN: Wheel him in . . .

HILL: I'll be in touch soon then.

KEN: Oh, before you go. Yesterday I refused to take a tranquilizer and Dr. Emerson came and gave me an injection. It made me pretty dopey. If I was like that when the psychiatrist came, he'd lock me up for life!

HILL: I'll mention it to him. Goodbye for now then.

KEN: Goodbye.

(*CROSS FADE on* DR. EMERSON's *office*)

(DR. EMERSON *is on the phone.* DR. TRAVERS *knocks on his door and looks in*)

DR. EMERSON: Can you find me Dr. Scott please?

(*He puts the phone down*)

DR. TRAVERS: You wanted to see me?

DR. EMERSON: Ah yes. If you can spare a moment.

DR. TRAVERS: What's the problem?

DR. EMERSON: Nasty one really. I have a road accident case, paralyzed from the neck down. He's naturally very depressed and wants to discharge himself. But with a neurogenic bladder and all the rest of it, he couldn't last a week out of here. I need time to get him used to the idea.

DR. TRAVERS: How long ago was the accident?

DR. EMERSON: Six months.

DR. TRAVERS: A long time.

DR. EMERSON: Yes, well there were other injuries but we've just about got him physically stabilized. The trouble is that he's got himself a solicitor and if I am to keep him here, I'll have to admit him compulsorily under the Mental Health Act. I wondered if you'd see him.

DR. TRAVERS: I'll see him of course, but my signature won't help you.

Dr. Emerson: Why not? You're the psychiatrist, aren't you?

Dr. Travers: Yes, but under the Act, you need two signatures and only one can come from a practitioner of the hospital where the patient is to be kept.

Dr. Emerson: Bloody hell!

Dr. Travers: Not to worry. I take it you regard this as an emergency.

Dr. Emerson: Of course I do.

Dr. Travers: Well, sign the application and then you've got three days to get another signature.

Dr. Emerson: There'll be no problem about that surely?

Dr. Travers: Depends upon whether he's clinically depressed or not.

Dr. Emerson: You haven't understood. He's suicidal. He's determined to kill himself.

Dr. Travers: I could name you several psychiatrists who wouldn't take that as evidence of insanity.

Dr. Emerson: Well, I could name several psychiatrists who *are* evidence of insanity. I've had a lot of experience in this kind of case. I'm sure, absolutely sure, I can win him around, given time–a few months . . .

Dr. Travers: I understand, Michael.

Dr. Emerson: . . . So you'll look at him, will you? . . . And get another chap in? . . .

Dr. Travers: Yes, I'll do that.

Dr. Emerson:

(*Twinkling*)

And . . . do me a favor, will you? Try and find an old codger like me, who believes in something better than suicide.

Dr. Travers:

(*Grinning*)

There's a chap at Ellertree . . . a very staunch Catholic, I believe. Would that suit you?

Dr. Emerson: Be Jasus–sounds just the man!

Dr. Travers: I'll see his notes and drop in on him

Dr. Emerson: Thank you very much, Paul . . . I'm very grateful–and Harrison will be too.

(Dr. Scott *comes in the room*)

Dr. Scott: Oh, sorry.

Dr. Travers: It's all right . . . I'm just off . . . I'll see him then, Michael, this afternoon.

(Dr. Travers *leaves*. Dr. Scott *looks at* Dr. Emerson *questioningly*)

Dr. Scott: You wanted me?

DR. EMERSON: Ah yes. Harrison's decided to discharge himself.

DR. SCOTT: Oh no, but I'm not surprised.

DR. EMERSON: So, Travers is seeing him now.

DR. SCOTT: Dr. Travers won't make him change his mind.

DR. EMERSON: I am committing him under Section 26.

DR. SCOTT: Oh, will Dr. Travers sign it?

DR. EMERSON: Evidently if I do, he can't, but he knows a chap over in Ellertree who probably will.

DR. SCOTT: I see.

DR. EMERSON: I have no choice, do you see, Clare? He's got himself a solicitor. It's the only way I can keep him here.

DR. SCOTT: Are you sure you should?

DR. EMERSON: Of course. No question.

DR. SCOTT: It's his life.

DR. EMERSON: But my responsibility.

DR. SCOTT: Only if he's incapable of making his own decision.

DR. EMERSON: But he isn't capable. I refuse to believe that a man with a mind as quick as his, a man with enormous mental resources, would calmly choose suicide.

DR. SCOTT: But he has done just that.

DR. EMERSON: And, therefore, I say he is unbalanced.

DR. SCOTT: But surely a wish to die is not *necessarily* a symptom of insanity? A man might want to die for perfectly sane reasons.

DR. EMERSON: No, Clare, a doctor cannot accept the choice for death; he's committed to life. When a patient is brought into my unit, he's in a bad way. I don't stand about thinking whether or not it's worth saving his life, I haven't the time for doubts. I get in there, do whatever I can to save life. I'm a doctor, not a judge.

DR. SCOTT: I hope you will forgive me sir, for saying this, but I think that is just how you are behaving–as a judge.

DR. EMERSON: You must, of course, say what you think–but I am the responsible person here.

DR. SCOTT: I know that sir.

(*She makes to go*)

DR. EMERSON: I'm sure it's not necessary for me to say this but I'd rather there was no question of misunderstanding later . . . Mr. Harrison is now physically stable. There is no reason why he should die; if he should die suddenly, I would think it necessary to order a post-mortem and to act on whatever was found.

DR. SCOTT: . . . Mr. Harrison is your patient, sir.

DR. EMERSON:

(*Smiling*)

Of course, of course. You make that sound a fate worse than death.

DR. SCOTT: Perhaps for him it is.

(*She goes out*)

(*CROSS FADE on* KEN's *room*)

(DR. TRAVERS *comes in*)

DR. TRAVERS: Mr. Harrison?

KEN: That's right.

DR. TRAVERS: Dr. Travers.

KEN: Are you a psychiatrist?

DR. TRAVERS: Yes.

KEN: For or against me . . . Or does that sound like paranoia?

DR. TRAVERS: You'd hardly expect me to make an instant diagnosis.

KEN: Did Dr. Emerson send you?

DR. TRAVERS: I work here, in the hospital.

KEN: Ah.

DR. TRAVERS: Would you describe yourself as suffering from paranoia?

KEN: No.

DR. TRAVERS: What would you say paranoia was?

KEN: Difficult. It depends on the person. A man whose feelings of security
    are tied to his own sense of what is right and can brook no denial. If he
    were, say, a sculptor, then we would describe his mental condition as
    paranoia. If, on the other hand, he was a doctor, we would describe it as
    professionalism.

DR. TRAVERS:

(*Laughing*)

You don't like doctors!

KEN: Do you like patients?

DR. TRAVERS: Some.

KEN: I like some doctors.

DR. TRAVERS: What's wrong with doctors then?

KEN: Speaking generally, I suppose that as a profession you've not learned
    that the level of awareness of the population has risen dramatically;
    that black magic is no longer much use and that people *can* and *want* to
    understand what's wrong with them and many of them can make deci-
    sions about their own lives.

DR. TRAVERS: What they need is information.

KEN: Of course, but as a rule, doctors dole out information like a kosher
    butcher gives out pork sausages.

DR. TRAVERS: That's fair. But you'd agree that patients need medical knowledge to make good decisions?

KEN: I would. Look at me, for example. I'm a sculptor, an airy-fairy artist, with no real hard knowledge and no capability to understand anything about my body. You're a doctor but I think I would hold my own with a competition in anatomy with *you*.

DR. TRAVERS: It's a long time since I did any anatomy.

KEN: Of course. Whereas I was teaching it every day up to six months ago. It wouldn't be fair.

DR. TRAVERS: Your knowledge of anatomy may be excellent, but what's your neurology like, or your dermatology, endocrinology, urology and so on.

KEN: Lousy, and in so far as these bear on my case, I should be grateful for information so that I can make a proper decision. But it is my decision. If you came to my studio to buy something, and look at all my work, and you say: "I want that bronze" and I say to you: "Look, you don't know anything about sculpture. The proportion of that is all wrong, the texture is boring and it should have been made in wood anyway. You are having the marble!" You'd think I was nuts. If you were sensible you'd ask for my professional opinion but if you were a mature adult, you'd reserve the right to choose for yourself.

DR. TRAVERS: But we're not talking about a piece of sculpture to decorate a room, but about your life.

KEN: That's right, Doctor. *My* life.

DR. TRAVERS: But your obvious intelligence weakens your case. I'm not saying that you would find life easy but you do have resources that an unintelligent person doesn't have.

KEN: That sounds like Catch 22. If you're clever and sane enough to put up an invincible case for suicide, it demonstrates you ought not to die.

(DR. TRAVERS *moves the stool near the bed*)

That's a disturbing tidiness compulsion you've got there.

DR. TRAVERS: I was an only child; enough of me. Have you any relation-ships outside the hospital? . . . You're not married, I see.

KEN: No. thank God.

DR. TRAVERS: A girl friend?

KEN: A fiancée, actually. I asked her not to visit me any more. About a fortnight ago.

DR. TRAVERS: She must have been upset.

KEN: Better that than a lifetime's sacrifice.

DR. TRAVERS: She wanted to . . . stay with you then?

KEN: Oh yes . . . Had it all worked out . . . But she's a young healthy woman. She wants babies–real ones. Not ones that never will learn to walk.

DR. TRAVERS: But if that's what she really wants.

KEN: Oh come on, Doctor. If that's what she really wants, there's plenty of other cripples who want help. I told her to go to release her, I hope, from the guilt she would feel if she did what she really wanted to.

DR. TRAVERS: That's very generous.

KEN: Balls. Really, Doctor, I did it for *me*. It would destroy *my* self-respect if I allowed myself to become the object with which people can safely exploit their masochist tendencies.

DR. TRAVERS: That's putting it very strongly.

KEN: Yes. Too strong. But you are beginning to sound like the chaplain. He was in here the other day. He seemed to think I should be quite happy to be God's chosen vessel into which people could pour their compassion . . . That it was all right being a cripple because it made other folk feel good when they helped me.

DR. TRAVERS: What about your parents?

KEN: Working class folk–they live in Scotland. I thought it would break my mother–I always thought of my father as a very tough egg. But it was the other way round. My father can only think with his hands. He used to stand around here–completely at a loss. My mother would sit there– just understanding. She knows what suffering's about. They were here a week ago–I got rid of my father for a while and told my mother what I was going to do. She looked at me for a minute. There were tears in her eyes. She said: "Aye lad, it's thy life . . . don't worry about your dad–I'll get him over it" . . . She stood up and I said: "What about you?" "What about me?" she said, "Do you think life's so precious to me, I'm frightened of dying?" . . . I'd like to think I was my mother's son.

DR. TRAVERS: . . . Yes, well, we shall have to see . . .

KEN: What about? You mean you haven't made up your mind?

DR. TRAVERS: . . . I shall have to do some tests . . .

KEN: What tests, for Christ's sake? I can tell you now, my time over a hundred meters is lousy.

DR. TRAVERS: You seem very angry.

KEN: Of course I'm angry . . . No, no . . . I'm . . . Yes. I am angry.

(*Breathing*)

But I am trying to hold it in because you'll just write me off as in a manic phase of a manic-depressive cycle.

DR. TRAVERS: You are very free with psychiatric jargon.

KEN: Oh, well then, you'll be able to say I'm an obsessive hypochondriac. (*Breathing*)

DR. TRAVERS: I certainly wouldn't do that, Mr. Harrison.

KEN: Can't you see what a trap I am in? Can anyone prove that they are sane? Could you?

DR. TRAVERS: ... I'll come and see you again.

KEN: No, don't come and see me again, because every time you come I'll get more and more angry, and more and more upset and depressed. And eventually you will destroy my mind.

DR. TRAVERS: I'm sorry if I upset you, Mr. Harrison.

(DR. TRAVERS *replaces the stool and exits. He crosses to the* SISTER's *office. Enter* DR. SCOTT *and* MR. HILL)

DR. SCOTT: I hate the idea. It's against all my training and instincts ...

HILL: Mine, too. But in this case, we're not dealing with euthanasia, are we?

DR. SCOTT: Something very close.

HILL: No. Something very far away. Suicide.

DR. SCOTT: Thank you for a lovely meal.

HILL: Not at all; I am glad you accepted. Tell me, what would you think, or rather feel, if there was a miracle and Ken Harrison was granted the use of his arms for just one minute and he used them to grab a bottle of sleeping tablets and swallowed the lot?

DR. SCOTT: It's irrational but ... I'd be very ... relieved.

HILL: It wouldn't go against your instincts? ... You wouldn't feel it was a wasted life and fight with stomach pumps and all that?

DR. SCOTT: No ... not if it was my decision.

HILL: You might even be sure there *was* a bottle of tablets handy and you not there.

DR. SCOTT: You make it harder and harder ... but yes, I might do that ...

HILL: Yes. Perhaps we ought to make suicide respectable again. Whenever anyone kills himself there's a whole legal rigmarole to go through–investigations, inquests and so on–and it all seems designed to find someone or something to *blame.* Can you ever recall a coroner saying something like: "We've heard all the evidence of how John Smith was facing literally insuperable odds and he made a courageous decision. I record a verdict of a noble death?"

DR. SCOTT: No ... It's been a ... very pleasant evening.

HILL: Thank you. For me too.

DR. SCOTT: I don't know if I've helped you though.

HILL: You have. I've made up my mind.

DR. SCOTT: You'll help him?

HILL: Yes . . . I hope you're not sorry.

DR. SCOTT: I'm pleased . . .

HILL: I'm sure it is morally wrong for anyone to try to hand the responsibility for their death to anyone else. And it's wrong to accept that responsibility, but Ken isn't trying to do that.

DR. SCOTT: I'm glad you've made up your mind . . . Good night.

(*They stop*)

HILL: I hope I see you again.

DR. SCOTT: I'm in the book . . . Goodnight.

HILL: Goodnight.

(*They exit.* NURSE SADLER *goes into* KEN's *room with a meal*)

KEN: You still on duty?

NURSE: We're very short-staffed . . .

(*She prepares to feed* KEN *with a spoon*)

It looks good tonight . . . Minced beef.

KEN: Excellent . . . and what wine shall we order then? How about a '48 claret. Yes, I think so . . . Send for the wine waiter.

NURSE: You are a fool, Mr. Harrison.

KEN: Is there any reason why I shouldn't have wine?

NURSE: I don't know. I'll ask Sister if you like . . .

KEN: After all, the hospital seems determined to depress my consciousness. But they'd probably think it's immoral if I enjoy it.

(NURSE SADLER *gives him a spoonful of mince*)

It's a bit salty.

NURSE: Do you want some water?

KEN: That would be good. Very nice . . . Not too full of body. Château Ogston Reservoir, I think, with just a cheeky little hint of Jeyes fluid from the sterilizer.

NURSE: We use Milton.

KEN: Oh dear . . . you'd better add to my notes. The final catastrophe. Mr. Harrison's palate is failing; rush up the emergency taste resuscitation unit.

(*In a phony American accent*)

"Nurse, give me orange . . . No response . . . Quick the lemon . . . God! Not a flicker . . . We're on the tightrope . . . Nurse pass the ultimate . . . Quick, there's no time to lose . . . Pass the hospital mince." That would bring people back from the dead. Don't tell Emerson that or he'll try it. I don't want any more of that.

(NURSE SADLER *exits.* DR. SCOTT *comes in*)

KEN: Sister.

DR. SCOTT: No, it's me. Still awake?

KEN: Yes.

DR. SCOTT: It's late.

KEN: What time is it?

DR. SCOTT: Half past eleven.

KEN: The Night Sister said I could have the light for half an hour. I couldn't sleep. I wanted to think.

DR. SCOTT: Yes.

KEN: You look lovely.

DR. SCOTT: Thank you.

KEN: Have you been out?

DR. SCOTT: For a meal.

KEN: Nice. Good company?

DR. SCOTT: You're fishing.

KEN: That's right.

DR. SCOTT: Yes, it was good company.

KEN: A colleague?

DR. SCOTT: No. Actually it was Philip Hill, your solicitor.

KEN: Well, well, well . . . The randy old devil. He didn't take long to get cracking, did he?

DR. SCOTT: It was just a dinner.

KEN: I know I engaged him to act for me. I didn't realize he would see his duties so comprehensively.

DR. SCOTT: It was just a dinner!

KEN: Well, I hope my surrogate self behaved myself.

DR. SCOTT: You were a perfect gentleman.

KEN: Mm . . . then perhaps I'd better engage another surrogate.

DR. SCOTT: Do you mind really?

KEN: . . . No. Unless you convinced him that Emerson was right.

DR. SCOTT: . . . I didn't try.

KEN: Thank you.

DR. SCOTT: I think you are enjoying all this.

KEN: I suppose I am in a way. For the first time in six months I feel like a human being again.

DR. SCOTT: Yes.

(*A pause*)

Isn't that the whole point Ken, that . . .

KEN: You called me Ken.

DR. SCOTT: Do you mind?

KEN: Oh! No, I liked it. I'll just chalk it up as another credit for today.

DR. SCOTT: I was saying, isn't that just the point; isn't that what this fight has shown you? That you are a human being again. You're not fighting for death. I don't think you want to win.

KEN: That was what I had to think about.

DR. SCOTT: And you have . . . Changed your mind?

KEN: . . . No. I know I'm enjoying the fight and I had to be sure that I wanted to win, really get what I'm fighting for, and not just doing it to convince myself I'm still alive.

DR. SCOTT: And are you sure?

KEN: Yes, quite sure; for me life is over. I want it recognized because I can't do the things that I want to do. That means I can't say the things I want to say. Is that a better end? You understand, don't you?

(NURSE SADLER *comes in with a feeding cup*)

NURSE: I didn't know you were here, Doctor.

DR. SCOTT: Yes, I'm just going.

KEN: See what I mean, Doctor. Here is my substitute mum, with her porcelain pap. This isn't for me.

DR. SCOTT: No . . .

KEN: So tomorrow, on with the fight!

DR. SCOTT: Goodnight . . . and good luck.

(*FADE*)

KERSHAW: So our psychiatrist is prepared to state that Harrison is sane.

HILL: Yes, he was sure. I'll have his written report tomorrow. He said he could understand the hospital fighting to save their patient from himself, but no matter how much he sympathized with them and how much he wished he could get Harrison to change his mind, nevertheless, he was sane and knew exactly what he was doing and why he was doing it.

KERSHAW: And you say that the hospital is holding him here under Section 26.

HILL: Yes, they rang me this morning. They got another chap in from Ellertree to sign it as well as Emerson.

KERSHAW: Hm . . . Tricky. There's no precedent for this, you know. Fascinating.

HILL: Yes.

KERSHAW: And you're sure in your mind he knows what he's doing?

HILL: Yes.

KERSHAW: . . . Well . . . Let's see him, shall we?

HILL: Here's the Sister's office.

KERSHAW: Is she your standard gorgon?

HILL: Only on the outside. But under that iron surface beats a heart of stainless steel.

(*They go into* SISTER*'s office*)

HILL: Good morning, Sister.

SISTER: Morning, Mr. Hill.

HILL: This is a colleague, Mr. Kershaw.

SISTER: Good morning.

KERSHAW: Good morning.

HILL: Is it all right to see Mr. Harrison? . . .

SISTER: Have you asked Dr. Emerson?

HILL: Oh yes . . . before we came . . .

SISTER: I see . . .

HILL: You can check with him . . .

SISTER: . . . I don't think that's necessary . . . However, I'm afraid I shall have to ask you if I can stay with Mr. Harrison whilst you interview him.

HILL: Why?

SISTER: We are very worried about Mr. Harrison's mental condition as you know. Twice recently he has . . . got excited . . . and his breathing function has not been able to cope with the extra demands. Dr. Emerson has ordered that at any time Mr. Harrison is subjected to stress, someone must be there as a precaution.

HILL: . . . I see.

(*He glances at* MR. KERSHAW, *who shrugs*)

Very well.

SISTER: This way, gentlemen.

(*They go into* KEN*'s room*)

HILL: Good morning, Mr. Harrison.

KEN: Morning.

HILL: I've brought along Mr. Kershaw. He is the barrister who is advising us.

KERSHAW: Good morning, Mr. Harrison.

HILL: Your doctor has insisted that Sister remains with us–to see you don't get too excited.

KEN: Oh! Sister, you know very well that your very presence always excites me tremendously. It must be the white apron and black stockings. A perfect mixture of mother and mistress.

(SISTER *grins a little sheepishly and takes a seat at the head of the bed.* KEN *strains his head to look at her.* SISTER *turns back the covers*)

Sister, what are you doing! Oh. Just for a minute there, Sister . . .

(SISTER *takes his pulse*)

HILL: . . . Well . . .

SISTER: Just a moment Mr. Hill . . .

(*She finishes taking the pulse*)

Very well.

KEN: So, Mr. Kershaw, what is your advice?

(MR. KERSHAW *pauses.* MR. HILL *makes to speak but* MR. KERSHAW *stops him with a barely perceptible shake of the head. A longer pause*)

KERSHAW: . . . If you succeed in your aim, you will be dead within a week.

KEN: I know.

KERSHAW: . . . I am informed that without a catheter the toxic substance will build up in your bloodstream and you will be slowly poisoned by your own blood.

KEN:

(*Smiles*)

. . . You should have brought along a tape-recorder. That speech would be much more dramatic with sound effects!

KERSHAW:

(*Relaxing and smiling*)

I had to be sure you know what you are doing.

KEN: I know.

KERSHAW: And you have no doubt whatsoever; no slightest reservations? . . .

KEN: None at all.

KERSHAW: Let's look at the possibilities. You are now being held under the Mental Health Act Section 26, which means they can keep you here and give you any treatment they believe you need. Under the law we can appeal to a tribunal.

KEN: How long will that take?

KERSHAW: . . . Up to a year.

KEN: A year! A year! Oh God, can't it be quicker than that?

KERSHAW: It might be quicker, but it could be a year.

KEN: Jesus Christ! I really would be crazy in a year.

KERSHAW: That's the procedure.

KEN: I couldn't stay like this for another year, I couldn't.

HILL: We could always try habeas corpus.

KERSHAW: That would depend if we could find someone.

KEN: Habeas corpus? What's that? I thought it was something to do with criminals.

KERSHAW: Well, it usually is, Mr. Harrison. Briefly, it's against the law to deprive anyone of their liberty without proper cause. If anyone is so deprived, they or a friend can apply for a writ of habeas corpus, which is the Latin for "you may have the body."

KEN: Particularly apt in my case.

KERSHAW: . . . The people who are doing the detaining have to produce the . . . person, before the judge and if they can't give a good enough reason for keeping him, the judge will order that he be released.

KEN: It sounds as if it will take as long as that tribunal you were talking about.

KERSHAW: No. Habeas corpus is one of the very few legal processes that move very fast. We can approach any judge at any time even when the courts aren't sitting and he will see that it's heard straight away–in a day or so usually.

HILL: If you could find a judge to hear it.

KEN: Why shouldn't a judge hear it?

KERSHAW: Habeas corpus itself is fairly rare. This would be rarer.

KEN: Will I have to go to court?

KERSHAW: I doubt it. The hearing can be in court or in private, in the judge's Chambers as we say. The best thing to do in this case is for Mr. Hill and I to find a judge, issue the writ, then I'll get together with the hospital's barrister and we'll approach the judge together and suggest we hold the subsequent hearing here.

KEN: In this room?

KERSHAW: I expect the judge will agree. If he ordered you to be produced in court and anything happened to you, it would be a classical case of prejudging the issue.

KEN: I wouldn't mind.

KERSHAW: But the judge would feel rather foolish. I should think it would be in a few days.

KEN: Thank you. It'll be an unusual case for you–making a plea for the defendant's death.

KERSHAW: I'll be honest with you. It's a case I could bear to lose.

KEN: If you do–it's a life sentence for me.

KERSHAW: Well, we shall see. Good morning, Mr. Harrison.

(*They go out with the* SISTER. *They pause at the* SISTER's *office*)

HILL: Thank you very much, Sister . . . I'm very sorry about all this. I do realize it must be upsetting for you.

SISTER: Not at all, Mr. Hill. As I have a stainless steel heart, it's easy to keep it sterilized of emotion. Good morning.

(*She goes into her room.* HILL *and* KERSHAW *go out*)

(*CROSS FADE on* KEN's *room*)

(JOHN *and* NURSE SADLER *are setting chairs for the hearing.* JOHN *begins to sing "Dry Bones"*)

NURSE: John!

JOHN: What's the matter?

(NURSE SADLER *is confused*)

NURSE: Nothing of course ... silly ...

(KEN *picks up the vibes between the two*)

KEN: Hello, hello ... What have we here? Don't tell me that Cupid has donned his antiseptic gown and is flying the corridors of the hospital, shooting his hypodermic syringes into maidens' hearts ...

NURSE: No!

KEN: John?

JOHN: Honestly, your honor, I'm not guilty. I was just walking down the corridor when I was struck dumb by the beauty of this nurse.

NURSE: Don't be an idiot, John ... We need an extra chair ... Can you go and find one please?

JOHN: Your wishes, oh queen, are my command.

(*He bows and goes out*)

NURSE: He is a fool.

KEN: He isn't. He's been bloody good to me. Have you been out with him? ... It's none of my business, of course.

NURSE: We went to a club of his last night ... He plays in a band, you know.

KEN: Yes, I know.

NURSE: They're really good. They should go a long way ... Still, I shouldn't be going on like this.

KEN: Why not? ... Because I'm paralyzed? Because I can't go dancing?

NURSE: Well ...

KEN: The other day I was low and said to John, who was shaving me, I was useless, what could I do? I served no purpose and all the rest of the whining miseries. John set about finding things I could do. He said, first, because I could move my head from side to side

(KEN *does so*)

I could be a tennis umpire; then as my head was going, I could knock a pendulum from side to side and keep a clock going. Then he said I could be a child-minder and because kids were always doing what they shouldn't I could be perpetually shaking my head. He went on and on getting more and more fantastic–like radar scanners. I laughed so much that the Sister had to rush in and give me oxygen.

NURSE: He is funny.

KEN: He's more than that. He's free!

NURSE: Free?

KEN: Free of guilt. Most everybody here feels guilt about me–including you. That's why you didn't want to tell me what a fantastic time you had dancing. So everybody makes me feel worse because I make them feel guilty. But not John. He's sorry for me but he knows bloody well it isn't his fault. He's a tonic.

(JOHN *comes back carrying* SISTER's *armchair*)

NURSE: John! Did Sister say you could have that chair?

JOHN: She wasn't there . . .

NURSE: She'll kill you; no one ever sits in her chair.

JOHN: Why? Is it contaminated or something? I just thought that if the poor old judge had to sit here listening to that miserable bugger moaning on about wanting to die, the least we could do was to make him comfortable.

KEN:

(*Laughing to* NURSE SADLER)

See?

(JOHN *sits in the chair and assumes a grave face*)

JOHN: Now, this is a very serious case. The two charges are proved . . . Firstly, this hospital has been found guilty of using drugs to make people happy. That's terrible. Next and most surprising of all, this hospital, in spite of all their efforts to the contrary, are keeping people alive! We can't have that.

(*Footsteps outside*)

NURSE: Sister's coming!

(JOHN *jumps up and stands between the chair and the door.* SISTER *comes in and as she approaches the bed with her back to the chair,* JOHN *slips out of the room*)

KEN: Well now, we have some very important visitors today, Sister.

SISTER: Indeed we have.

KEN: Will you be here?

SISTER: No.

KEN: I feel a bit like a traitor.

SISTER: . . . We all do what we've got to.

KEN: That's right, but not all of us do it as well as you Sister . . .

SISTER:

(*Rapidly*)

. . . Thank you.

(*She moves quickly to go.* DR. SCOTT *comes in*)

DR. SCOTT: Good morning, Sister.

SISTER:

(*Brightly*)

Good morning.

(*She goes quickly without noticing the chair.* DR. SCOTT *watches her go*)

KEN: I've upset her, I'm afraid.

DR. SCOTT: You shouldn't do that. She is a marvelous Sister. You ought to see some of the others.

KEN: That's what I told her.

DR. SCOTT: Oh, I see. Well, I should think that's just about the one way past her defenses. How are you this morning?

KEN: Fine.

DR. SCOTT: And you're going ahead with it?

KEN: Of course.

DR. SCOTT: Of course.

KEN: I haven't had any tablets, yesterday or today.

DR. SCOTT: No.

KEN: Thank you.

DR. SCOTT: Thank the Judge. He ordered it.

KEN: Ah!

(DR. EMERSON: *comes in*)

DR. EMERSON: Good morning, Mr. Harrison.

KEN: Morning, Doctor.

DR. EMERSON: There's still time.

KEN: No, I want to go on with it . . . unless you'll discharge me.

DR. EMERSON: I'm afraid I can't do that. The Judge and lawyers are conferring. I thought I'd just pop along and see if you were all right. We've made arrangements for the witnesses to wait in the Sister's office. I am one, so I should be grateful if you would remain here, with Mr. Harrison.

DR. SCOTT: Of course.

DR. EMERSON: Well, I don't want to meet the Judge before I have to. I wish you the best of luck, Mr. Harrison, so that we'll be able to carry on treating you.

KEN:

(*Smiling*)

Thank you for your good wishes.

(DR. EMERSON *nods and goes out*)

DR. SCOTT: If I didn't know *you* I'd say *he* was the most obstinate man I've ever met.

(*As* DR. EMERSON *makes for his office,* MR. HILL *comes down the corridor*)

HILL: Good morning.

DR. EMERSON: Morning.

(MR. HILL *stops and calls after* DR. EMERSON)

HILL: Oh, Dr. Emerson . . .

DR. EMERSON: Yes?

HILL: I don't know . . . I just want to say how sorry I am that you have been forced into such a . . . distasteful situation.

DR. EMERSON: It's not over yet, Mr. Hill. I have every confidence that the law is not such an ass that it will force me to watch a patient of mine die unnecessarily.

HILL: We are just as confident that the law is not such an ass that it will allow anyone arbitrary power.

DR. EMERSON: My power isn't arbitrary; I've earned it with knowledge and skill and it's also subject to the laws of nature.

HILL: And to the laws of the state.

DR. EMERSON: If the state is so foolish as to believe it is competent to judge a purely professional issue.

HILL: It's always doing that. Half the civil cases in the calendar arise because someone is challenging a professional's opinion.

DR. EMERSON: I don't know about other professions but I do know this one, medicine, is being seriously threatened because of the intervention of law. Patients are becoming so litigious that doctors will soon be afraid to offer any opinion or take any action at all.

HILL: Then they will be sued for negligence.

DR. EMERSON: We can't win.

HILL: Everybody wins. You wouldn't like to find yourself powerless in the hands of, say, a lawyer or a . . . bureaucrat. I wouldn't like to find myself powerless in the hands of a doctor.

DR. EMERSON: You make one sound as if I were some sort of Dracula . . .

HILL: No! . . . I for one certainly don't doubt your good faith but in spite of that I wouldn't like to place *anyone* above the law.

DR. EMERSON: I don't want to be above the law; I just want to be under laws that take full account of professional opinion.

HILL: I'm sure it will do that, Dr. Emerson. The question is, whose professional opinion?

DR. EMERSON: We shall see.

(MR. ANDREW EDEN, *the hospital's barrister, and* MR. HILL *and* MR. KERSHAW *come into* KEN's *room*)

HILL: Morning, Mr. Harrison. This is Mr. Eden who will be representing the hospital.

KEN: Hello.

(*They settle themselves into the chairs. The* SISTER *enters with the* JUDGE)

SISTER: Mr. Justice Millhouse.

JUDGE: Mr. Kenneth Harrison?

KEN: Yes, my Lord.

JUDGE: This is an informal hearing which I want to keep as brief as possible. You are, I take it, Dr. Scott?

DR. SCOTT: Yes, my Lord.

JUDGE: I should be grateful, Doctor, if you would interrupt the proceedings at any time you think it necessary.

DR. SCOTT: Yes, my Lord.

JUDGE: I have decided in consultation with Mr. Kershaw and Mr. Hill that we shall proceed thus. I will hear a statement from Dr. Michael Emerson as to why he believes Mr. Harrison is legally detained, and then a statement from Dr. Richard Barr, who will support the application. We have decided not to subject Mr. Harrison to examination and cross-examination.

KEN: But I . . .

JUDGE:

(*Sharply*)

Just a moment, Mr. Harrison. If, as appears likely, there remains genuine doubt as to the main issue, I shall question Mr. Harrison myself. Dr. Scott, I wonder if you would ask Dr. Emerson to come in.

DR. SCOTT: Yes, my Lord.

(*She goes out*)

Would you come in now, sir?

(SISTER *and* DR. EMERSON *come into* KEN's *room*)

JUDGE: Dr. Emerson, I would like you to take the oath.

(*The* JUDGE *hands* DR. EMERSON *a card with the oath written on it*)

DR. EMERSON: I swear the evidence that I give shall be the truth, the whole truth and nothing but the truth.

JUDGE: Stand over there, please.

(*The* JUDGE *nods to* MR. EDEN)

EDEN: You are Dr. Michael Emerson?

DR. EMERSON: I am.

EDEN: And what is your position here?

DR. EMERSON: I am a consultant physician and in charge of the intensive care unit.

EDEN: Dr. Emerson, would you please give a brief account of your treatment of this patient.

DR. EMERSON:

(*Referring to notes*)

Mr. Harrison was admitted here on the afternoon of October 9th, as an emergency following a road accident. He was suffering from a fractured left tibia and right tibia and fibia, a fractured pelvis, four fractured ribs, one of which had punctured the lung, and a dislocated fourth vertebra, which had ruptured the spinal cord. He was extensively bruised and had minor lacerations. He was deeply unconscious and remained so for thirty hours. As a result of treatment all the broken bones and ruptured tissue have healed with the exception of a severed spinal cord and this, together with a mental trauma, is now all that remains of the initial injury.

EDEN: Precisely, Doctor. Let us deal with those last two points. The spinal cord. Will there be any further improvement in that?

DR. EMERSON: In the present state of medical knowledge, I would think not.

EDEN: And the mental trauma you spoke of?

DR. EMERSON: It's impossible to injure the body to the extent that Mr. Harrison did and not affect the mind. It is common in these cases that depression and the tendency to make wrong decisions goes on for months, even years.

EDEN: And in your view Mr. Harrison is suffering from such a depression?

DR. EMERSON: Yes.

EDEN: Thank you, Doctor.

JUDGE: Mr. Kershaw?

KERSHAW: Doctor. Is there any objective way you could demonstrate this trauma? Are there, for example, the results of any tests, or any measurements you can take to show it to us?

DR. EMERSON: No.

KERSHAW: Then how do you distinguish between a medical syndrome and a sane, even justified, depression?

DR. EMERSON: By using my thirty years' experience as a physician, dealing with both types.

KERSHAW: No more questions, my Lord.

JUDGE: Mr. Eden, do you wish to re-examine?

EDEN: No, my Lord.

JUDGE: Thank you, Doctor. Would you ask Dr. Barr if he would step in please?

(DR. EMERSON goes out)

DR. EMERSON: It's you now, Barr.

(SISTER brings DR. BARR into KEN's room)

SISTER: Dr. Barr.

JUDGE: Dr. Barr, will you take the oath please.

(He does so)

Mr. Kershaw.

KERSHAW: You are Dr. Richard Barr?

DR. BARR: I am.

KERSHAW: And what position do you hold?

DR. BARR: I am a consultant psychiatrist at Norwood Park Hospital.

KERSHAW: That is primarily a mental hospital is it not?

DR. BARR: It is.

KERSHAW: Then you must see a large number of patients suffering from depressive illness.

DR. BARR: I do, yes.

KERSHAW: You have examined Mr. Harrison?

DR. BARR: I have, yes.

KERSHAW: Would you say that he was suffering from such an illness?

DR. BARR: No, I would not.

KERSHAW: Are you quite sure, Doctor?

DR. BARR: Yes, I am.

KERSHAW: The court has heard evidence that Mr. Harrison is depressed. Would you dispute that?

DR. BARR: No, but depression is not necessarily an illness. I would say that Mr. Harrison's depression is reactive rather than endogenous. That is to say, he is reacting in a perfectly rational way to a very bad situation.

KERSHAW: Thank you, Dr. Barr.

JUDGE: Mr. Eden?

EDEN: Dr. Barr. Are there any objective results that you could produce to prove Mr. Harrison is capable?

DR. BARR: There are clinical symptoms of endogenous depression, of course, disturbed sleep patterns, loss of appetite, lassitude, but, even if they were present, they would be masked by the physical condition.

EDEN: So how can you be sure this *is* in fact just a reactive depression?

DR. BARR: Just by experience, that's all, and by discovering when I talk to him that he has a remarkably incisive mind and is perfectly capable of understanding his position and of deciding what to do about it.

EDEN: One last thing, Doctor, do you think Mr. Harrison has made the right decision?

KERSHAW:

(*Quickly*)

Is that really relevant, my Lord? After all . . .

JUDGE: Not really . . .

DR. BARR: I should like to answer it though.

JUDGE: Very well.

DR. BARR: No, I thought he made the wrong decision.

(*To* KEN)

Sorry.

EDEN: No more questions, my Lord.

JUDGE: Do you wish to re-examine, Mr. Kershaw?

KERSHAW: No, thank you, my Lord.

JUDGE: That will be all, Dr. Barr.

(DR. BARR *goes out. The* JUDGE *stands*)

JUDGE: Do you feel like answering some questions?

KEN: Of course.

JUDGE: Thank you.

KEN: You are too kind.

JUDGE: Not at all.

KEN: I mean it. I'd prefer it if you were a hanging judge.

JUDGE: There aren't any any more.

KEN: Society is now much more sensitive and humane?

JUDGE: You could put it that way.

KEN: I'll settle for that.

JUDGE: I would like you to take the oath. Dr. Scott, his right hand, please.

(KEN *takes the oath*)

The consultant physician here has given evidence that you are not capable
    of making a rational decision.

KEN: He's wrong.

JUDGE: When then do you think he came to that opinion?

KEN: He's a good doctor and won't let a patient die if he can help it.

JUDGE: He found that you were suffering from acute depression.

KEN: Is that surprising? I am almost totally paralyzed. I'd be insane if I
    weren't depressed.

JUDGE: But there is a difference between being unhappy and being
    depressed in the medical sense.

KEN: I would have thought that my psychiatrist answered that point.

JUDGE: But, surely, wishing to die must be strong evidence that the depres-
    sion has moved beyond a mere unhappiness into a medical realm?

KEN: I don't wish to die.

JUDGE: Then what is this case all about?

KEN: Nor do I wish to live at any price. Of course I want to live, but as far as
    I am concerned I'm dead already. I merely require the doctors to recog-
    nize the fact. I cannot accept this condition constitutes life in any real
    sense at all.

JUDGE: Certainly, you're alive legally.

KEN: I think I could challenge even that.

JUDGE: How?

KEN: Any reasonable definition of life must include the idea of its being self-supporting. I seem to remember something in the papers–when all the heart transplant controversy was on–about it being all right to take someone's heart if they require constant attention from respirators and so on to keep them alive.

JUDGE: There also has to be absolutely no brain activity at all. Yours is certainly working.

KEN: It is and sanely.

JUDGE: That is the question to be decided.

KEN: My Lord, I am not asking anyone to kill me. I am only asking to be discharged from this hospital.

JUDGE: It comes to the same thing.

KEN: Then that proves my point; not just the fact that I will spend the rest of my life in hospital, but that whilst I am here, everything is geared just to keeping my brain active, with no real possibility of it ever being able to direct anything. As far as I can see, that is an act of deliberate cruelty.

JUDGE: Surely, it would be more cruel if society let people die, when it could, with some effort, keep them alive.

KEN: No, not *more* cruel, *just* as cruel.

JUDGE: Then why should the hospital let you die–if it is just as cruel?

KEN: The cruelty doesn't reside in saving someone or allowing them to die. It resides in the fact that the choice is removed from the man concerned.

JUDGE: But a man who is very desperately depressed is not capable of making a reasonable choice.

KEN: As you said, my Lord, that is the question to be decided.

JUDGE: All right. You tell me why it is a reasonable choice that you decided to die.

KEN: It is a question of dignity. Look at me here. I can do nothing, not even the basic primitive functions. I cannot even urinate, I have a permanent catheter attached to me. Every few days my bowels are washed out. Every few hours two nurses have to turn me over or I would rot away from bedsores. Only my brain functions unimpaired but even that is futile because I can't act on any conclusions it comes to. This hearing proves that. Will you please listen.

JUDGE: I am listening.

KEN: I choose to acknowledge the fact that I am in fact dead and I find the hospital's persistent effort to maintain this shadow of life an indignity and it's inhumane.

JUDGE: But wouldn't you agree that many people with appalling physical handicaps have overcome them and lived essentially creative, dignified lives?

KEN: Yes, I would, but the dignity starts with their choice. If I choose to live, it would be appalling if society killed me. If I choose to die, it is equally appalling if society keeps me alive.

JUDGE: I cannot accept that it is undignified for society to devote resources to keeping someone alive. Surely it enhances that society.

KEN: It is not undignified if the man wants to stay alive, but I must restate that the dignity starts with his choice. Without it, it is degrading because technology has taken over from human will. My Lord, if I cannot be a man, I do not wish to be a medical achievement. I'm fine . . . I am fine.

JUDGE: It's all right. I have no more questions.

(*The* JUDGE *stands up and walks to the window. He thinks a moment*)

JUDGE: This is a most unusual case. Before I make a judgment I want to state that I believe all the parties have acted in good faith. I propose to consider this for a moment. The law on this is fairly clear. A deliberate decision to embark on a course of action that will lead inevitably to death is not *ipso facto* evidence of insanity. If it were, society would have to reward many men with a dishonorable burial rather than a posthumous medal for gallantry. On the other hand, we do have to bear in mind that Mr. Harrison has suffered massive physical injuries and it is possible that his mind is affected. Any judge in his career will have met men who are without doubt insane in the meaning of the Act and yet appear in the witness box to be rational. We must, in this case, be most careful not to allow Mr. Harrison's obvious wit and intelligence to blind us to the fact that he could be suffering from a depressive illness . . . and so we have to face the disturbing fact of the divided evidence . . . and bear in mind that, however much we may sympathize with Mr. Harrison in his cogently argued case to be allowed to die, the law instructs us to ignore it if it is the product of a disturbed or clinically depressed mind . . . However, I am satisfied that Mr. Harrison is a brave and cool man who is in complete control of his mental faculties and I shall therefore make an order for him to be set free.

(*A pause. The* JUDGE *walks over to* KEN)

Well, you got your hanging judge!

KEN: I think not, my Lord. Thank you.

(*The* JUDGE *nods and smiles*)

JUDGE: Goodbye.

(*He turns and goes. He meets* DR. EMERSON *in the* SISTER'S *room. While he talks to him, everyone else, except* DR. SCOTT, *comes out*)

Ah, Dr. Emerson.

DR. EMERSON: My Lord?

JUDGE: I'm afraid you'll have to release your patient.

DR. EMERSON: I see.

JUDGE: I'm sorry. I understand how you must feel.

DR. EMERSON: Thank you.

JUDGE: If ever I have to have a road accident, I hope it's in this town and I finish up here.

DR. EMERSON: Thank you again.

JUDGE: Goodbye.

(*He walks down the corridor.* DR. EMERSON *stands a moment, then slowly goes back to the room.* KEN *is looking out of the window.* DR. SCOTT *is sitting by the bed*)

DR. EMERSON: Where will you go?

KEN: I'll get a room somewhere.

DR. EMERSON: There's no need.

KEN: Don't let's . . .

DR. EMERSON: We'll stop treatment, remove the drips. Stop feeding you if you like. You'll be unconscious in three days, dead in six at most.

KEN: There'll be no last minute resuscitation?

DR. EMERSON: Only with your express permission.

KEN: That's very kind; why are you doing it?

DR. EMERSON: Simple! You might change your mind.

(KEN *smiles and shakes his head*)

KEN: Thanks. I won't change my mind, but I'd like to stay.

(DR. EMERSON *nods and goes.* DR. SCOTT *stands and moves to the door. She turns and moves to* KEN *as if to kiss him*).

KEN: Oh, don't, but thank you.

(DR. SCOTT *smiles weakly and goes out*)

(*The lights are held for a long moment and then snap out*)

The Elephant Man

৪১

Bernard Pomerance

Introduction

The Elephant Man, by Bernard Pomerance, recreates the real-life experience of
John Merrick, who lived in London during the Victorian Age. Suffering from
what appears to be neurofibromatosis, Merrick is markedly disfigured and
regarded by society as a freak, frequently being put on display in the popular
exhibitions of the day. While cast aside from the community of upright citizens, individuals of various anomalies were prized for the entertainment they
provided. Led by Queen Victoria, who, among her other amusements, was
delighted to view P. T. Barnum's famous attraction Tom Thumb on at least three
occasions, the curious public flocked to the sideshows to see the oddities—but
only at a distance. In Merrick's case, his hydrocephalic head, fibrous tumors,
dangling flesh, and other physical deformities earned him the appellation "the
elephant man." The name suited the purposes of the presenter who exhibited
him before the gullible crowd and offered a fascinating tale of the history of the
person on view, including medically impossible explanations for his appearance. Merrick offers his own narrative to explain his condition. He relates that
his pregnant mother was knocked down by an elephant at a circus. He has his
doubts, though, an indication that the common view linking disability and
defective cognition is erroneous. A policeman in the play—presumably the
common man—reasons, "People who think right don't look like that then, do
they?" (14). Merrick replies by his actions during the course of the play as he
reveals his intelligence, acute sensitivity, and creative imagination.

The body viewed by the policeman repulses the ordinary man, leading
him to shun the afflicted man. Yet another gaze, "the clinical gaze," authorizes
a medical view. In Scene 3 the audience is witness to a lecture delivered by
Frederick Treves, an idealistic young surgeon who rescues Merrick from a
life of brutality and abuse. The subject of Treves's talk is the physical state of
"the elephant man." With the actor playing the role of Merrick present, the

physician illustrates his lecture with projected slides of the real Merrick. A follow-up paper is to be submitted to the London Pathological Society.

Assuming the expected paternalistic attitude toward his patient, Treves proceeds to transform Merrick into a scientific object with a view to a bolder transformation. The physician accepts the limitations of medical science to restore his patient to health. In the century to follow, Merrick's condition would be identified, labeled, and treated; and the achievements of a new specialty, plastic and reconstructive surgery, would provide enormous emotional benefits to the afflicted. Denied such knowledge, Treves can seek only an alternative course. He sets out on a social experiment: since he cannot alter his patient's body, he will change his environment. The first step is to house the patient within the controlled setting of the hospital. His aim is to negate the damage caused by Merrick's exclusion from communal life. To this end the doctor introduces the withdrawn man to various well-intentioned upper-class Victorians brought in for arranged and cordial visits with the subject. In effect, Treves reconstructs a social context for Merrick, creating a world of warmth and good fellowship in sharp contrast to the harsh reality he had known.

Treves's motive in socializing Merrick springs primarily from his conviction that science can demythologize the aberrations of nature. In carrying out his research, he has every reasonable expectation that the discomforts to his subject in the controlled environment he has created are minimal compared to the exploitation and abuse Merrick has experienced elsewhere. The situation appears to be one in which the risk of intervention is minor compared to the alternative. In addition, Treves acts with the full consent of his patient. Although the play is set in Victorian times, one may well commend Treves for conforming to current guidelines for the protection of human subjects in biomedical and behavioral research. In the absence of regulations, the doctor has acted out of a responsible physician's inclination to relieve suffering. Very much to Treves's credit is his patient's sensitivity to his good intentions to the point of becoming a willing subject in his hands. Well in advance of any legalistically grounded views regarding informed consent, Merrick agrees to participate in his treatment out of pure faith in his rescuer. Treves believes firmly that he can transform his patient into a reasonable facsimile of an upper-class Englishman of the Victorian age. And Merrick participates eagerly in the experiment, quick to identify with two prominent Victorian gentlemen, the "Prince" and the "Irishman" (the Prince of Wales and Charles Stewart Parnell), both of whom kept mistresses, a notion that appeals to Merrick. His wish to be similarly advantaged shocks his physician, who fails seriously in not recognizing that the man he has been treating as a child has normal sexual needs. His admonishment of Merrick's curiosity regarding sexuality and women—"Are you not ashamed? Do you know what you are? Don't you know what is forbidden?"—forces Merrick to a jolting awareness of self (50).

The dream that has sustained "the elephant man" is that he could, with Treves's help, become like everyone else. More perceptive than his benefactor, he comes to realize that his existence is only an approximation of the life he longs for. Each encounter with his visitors only confirms the great distance that separates him from others. Although saved from a life of brutality, Merrick is isolated within an environment where normalcy and freedom are illusory. What remains to him is his imagination and artistic sensibility. With his one good hand he completes a model of St. Phillip's Church, a building glimpsed from his hospital window. The miniature cathedral, unlike his body, is a perfect structure to house his soul that alone makes him like other men. The single right he can exercise is his freedom to create. He acts—for the first time in his life—as subject not object. With his project completed, he lies down to sleep. The normal action causes the weight of his enormous head to crush his trachea. Merrick's action is total withdrawal from the society that has marginalized him. For Treves, the outcome is equally grave. Having begun to question the ethics of obliging Merrick to conform to society's conception of normalcy, he ends by experiencing a crisis of conscience in which he loses faith in the power of science to cure his world.

What has altered the doctor's outlook to the point where he begins to doubt his early premise is his increased awareness of his patient's true nature. Having acted always out of the purest motives, he has sought simply to ameliorate suffering and to advance knowledge. His intervention was accomplished to improve Merrick's welfare. The principle he adhered to demands that the interests of an incompetent patient be protected. On the basis of his initial assessment of Merrick, Treves has reached the expected conclusion that he possesses the professional competence to judge what is best for his patient. He errs in confusing Merrick's vulnerability with incompetence. Merrick is keenly aware of his situation and, once given the hope of rehabilitation, most eager to exercise his autonomy. The paternalism Treves exercises runs counter to Merrick's view of their relationship. To the extent that the patient is able to characterize his association with his physician, he thinks in terms of a contractual arrangement. Fearing for his security, he startles a sympathetic observer with the egalitarian tone of his question, "Will Frederick keep his word with me, his contract?" (45). While Treves is acting to promote his patient's well-being, Merrick is straining for independence. The experiment does not succeed due to Treves's failure to calculate the risks in relation to the benefits he sees so clearly, the greatest risk being to the patient's sense of personhood. That sense, with its accompanying feelings of worth and dignity, is awakened by Treves when the physician takes

Merrick off the streets. Tragically, he is incapable of completing the process that would lead to his patient's total rehabilitation. His accomplishment, though he cannot recognize it, is to aid in the accumulation of data, a first step toward reaching a solution to the problem that causes him to despair.

The sort of moral growth Treves achieves is that which results from one physician's interaction with a unique patient. Despite preconceived notions, he is able to modify his initial approach due to Merrick's response. One can only speculate what the outcome of their tale would have been had more meaningful communication taken place between them. But any possibility of dialogue is precluded by a number of factors: Treves's view of himself in relation to Merrick, the necessity of maintaining scientific objectivity, and Merrick's own naive expectations that his benefactor can accomplish the impossible.

In presenting the hypocrisy and brutality beneath the surface of a society much removed from our own in time and sophistication, Pomerance removes the matter from immediate experience. Yet the audience is challenged in every scene of his drama to measure its own values and cultural assumptions against those of the Victorians and determine what, if any, essential differences exist between them.

Works Cited

Pomerance, Bernard. *The Elephant Man.* New York: Grove, 1979.

THE ELEPHANT MAN

By Bernard Pomerance

Introductory Note

The Elephant Man was suggested by the life of John Merrick, known as The Elephant Man. It is recounted by Sir Frederick Treves in *The Elephant Man and Other Reminiscences,* Cassell and Co. Ltd., 1923. This account is reprinted in *The Elephant Man, A Study in Human Dignity,* by Ashley Montagu (Ballantine Books, 1973), to whom much credit is due for reviving contemporary interest in the story. My own knowledge of it came via my brother Michael, who told me the story, provided me with xeroxes of Treves' memoirs until I came on my own copy, and sent me the Montagu book. In Montagu's book are included photographs of Merrick as well as of Merrick's model of St. Phillip's Church. Merrick's bones are still at London Hospital.

I believe the building of the church model constitutes some kind of central metaphor, and the groping toward conditions where it can be built and the building of it are the action of the play. It does not, and should not, however, dominate the play visually, as I originally believed.

Merrick's face was so deformed he could not express any emotion at all. His speech was very difficult to understand without practice. Any attempt to reproduce his appearance and his speech naturalistically–*if* it were possible– would seem to me not only counterproductive, but, the more remarkably successful, the more distracting from the play. For how he appeared, let slide projections suffice.

If the pinheaded women are two actresses, then the play, in a pinch, can be performed with seven players, five men, two women.

No one with any history of back trouble should attempt the part of MER- RICK *as contorted. Anyone playing the part of* MERRICK *should be advised to consult a physician about the problems of sustaining any unnatural or twisted position. –B.P.*

1884–1890. London. One scene is in Belgium.

CHARACTERS

FREDERICK TREVES, a surgeon and teacher
CARR GOMM, administrator of the London Hospital
ROSS, Manager of the Elephant Man
JOHN MERRICK, the Elephant Man
Three PINHEADS, three women freaks whose heads are pointed
BELGIAN POLICEMAN
LONDON POLICEMAN
MAN, at a fairground in Brussels
CONDUCTOR, of Ostend-London boat train
BISHOP WALSHAM HOW
PORTER, at the London Hospital
SNORK, also a porter
MRS. KENDAL, an actress
DUCHESS
COUNTESS
PRINCESS ALEXANDRA
LORD JOHN
NURSE, MISS SANDWICH

Scene I

He Will Have 100 Guinea Fees Before He's Forty

The London Hospital, Whitechapel Rd. Enter GOMM, *enter* TREVES.
TREVES: Mr. Carr Gomm? Frederick Treves. Your new lecturer in anatomy.
GOMM: Age thirty-one. Books on Scrofula and Applied Surgical Anatomy–
   I'm happy to see you rising, Mr. Treves. I like to see merit credited,
   and your industry, accomplishment, and skill all do you credit. Ignore
   the squalor of Whitechapel, the general dinginess, neglect and poverty
   without, and you will find a continual medical richesse in the London
   Hospital. We study and treat the widest range of diseases and disorders,
   and are certainly the greatest institution of our kind in the world. The
   Empire provides unparalleled opportunities for our studies, as places
   cruel to life are the most revealing scientifically. Add to our reputation by
   going further, and that'll satisfy. You've bought a house?
TREVES: On Wimpole Street.
GOMM: Good. Keep at it, Treves. You'll have an FRS and 100 guinea fees
   before you're forty. You'll find it is an excellent consolation prize.
TREVES: Consolation? I don't know what you mean.
GOMM: I know you don't. You will *(Exits.)*
TREVES: A happy childhood in Dorset.
A scientist in an age of science.
In an English age, an Englishman. A teacher and a doctor at the London.
   Two books published by my thirty-first year. A house. A wife who loves
   me, and my god, 100 guinea fees before I'm forty.
Consolation for what?
As of the year AD 1884, I, Freddie Treves, have excessive blessings. Or so it
   seems to me.
Blackout.

Scene II

Art Is As Nothing To Nature

*Whitechapel Rd. A storefront. A large advertisement of a creature with an
   elephant's head.* ROSS, *his manager.*
ROSS: Tuppence only, step in and see: This side of the grave, John Merrick has no hope nor expectation of relief. In every sense his situation
   is desperate. His physical agony is exceeded only by his mental anguish,
   a despised creature without consolation. Tuppence only, step in and

see! To live with his physical hideousness, incapacitating deformities and unremitting pain is trial enough, but to be exposed to the cruelly lacerating expressions of horror and disgust by all who behold him–is even more difficult to bear. Tuppence only, step in and see! For in order to survive, Merrick forces himself to suffer these humiliations, I repeat, humiliations, in order to survive, thus he exposes himself to crowds who pay to gape and yawp at this freak of nature, the Elephant Man.

Enter TREVES *who looks at advertisement.*

ROSS: See Mother Nature uncorseted and in malignant rage! Tuppence.

TREVES: This sign's absurd. Half-elephant, half-man is not possible. Is he foreign?

ROSS: Right, from Leicester. But nothing to fear.

TREVES: I'm at London across the road. I would be curious to see him if there is some genuine disorder. If he is a mass of papier-maché and paint however–

ROSS: Then pay me nothing. Enter, sir. Merrick, stand up. Ya bloody donkey, up, up.

They go in, then emerge. TREVES *pays.*

TREVES: I must examine him further at the hospital. Here is my card. I'm Treves. I will have a cab pick him up and return him. My card will gain him admittance.

ROSS: Five bob he's yours for the day.

TREVES: I wish to examine him in the interest of science, you see.

ROSS: Sir, I'm Ross. I look out for him, get him his living. Found him in Leicester workhouse. His own ma put him there age of three. Couldn't bear the sight, well you can see why. We–he and I–are in business. He is our capital, see. Go to a bank. Go anywhere. Want to borrow capital, you pay interest. Scientists even. He's good value though. You won't find another like him.

TREVES: Fair enough. (*He pays.*)

ROSS: Right. Out here, Merrick. Ya bloody donkey, out!

Lights fade out.

SCENE III

Who Has Seen The Like Of This?

TREVES *lectures.* MERRICK *contorts himself to approximate projected slides of the real Merrick.*

TREVES: The most striking feature about him was his enormous head. Its circumference was about that of a man's waist. From the brow there projected a huge bony mass like a loaf, while from the back of his head hung a bag of spongy fungous-looking skin, the surface of which was comparable to brown cauliflower. On the top of the skull were a few long lank hairs. The osseous growth on the forehead, at this stage about the size of a tangerine, almost occluded one eye. From the upper jaw there projected another mass of bone. It protruded from the mouth like a pink stump, turning the upper lip inside out, and making the mouth a wide slobbering aperture. The nose was merely a lump of flesh, only recognizable as a nose from its position. The deformities rendered the face utterly incapable of the expression of any emotion whatsoever. The back was horrible because from it hung, as far down as the middle of the thigh, huge sack-like masses of flesh covered by the same loathsome cauliflower stain. The right arm was of enormous size and shapeless. It suggested but was not elephantiasis, and was overgrown also with pendant masses of the same cauliflower-like skin. The right hand was large and clumsy–a fin or paddle rather than a hand. No distinction existed between the palm and back, the thumb was like a radish, the fingers like thick tuberous roots. As a limb it was useless. The other arm was remarkable by contrast. It was not only normal, but was moreover a delicately shaped limb covered with a fine skin and provided with a beautiful hand which any woman might have envied. From the chest hung a bag of the same repulsive flesh. It was like a dewlap suspended from the neck of a lizard. The lower limbs had the characters of the deformed arm. They were unwieldy, dropsical-looking, and grossly misshapen. There arose from the fungous skin growths a very sickening stench which was hard to tolerate. To add a further burden to his trouble, the wretched man when a boy developed hip disease which left him permanently lame, so that he could only walk with a stick. (*To* MERRICK) Please. (MERRICK *walks.* He was thus denied all means of escape from his tormentors.

VOICE: Mr. Treves, you have shown a profound and unknown disorder to us. You have said when he leaves here it is for his exhibition again. I do not think it ought to be permitted. It is a disgrace. It is a pity and a disgrace. It is an indecency in fact. It may be a danger in ways we do not know. Something ought to be done about it.

TREVES: I am a doctor. What would you have me do?

VOICE: Well. I know what to do. *I* know.

Silence. A policeman enters as lights fade out.

Scene IV

This Indecency May Not Continue

Music. A fair. Pinheads *huddling together, holding a portrait of Leopold, King of the Congo. Enter* Man.

Man: Now, my pinheaded darlings, your attention please. Every freak in Brussels Fair is doing something to celebrate Leopold's fifth year as King of the Congo. Him. Our King. Our Empire. (*They begin reciting.*) No, don't recite yet, you morons. I'll say when. And when you do, get it *right.* You don't, it's back to the asylum. Know what that means, don't you? They'll cut your heads. They'll spoon out your little brains, replace 'em in the dachshund they were nicked from. Cut you. Yeah. Be back with customers. Come see the Queens of the Congo! (*Exits.*)

Enter Merrick, Ross.

Merrick: Cosmos? Cosmos?

Ross: Congo. Land of darkness. Hobo! (*Sees* Pins.) Look at them, lad. It's freer on the continent. Loads of indecency here, no one minds. You won't get coppers sent round to roust you out like London. Reckon in Brussels here's our fortune. You have a little tête-à-tête with this lot while I see the coppers about our license to exhibit. Be right back. (*Exits.*)

Merrick: I come from England.

Pins: Allo!

Merrick: At home they chased us. Out of London. Police. Someone complained. They beat me. You have no trouble? No?

Pins: Allo! Allo!

Merrick: Hello. In Belgium we make money. I look forward to it. Happiness, I mean. You pay your police? How is it done?

Pins: Allo! Allo!

Merrick: We do a show together sometime? Yes? I have saved forty-eight pounds. Two shillings. Nine pence. English money. Ross takes care of it.

Pins: Allo! Allo!

Merrick: Little vocabulary problem, eh? Poor things. Looks like they put your noses to the grindstone and forgot to take them away.

Man *enters.*

Man: They're coming.

(*People enter to see the girls' act.*)

Now.

Pins: (*dancing and singing*)

We are the Queens of the Congo,

The Beautiful Belgian Empire.

Our niggers are bigger

Our miners are finer

Empire, Empire, Congo and power

Civilizuzu's finest hour

Admire, perspire, desire, acquire

Or we'll set you on fire!

MAN: You cretins! Sorry, they're not ready yet. Out please.

(*People exit.*)

Get those words right, girls! Or you know what.

MAN *exits.* PINS *weep.*

MERRICK: Don't cry. You sang nicely. Don't cry. There there.

Enter ROSS *in grip of two* POLICEMEN.

ROSS: I was promised a permit. I lined a tour up on that!

POLICEMEN: This is a brutal, indecent, and immoral display. It is a public indecency, and it is forbidden here.

ROSS: What about them with their perfect cone heads?

POLICEMEN: They are ours.

ROSS: Competition's good for business. Where's your spirit of competition?

POLICEMEN: Right here. (*Smacks* MERRICK.)

ROSS: Don't do that, you'll kill him!

POLICEMEN: Be better off dead. Indecent bastard.

MERRICK: Don't cry girls. Doesn't hurt.

PINS: Indecent, indecent, indecent, indecent!!

POLICEMEN *escort* MERRICK *and* ROSS *out, i.e., forward. Blackout except spot on* MERRICK *and* ROSS.

MERRICK: Ostend will always mean bad memories. Won't it, Ross?

ROSS: I've decided. I'm sending you back, lad. You're a flop. No, you're a liability. You ain't the moneymaker I figured, so that's it.

MERRICK: Alone?

ROSS: Here's a few bob, have a nosh. I'm keeping the rest. For my trouble. I deserve it, I reckon. Invested enough with you. Pick up your stink if I stick around. Stink of failure. Stink of lost years. Just stink, stink, stink, stink, stink.

Enter CONDUCTOR.

CONDUCTOR: This the one?

ROSS: Just see him to Liverpool St. Station safe, will you? Here's for your trouble.

MERRICK: Robbed.

CONDUCTOR: What's he say?

Ross: Just makes sounds. Fella's an imbecile.

Merrick: Robbed.

Ross: Bon voyage, Johnny. His name is Johnny. He knows his name, that's all, though.

Conductor: Don't follow him, Johnny. Johnny, come on boat now. Conductor find Johnny place out of sight. Johnny! Johnny! Don't struggle, Johnny. Johnny come on.

Merrick: Robbed! Robbed!

Fadeout on struggle.

Scene V

Police Side With Imbecile Against The Crowd

Darkness. Uproar, shouts.

Voice: Liverpool St. Station!

Enter Merrick, Conductor, Policeman.

Policeman: We're safe in here. I barred the door.

Conductor: They wanted to rip him to pieces. I've never seen anything like it. It was like being Gordon at bleedin' Khartoum.

Policeman: Got somewhere to go in London, lad? Can't stay here.

Conductor: He's an imbecile. He don't understand. Search him.

Policeman: Got any money?

Merrick: Robbed.

Policeman: What's that?

Conductor: He just makes sounds. Frightened sounds is all he makes. Go through his coat.

Merrick: Je-sus

Policeman: Don't let me go through your coat, I'll turn you over to that lot! Oh, I was joking, don't upset yourself.

Merrick: Joke? Joke?

Policeman: Sure, croak, croak, croak, croak.

Merrick: Je-sus.

Policeman: Got a card here. You Johnny Merrick? What's this old card here, Johnny? Someone give you a card?

Conductor: What's it say?

Policeman: Says Mr. Frederick Treves, Lecturer in Anatomy, the London Hospital.

CONDUCTOR: I'll go see if I can find him, it's not far. (*Exits.*)

POLICEMAN: What's he do, lecture you on your anatomy? People who think right don't look like that then, do they? Yeah, glung, glung, glung, glung.

MERRICK: Jesus. Jesus.

CONDUCTOR: Sure, Treves, Treves, Treves, Treves.

Blackout, then lights go up as CONDUCTOR *leads* TREVES *in.*

TREVES: What is going on here? Look at that mob, have you no sense of decency. I am Frederick Treves. This is my card.

POLICEMAN: This poor wretch here had it. Arrived from Ostend.

TREVES: Good Lord, Merrick? John Merrick? What has happened to you?

MERRICK: Help me!

Fadeout.

SCENE VI

Even On The Niger And Ceylon, Not This

The London Hospital. MERRICK *in bathtub.* TREVES *outside. Enter* MISS SANDWICH.

TREVES: You are? Miss Sandwich?

SANDWICH: Sandwich. Yes.

TREVES: You have had experience in missionary hospitals in the Niger.

SANDWICH: And Ceylon.

TREVES: I may assume you've seen–

SANDWICH: The tropics. Oh those diseases. The many and the awful scourges our Lord sends, yes, sir.

TREVES: I need the help of an experienced nurse, you see.

SANDWICH: Someone to bring him food, take care of the room. Yes, I understand. But it is somehow difficult.

TREVES: Well, I have been let down so far. He really is–that is, the regular sisters–well, it is not part of their job and they will not do it. Be ordinarily kind to Mr. Merrick. Without–well–panicking. He is quite beyond ugly. You understand that? His appearance has terrified them.

SANDWICH: The photographs show a terrible disease.

TREVES: It is a disorder, not a disease; it is in no way contagious though we don't in fact know what it is. I have found however that there is a deep superstition in those I've tried, they actually believe he somehow brought it on himself, this thing, and of course it is not that at all.

SANDWICH: I am not one who believes it is ourselves who attain grace or bring chastisement to us, sir.

TREVES: Miss Sandwich, I am hoping not.

SANDWICH: Let me put your mind to rest. Care for lepers in the East, and you have cared, Mr. Treves. In Africa, I have seen dreadful scourges quite unknown to our more civilized climes. What at home could be worse than a miserable and afflicted rotting black?

TREVES: I imagine.

SANDWICH: Appearances do not daunt me.

TREVES: It is really that that has sent me outside the confines of the London seeking help.

SANDWICH: "I look unto the hills whence cometh my help." I understand: I think I will be satisfactory.

Enter PORTER *with tray.*

PORTER: His lunch. (*Exits.*)

TREVES: Perhaps you would be so kind as to accompany me this time. I will introduce you.

SANDWICH: Allow me to carry the tray.

TREVES: I will this time. You are ready.

SANDWICH: I am.

TREVES: He is bathing to be rid of his odor.

(*They enter to* MERRICK.)

John, this is Miss Sandwich. She–

SANDWICH: I– (*unable to control herself*) Oh my good God in Heaven. (*Bolts room.*)

TREVES: (*puts* MERRICK's *lunch down*) I am sorry. I thought–

MERRICK: Thank you for saving the lunch this time.

TREVES: Excuse me.

(*Exits to* MISS SANDWICH.)

You have let me down, you know. I did everything to warn you and still you let me down.

SANDWICH: You didn't say.

TREVES: But I–

SANDWICH: Didn't! You said–just words!

TREVES: But the photographs.

SANDWICH: Just pictures. No one will do this. I am sorry. (Exits.)

TREVES: Yes. Well. This is not helping him.

Fadeout.

SCENE VII

The English Public Will Pay For Him To Be Like Us

The London Hospital. MERRICK *in a bathtub reading.* TREVES, BISHOP
　How *in foreground.*

BISHOP: With what fortitude he bears his cross! It is remarkable. He has
　made the acquaintance of religion and knows sections of the Bible by
　heart. Once I'd grasped his speech, it became clear he'd certainly had
　religious instruction at one time.

TREVES: I believe it was in the workhouse, Dr. How.

BISHOP: They are awfully good about that sometimes. The psalms he loves,
　and the book of Job perplexes him, he says, for he cannot see that a just
　God must cause suffering, as he puts it, merely then to be merciful. Yet
　that Christ will save him he does not doubt, so he is not resentful.

Enter GOMM.

GOMM: Christ had better; be damned if we can.

BISHOP: Ahem. In any case Dr. Treves, he has a religious nature, further
　instruction would uplift him and I'd be pleased to provide it. I plan to
　speak of him from the pulpit this week.

GOMM: I see our visiting bather has flushed the busy Bishop How from his
　cruciform lair.

BISHOP: Speak with Merrick, sir. I have spoken to him of Mercy and Jus-
　tice. There's a true Christian in the rough.

GOMM: This makes my news seem banal, yet yes: Frederick, the response
　to my letter to the *Times* about Merrick has been staggering. The English
　public has been so generous that Merrick may be supported for life with-
　out a penny spent from Hospital funds.

TREVES: But that is excellent.

BISHOP: God bless the English public.

GOMM: Especially for not dismembering him at Liverpool St. Station. Fred-
　die, the London's no home for incurables, this is quite irregular, but for
　you I permit it–though god knows what you'll do.

BISHOP: God does know, sir, and Darwin does not.

GOMM: He'd better, sir; he deformed him.

BISHOP: I had apprehensions coming here. I find it most fortunate Merrick
　is in the hands of Dr. Treves, a Christian, sir.

GOMM: Freddie is a good man and a brilliant doctor, and that is fortunate
　indeed.

TREVES: I couldn't have raised the funds though, Doctor.

BISHOP: Don't let me keep you longer from your duties, Mr. Treves. Yet, Mr. Gomm, consider: is it science, sir, that motivates us when we transport English rule of law to India or Ireland? When good British churchmen leave hearth and home for missionary hardship in Africa, is it science that bears them away? Sir it is not. It is Christian duty. It is the obligation to bring our light and benefices to benighted man. That motivates us, even as it motivates Treves toward Merrick, sir, to bring salvation where none is. Gordon was a Christian, sir, and died at Khartoum for it. Not for science, sir.

GOMM: You're telling me, not for science.

BISHOP: Mr. Treves, I'll visit Merrick weekly if I may.

TREVES: You will be welcome, sir, I am certain.

BISHOP: Then good day, sirs. (*Exits.*)

GOMM: Well, Jesus my boy, now we have the money, what do you plan for Merrick?

TREVES: Normality as far as is possible.

GOMM: So he will be like us? Ah. (*Smiles.*)

TREVES: Is something wrong, Mr. Gomm? With us?

Fadeout.

SCENE VIII

Mercy And Justice Elude Our Minds And Actions

MERRICK *in bath.* TREVES, GOMM.

MERRICK: How long is as long as I like?

TREVES: You may stay for life. The funds exist.

MERRICK: Been reading this. About homes for the blind. Wouldn't mind going to one when I have to move.

TREVES: But you do not have to move; and you're not blind.

MERRICK: I would prefer it where no one stared at me.

GOMM: No one will bother you here.

TREVES: Certainly not. I've given instructions.

PORTER *and* SNORK *peek in.*

PORTER: What'd I tell you?

SNORK: Gawd almighty. Oh, Mr. Treves. Mr. Gomm.

TREVES: You were told not to do this. I don't understand. You must not lurk about. Surely you have work.

PORTER: Yes, sir.

TREVES: Well, it is infuriating. When you are told a thing, you must listen. I won't have you gaping in on my patients. Kindly remember that.

PORTER: Isn't a patient, sir, is he?

TREVES: Do not let me find you here again.

PORTER: Didn't know you were here, sir. We'll be off now.

GOMM: No, no, Will. Mr. Treves was precisely saying no one would intrude when you intruded.

TREVES: He is warned now. Merrick does not like it.

GOMM: He was warned before. On what penalty, Will?

PORTER: That you'd sack me, sir.

GOMM: You are sacked, Will. You, his friend, you work here?

SNORK: Just started last week, sir.

GOMM: Well, I hope the point is taken now.

PORTER: Mr. Gomm–I ain't truly sacked, am I?

GOMM: Will, yes. Truely sacked. You will never be more truly sacked.

PORTER: It's not me. My wife ain't well. My sister has got to take care of our kids, and of her. Well.

GOMM: Think of them first next time.

PORTER: It ain't as if I interfered with his medicine.

GOMM: That is exactly what it is. You may go.

PORTER: Just keeping him to look at in private. That's all. Isn't it?

SNORK *and* PORTER *exit.*

GOMM: There are priorities, Frederick. The first is discipline. Smooth is the passage to the tight ship's master. Merrick, you are safe from prying now.

TREVES: Have we nothing to say, John?

MERRICK: If all that'd stared at me'd been sacked–there'd be whole towns out of work.

TREVES: I meant, "Thank you, sir."

MERRICK: "Thank you sir."

TREVES: We always do say please and thank you, don't we?

MERRICK: Yes, sir. Thank you.

TREVES: If we want to properly be like others.

MERRICK: Yes, sir, I want to.

TREVES: Then it is for our own good, is it not?

MERRICK: Yes, sir. Thank you, Mr. Gomm.

GOMM: Sir, you are welcome. (*Exits.*)

TREVES: You are happy here, are you not, John?

MERRICK: Yes.

TREVES: The baths have rid you of the odor, have they not?

MERRICK: First chance I had to bathe regular. Ly.

TREVES: And three meals a day delivered to your room?

MERRICK: Yes, sir.

TREVES: This is your Promised Land, is it not? A roof. Food. Protection. Care. Is it not?

MERRICK: Right, Mr. Treves.

TREVES: I will bet you don't know what to call this.

MERRICK: No, sir, I don't know.

TREVES: You call it, Home.

MERRICK: Never had a home before.

TREVES: You have one now. Say it, John: Home.

MERRICK: Home.

TREVES: No, no, really say it. I have a home. This is my. Go on.

MERRICK: I have a home. This is my home. This is my home. I have a home. As long as I like?

TREVES: That is what home is.

MERRICK: That is what is home.

TREVES: If I abide by the rules I will be happy.

MERRICK: Yes, sir.

TREVES: Don't be shy.

MERRICK: If I abide by the rules I will be happy.

TREVES: Very good. Why?

MERRICK: Why what?

TREVES: Will you be happy?

MERRICK: Because it is my home?

TREVES: No, no. Why do rules make you happy?

MERRICK: I don't know.

TREVES: Of course you do.

MERRICK: No, I really don't.

TREVES: Why does anything make you happy?

MERRICK: Like what? Like what?

TREVES: Don't be upset. Rules make us happy because they are for our own good.

MERRICK: Okay.

TREVES: Don't be shy, John. You can say it.

MERRICK: This is my home?

TREVES: No. About rules making us happy.

MERRICK: They make us happy because they are for our own good.

TREVES: Excellent. Now: I am submitting a follow-up paper on you to the London Pathological Society. It would help if you told me what you recall about your first years, John. To fill in gaps.

MERRICK: To fill in gaps. The workhouse where they put me. They beat you there like a drum. Boom boom: scrape the floor white. Shine the pan, boom boom. It never ends. The floor is always dirty. The pan is always tarnished. There is nothing you can do about it. You are always attacked anyway. Boom boom. Boom boom. Boom boom. Will the children go to the workhouse?

TREVES: What children?

MERRICK: The children. The man he sacked.

TREVES: Of necessity Will will find other employment. You don't want crowds staring at you, do you?

MERRICK: No.

TREVES: Then Mr. Gomm was merciful. You yourself are proof. Is it not so? (*Pause.*) Well? Is it not so?

MERRICK: If your mercy is so cruel, what do you have for justice?

TREVES: I am sorry. It is just the way things are.

MERRICK: Boom boom. Boom boom. Boom boom.

Fadeout.

SCENE IX

Most Important Are Women

MERRICK *asleep, head on knees.* TREVES, MRS. KENDAL *foreground.*

TREVES: You have seen the photographs of John Merrick, Mrs. Kendal. You are acquainted with his appearance.

MRS. KENDAL: He reminds me of an audience I played Cleopatra for in Brighton once. All huge grim head and grimace and utterly unable to clap.

TREVES: Well. My aim's to lead him to as normal a life as possible. His terror of us all comes from having been held at arm's length from society. I am determined that shall end. For example, he loves to meet people and converse. I am determined he shall. For example, he had never seen the inside of any normal home before. I had him to mine, and what a reward, Mrs. Kendal; his astonishment, his joy at the most ordinary things. Most critical I feel, however, are women. I will explain. They have always shown the greatest fear and loathing of him. While he adores them of course.

MRS. KENDAL: Ah. He is intelligent.

TREVES: I am convinced they are the key to retrieving him from his exclusion. Though, I must warn you, women are not quite real to him–more
creatures of his imagination.

MRS. KENDAL: Then he is already like other men, Mr. Treves.

TREVES: So I thought, an actress could help. I mean, unlike most women,
you won't give in, you are trained to hide your true feelings and assume
others.

MRS. KENDAL: You mean unlike most women I am famous for it, that is
really all.

TREVES: Well. In any case. If you could enter the room and smile and wish
him good morning. And when you leave, shake his hand, the left one
is usable, and really quite beautiful, and say, "I am very pleased to have
made your acquaintance, Mr. Merrick."

MRS. KENDAL: Shall we try it? Left hand out please. (*Suddenly radiant*) I
am *very* pleased to have made your acquaintance Mr. Merrick. I am very
pleased to have made your acquaintance Mr. Merrick. I am very pleased
to have made your *acquaintance* Mr. Merrick. I *am* very pleased to have
made *your* acquaintance Mr. Merrick. Yes. That one.

TREVES: By god, they are all splendid. Merrick will be so pleased. It will be
the day he becomes a man like other men.

MRS. KENDAL: Speaking of that, Mr. Treves.

TREVES: Frederick, please.

MRS. KENDAL: Freddie, may I commit an indiscretion?

TREVES: Yes?

MRS. KENDAL: I could not but help noticing from the photographs that–
well–of the unafflicted parts–ah, how shall I put it? (*Points to photograph.*)

TREVES: Oh. I see! I quite. Understand. No, no, no, it is quite normal.

MRS. KENDAL: I thought as much.

TREVES: Medically speaking, uhm, you see the papillomatous extru-
sions which disfigure him, uhm, seem to correspond quite regularly to
the osseous deformities, that is, excuse me, there is a link between the
bone disorder and the skin growths, though for the life of me I have not
discovered what it is or why it is, but in any case this–part–it would be
therefore unlikely to be afflicted because well, that is, well, there's no
bone in it. None at all. I mean.

MRS. KENDAL: Well. Learn a little every day don't we?

TREVES: I am horribly embarrassed.

MRS. KENDAL: Are you? Then he must be lonely indeed.

Fadeout.

SCENE X

When The Illusion Ends He Must Kill Himself

MERRICK *sketching. Enter* TREVES, MRS. KENDAL.

TREVES: He is making sketches for a model of St. Phillip's church. He wants someday to make a model, you see. John, my boy, this is Mrs. Kendal. She would very much like to make your acquaintance.

MRS. KENDAL: Good morning Mr. Merrick.

TREVES: I will see to a few matters. I will be back soon. (*Exits.*)

MERRICK: I planned so many things to say. I forget them. You are so beautiful.

MRS. KENDAL: How charming, Mr. Merrick.

MERRICK: Well. Really that was what I planned to say. That I forgot what I planned to say. I couldn't think of anything else I was so excited.

MRS. KENDAL: Real charm is always planned, don't you think?

MERRICK: Well. I do not know why I look like this, Mrs. Kendal. My mother was so beautiful. She was knocked down by an elephant in a circus while she was pregnant. Something must have happened, don't you think?

MRS. KENDAL: It may well have.

MERRICK: It may well have. But sometimes I think my head is so big because it is so full of dreams. Because it is. Do you know what happens when dreams cannot get out?

MRS. KENDAL: Why, no.

MERRICK: I don't either. Something must. (*Silence.*) Well. You are a famous actress.

MRS. KENDAL: I am not unknown.

MERRICK: You must display yourself for your living then. Like I did.

MRS. KENDAL: That is not myself, Mr. Merrick. That is an illusion. This is myself.

MERRICK: This is myself too.

MRS. KENDAL: Frederick says you like to read. So: books.

MERRICK: I am reading *Romeo and Juliet* now.

MRS. KENDAL: Ah. Juliet. What a love story. I adore love stories.

MERRICK: I like love stories too. If I had been Romeo, guess what.

MRS. KENDAL: What?

MERRICK: I would not have held the mirror to her breath.

MRS. KENDAL: You mean the scene where Juliet appears to be dead and he holds a mirror to her breath and sees–

MERRICK: Nothing. How does it feel when he kills himself because he just sees nothing?

MRS. KENDAL: Well. My experience as Juliet has been–particularly with an actor I will not name–that while I'm laying there dead dead dead, and he is lamenting excessively, I get to thinking that if this slab of ham does not part from the hamhock of his life toute suite, I am going to scream, pop off the tomb, and plunge a dagger into his scene-stealing heart. Romeos are very undependable.

MERRICK: Because he does not care for Juliet.

MRS. KENDAL: Not care?

MERRICK: Does he take her pulse? Does he get a doctor? Does he make sure? No. He kills himself. The illusion fools him because he does not care for her. He only cares about himself. If I had been Romeo, we would have got away.

MRS. KENDAL: But then there would be no play, Mr. Merrick.

MERRICK: If he did not love her, why should there be a play? Looking in a mirror and seeing nothing. That is not love. It was all an illusion. When the illusion ended he had to kill himself.

MRS. KENDAL: Why. That is extraordinary.

MERRICK: Before I spoke with people, I did not think of all these things because there was no one to bother to think them for. Now things just come out of my mouth which are true.

TREVES *enters.*

TREVES: You are famous, John. We are in the papers. Look. They have written up my report to the Pathological Society. Look–it is a kind of apotheosis for you.

MRS. KENDAL: Frederick, I feel Mr. Merrick would benefit by even more company than you provide; in fact by being acquainted with the best, and they with him. I shall make it my task if you'll permit. As you know, I am a friend of nearly everyone, and I do pretty well as I please and what pleases me is this task, I think.

TREVES: By god, Mrs. Kendal, you are splendid.

MRS. KENDAL: Mr. Merrick I must go now. I should like to return if I may. And so that we may without delay teach you about society, I would like to bring my good friend Dorothy Lady Neville. She would be most pleased if she could meet you. Let me tell her yes?

(MERRICK *nods yes.*)

Then until next time. I'm sure your church model will surprise us all. Mr. Merrick, it has been a very great pleasure to make your acquaintance.

TREVES: John. Your hand. She wishes to shake your hand

MERRICK: Thank you for coming.

MRS. KENDAL: But it was my pleasure. Thank you. (*Exits, accompanied by* TREVES.)

TREVES: What a wonderful success. Do you know he's never shook a woman's hand before?

As lights fade MERRICK *sobs soundlessly, uncontrollably.*

SCENE XI

He Does It With Just One Hand

Music. MERRICK *working on model of St. Phillip's church. Enter* DUCHESS. *At side* TREVES *ticks off a gift list.*

MERRICK: Your grace.

DUCHESS: How nicely the model is coming along, Mr. Merrick. I've come to say Happy Christmas, and that I hope you will enjoy this ring and remember your friend by it.

MERRICK: Your grace, thank you.

DUCHESS: I am very pleased to have made your acquaintance. (*Exits.*)

Enter COUNTESS.

COUNTESS: Please accept these silver-backed brushes and comb for Christmas, Mr. Merrick.

MERRICK: With many thanks, Countess.

COUNTESS: I am very pleased to have made your acquaintance. (*Exits.*)

Enter LORD JOHN.

LORD JOHN: Here's the silver-topped walking stick, Merrick. Make you a regular Piccadilly exquisite. Keep up the good work. Self-help is the best help. Example to us all.

MERRICK: Thank you, Lord John.

LORD JOHN: Very pleased to have made your acquaintance. (*Exits.*)

Enter TREVES *and* PRINCESS ALEXANDRA.

TREVES: Her Royal Highness Princess Alexandra.

PRINCESS: The happiest of Christmases, Mr. Merrick.

TREVES: Her Royal Highness has brought you a signed photograph of herself.

MERRICK: I am honored, your Royal Highness. It is the treasure of my possessions. I have written to His Royal Highness the Prince of Wales to thank him for the pheasants and woodcock he sent.

PRINCESS: You are a credit to Mr. Treves, Mr. Merrick. Mr. Treves, you are a credit to medicine, to England, and to Christendom. I am very pleased to have made your acquaintance.

PRINCESS, TREVES *exits. Enter* MRS. KENDAL.

MRS. KENDAL: Good news, John. Bertie says we may use the Royal Box whenever I like. Mrs. Keppel says it gives a unique perspective. And for Christmas, ivory-handled razors and toothbrush.

Enter TREVES.

TREVES: And a cigarette case, my boy, full of cigarettes!

MERRICK: Thank you. Very much.

MRS. KENDAL: Look Freddie, look. The model of St. Phillip's.

TREVES: It is remarkable, I know.

MERRICK: And I do it with just one hand, they all say.

MRS. KENDAL: You are an artist, John Merrick, an artist.

MERRICK: I did not begin to build at first. Not till I saw what St. Phillip's really was. It is not stone and steel and glass; it is an imitation of grace flying up and up from the mud. So I make my imitation of an imitation. But even in that is heaven to me, Mrs. Kendal.

TREVES: That thought's got a good line, John. Plato believed this was all a world of illusion and that artists made illusions of illusions of heaven.

MERRICK: You mean we are all just copies? Of originals?

TREVES: That's it.

MERRICK: Who made the copies?

TREVES: God. The Demi-urge.

MERRICK: (*goes back to work*) He should have used both hands shouldn't he?
Music. Puts another piece on St. Phillip's. Fadeout.

SCENE XII

Who Does He Remind You Of?

TREVES, MRS. KENDAL.

TREVES: Why all those toilet articles, tell me? He is much too deformed to use any of them.

MRS. KENDAL: Props of course. To make himself. As I make me.

TREVES: You? You think of yourself.

MRS. KENDAL: Well. He is gentle, almost feminine. Cheerful, honest within limits, a serious artist in his way. He is almost like me.

Enter BISHOP HOW.

BISHOP: He is religious and devout. He knows salvation must radiate to us or all is lost, which it's certainly not.

Enter GOMM.

GOMM: He seems practical, like me. He has seen enough of daily evil to be thankful for small goods that come his way. He knows what side his bread is buttered on, and counts his blessings for it. Like me.

Enter DUCHESS.

DUCHESS: I can speak with him of anything. For I know he is discreet. Like me.

All exit except TREVES.

TREVES: How odd. I think him curious, compassionate, concerned about the world, well, rather like myself, Freddie Treves, 1889 AD.

Enter MRS. KENDAL.

MRS. KENDAL: Of course he is rather odd. And hurt. And helpless not to show the struggling. And so am I.

Enter GOMM.

GOMM: He knows I use him to raise money for the London, I am certain. He understands I would be derelict if I didn't. He is wary of any promise, yet he fits in well. Like me.

Enter BISHOP HOW.

BISHOP: I as a seminarist had many of the same doubts. Struggled as he does. And hope they may be overcome.

Enter PRINCESS ALEXANDRA.

PRINCESS: When my husband His Royal Highness Edward Prince of Wales asked Dr. Treves to be his personal surgeon, he said, "Dear Freddie, if you can put up with the Elephant bloke, you can surely put up with me."

All exit, except TREVES. *Enter* LORD JOHN.

LORD JOHN: See him out of fashion, Freddie. As he sees me. Social contacts critical. Oh–by the way–ignore the bloody papers; all lies. (*Exits.*)

TREVES: Merrick visibly worse than 86–87. That, as he rises higher in the consolations of society, he gets visibly more grotesque is proof definitive he is like me. Like his condition, which I make no sense of, I make no sense of mine.

Spot on MERRICK *placing another piece on St. Phillip's. Fadeout.*

Scene XIII

Anxieties Of The Swamp

Merrick, *in spot, strains to listen:* Treves, Lord John *outside.*

Treves: But the papers are saying you broke the contracts. They are saying you've lost the money.

Lord John: Freddie, if I were such a scoundrel, how would I dare face investors like yourself. Broken contracts! I never considered them actual contracts–just preliminary things, get the old deal under way. An actual contract's something between gentlemen; and this attack on me shows they are no gentlemen. Now I'm only here to say the company remains a terribly attractive proposition. Don't you think? To recapitalize–if you could spare another–ah.

(*Enter* Gomm.)

Mr. Gomm. How good to see you. Just remarking how splendidly Merrick thrives here, thanks to you and Freddie.

Gomm: Lord John. Allow me: I must take Frederick from you. Keep him at work. It's in his contract. Wouldn't want him breaking it. Sort of thing makes the world fly apart, isn't it?

Lord John: Yes. Well. Of course, mmm.

Gomm: Sorry to hear you're so pressed. Expect we'll see less of you around the London now?

Lord John: Of course, I, actually–ah! Overdue actually. Appointment in the City. Freddie. Mr. Gomm. (*Exits.*)

Treves: He plain fooled me. He was kind to Merrick.

Gomm: You have risen fast and easily, my boy. You've forgot how to protect yourself. Break now.

Treves: It does not seem right somehow.

Gomm: The man's a moral swamp. Is that not clear yet? Is he attractive? Deceit often is. Friendly? Swindlers can be. Another loan? Not another cent. It may be your money, Freddie; but I will not tolerate laboring like a navvy that the London should represent honest charitable and com- passionate science, and have titled swindlers mucking up the pitch. He has succeeded in destroying himself so rabidly, you ought not doubt an instant it was his real aim all along. He broke the contracts, gambled the money away, lied, and like an infant in his mess, gurgles and wants to do it again. Never mind details, don't want to know. Break and be glad. Don't hesitate. Today. One-man moral swamp. Don't be sucked in.

Enter Mrs. Kendal.

Mrs. Kendal Have you seen the papers?

Treves: Yes.

Gomm: Yes, yes. A great pity. Freddie: today. (*Exits.*)

Mrs. Kendal: Freddie?

Treves: He has used us. I shall be all right. Come.

Mrs. Kendal, Treves *enter to* Merrick.

John: I shall not be able to stay this visit. I must, well, unravel a few things. Nurse Ireland and Snork are–?

Merrick: Friendly and respectful, Frederick.

Treves: I'll look in in a few days.

Merrick: Did I do something wrong?

Mrs. Kendal: No.

Treves: This is a hospital. Not a marketplace. Don't forget it, ever. Sorry. Not you. Me. (*Exits.*)

Mrs. Kendal: Well. Shall we weave today? Don't you think weaving might be fun? So many things are fun. Most men really can't enjoy them. Their loss, isn't it? I like little activities which engage me; there's something ancient in it, I don't know. Before all this. Would you like to try? John?

Merrick: Frederick said I may stay here for life.

Mrs. Kendal: And so you shall.

Merrick: If he is in trouble?

Mrs. Kendal: Frederick is your protector, John.

Merrick: If he is in trouble? (*He picks up small photograph.*)

Mrs. Kendal: Who is that? Ah, is it not your mother? She is pretty, isn't she?

Merrick: Will Frederick keep his word with me, his contract, Mrs. Kendal? If he is in trouble.

Mrs. Kendal: What? Contract? Did you say?

Merrick: And will you?

Mrs. Kendal: I? What? Will I?

Merrick *silent. Puts another piece on model. Fadeout.*

Scene XIV

Art Is Permitted But Nature Forbidden

Rain. Merrick *working.* Mrs. Kendal.

Merrick: The Prince has a mistress. (*Silence.*) The Irishman had one. Everyone seems to. Or a wife. Some have both. I have concluded I need a mistress. It is bad enough not to sleep like others.

MRS. KENDAL: Sitting up, you mean. Couldn't be very restful.

MERRICK: I have to. Too heavy to lay down. My head. But to sleep alone; that is worst of all.

MRS. KENDAL: The artist expresses his love through his works. That is civilization.

MERRICK: Are you very shocked?

MRS. KENDAL: Why should I be?

MERRICK: Others would be.

MRS. KENDAL: I am not others.

MERRICK: I suppose it is hopeless.

MRS. KENDAL: Nothing is hopeless. However it is unlikely.

MERRICK: I thought you might have a few ideas.

MRS. KENDAL: I can guess who has ideas here.

MERRICK: You don't know something. I have never even seen a naked woman.

MRS. KENDAL: Surely in all the fairs you worked.

MERRICK: I mean a real woman.

MRS. KENDAL: Is one more real than another?

MERRICK: I mean like the ones in the theater. The opera.

MRS. KENDAL: Surely you can't mean they are more real.

MERRICK: In the audience. A woman not worn out early. Not deformed by awful life. A lady. Someone kept up. Respectful of herself. You don't know what fairgrounds are like, Mrs. Kendal.

MRS. KENDAL: You mean someone like Princess Alexandra?

MERRICK: Not so old.

MRS. KENDAL: Ah. Like Dorothy.

MERRICK: She does not look happy. No.

MRS. KENDAL: Lady Ellen?

MERRICK: Too thin.

MRS. KENDAL: Then who?

MERRICK: Certain women. They have a kind of ripeness. They seem to stop at a perfect point.

MRS. KENDAL: My dear she doesn't exist.

MERRICK: That is probably why I never saw her.

MRS. KENDAL: What would your friend Bishop How say of all this I wonder?

MERRICK: He says I should put these things out of my mind.

MRS. KENDAL: Is that the best he can suggest?

MERRICK: I put them out of my mind. They reappeared, snap.

MRS. KENDAL: What about Frederick?

MERRICK: He would be appalled if I told him.

MRS. KENDAL: I am flattered. Too little trust has maimed my life. But that is another story.

MERRICK: What a rain. Are we going to read this afternoon?

MRS. KENDAL: Yes. Some women are lucky to look well, that is all. It is a rather arbitrary gift; it has no really good use, though it has uses, I will say that. Anyway it does not signify very much.

MERRICK: To me it does.

MRS. KENDAL: Well. You are mistaken.

MERRICK: What are we going to read?

MRS. KENDAL: Trust is very important you know. I trust you.

MERRICK: Thank you very much. I have a book of Thomas Hardy's here. He is a friend of Frederick's. Shall we read that?

MRS. KENDAL: Turn around a moment. Don't look.

MERRICK: Is this a game?

MRS. KENDAL: I would not call it a game. A surprise. (*She begins undressing.*)

MERRICK: What kind of a surprise?

MRS. KENDAL: I saw photographs of you. Before I met you. You didn't know that, did you?

MERRICK: The ones from the first time, in '84? No, I didn't.

MRS. KENDAL: I felt it was–unjust. I don't know why. I cannot say my sense of justice is my most highly developed characteristic. You may turn around again. Well. A little funny, isn't it?

MERRICK: It was the most beautiful sight I have seen. Ever.

MRS. KENDAL: If you tell anyone, I shall not see you again, we shall not read, we shall not talk, we shall do nothing. Wait. (*Undoes her hair.*) There. No illusions. Now. Well? What is there to say? "I am extremely pleased to have made your acquaintance?"

Enter TREVES.

TREVES: For God's sakes. What is going on here? What is going on?

MRS. KENDAL: For a moment, Paradise, Freddie. (*She begins dressing.*)

TREVES: But–have you no sense of decency? Woman, dress yourself quickly.

(*Silence.* MERRICK *goes to put another piece on St. Phillip's.*)

Are you not ashamed? Do you know what you are? Don't you know what is forbidden?

Fadeout.

SCENE XV

Ingratitude

ROSS *in* MERRICK's *room.*

ROSS: I come actually to ask your forgiveness.

MERRICK: I found a good home, Ross. I forgave you.

ROSS: I was hoping we could work out a deal. Something new maybe.

MERRICK: No.

ROSS: See, I was counting on it. That you were kindhearted. Like myself.
Some things don't change. Got to put your money on the things that don't, I
figure. I figure from what I read about you, you don't change. Dukes, Ladies
coming to see you. Ask myself why? Figure it's same as always was. Makes
'em feel good about themselves by comparison. Them things don't change.
There but for the grace of. So I figure you're selling the same service as
always. To better clientele. Difference now is you ain't charging for it.

MERRICK: You make me sound like a whore.

ROSS: You are. I am. They are. Most are. No disgrace, John. Disgrace is to
be a stupid whore. Give it for free. Not capitalize on the interest in you.
Not to have a manager then is stupid.

MERRICK: You see this church. I am building it. The people who visit are
friends. Not clients. I am not a dog walking on its hind legs.

ROSS: I was thinking. Charge these people. Pleasure of the Elephant Man's
company. Something. Right spirit is everything. Do it in the right spirit,
they'd pay happily. I'd take ten percent. I'd be okay with ten percent.

MERRICK: Bad luck's made you daft.

ROSS: I helped you, John. Discovered you. Was that daft? No. Only daftness
was being at a goldmine without a shovel. Without proper connections.
Like Treves has. What's daft? Ross sows, Treves harvests? It's not fair, is it
John? When you think about it. I do think about it. Because I'm old. Got
something in my throat. You may have noticed. Something in my lung
here too. Something in my belly I guess too. I'm not a heap of health, am
I? But I'd do well with ten percent. I don't need more than ten percent.
Ten percent'd give me a future slightly better'n a cobblestone. This lot
would pay, if you charged in the right spirit. I don't ask much.

MERRICK: They're the cream, Ross. They know it. Man like you tries to
make them pay, they'll walk away.

ROSS: I'm talking about doing it in the right spirit.

MERRICK: They are my friends. I'd lose everything. For you. Ross, you lived
your life. You robbed me of forty-eight pounds, nine shillings, tuppence.

You left me to die. Be satisfied Ross. You've had enough. You kept me like an animal in darkness. You come back and want to rob me again. Will you not be satisfied? Now I am a man like others, you want me to return?

ROSS: Had a woman yet?

MERRICK: Is that what makes a man?

ROSS: In my time it'd do for a start.

MERRICK: Not what makes this one. Yet I am like others.

ROSS: Then I'm condemned. I got no energy to try nothing new. I may as well go to the dosshouse straight. Die there anyway. Between filthy dosshouse rags. Nothing in the belly but acid. I don't like pain, John. The future gives pain sense. Without a future–(*Pauses*) Five percent? John?

MERRICK: I'm sorry, Ross. It's just the way things are.

ROSS: By god. Then I am lost.

Fadeout.

SCENE XVI

No Reliable General Anesthetic Has Appeared Yet

TREVES, *reading, makes notes.* MERRICK *works.*

MERRICK: Frederick–do you believe in heaven? Hell? What about Christ? What about God? I believe in heaven. The Bible promises in heaven the crooked shall be made straight.

TREVES: So did the rack, my boy. So do we all.

MERRICK: You don't believe?

TREVES: I will settle for a reliable general anesthetic at this point. Actually, though–I had a patient once. A woman. Operated on her for–a woman's thing. Used ether to anesthetize. Tricky stuff. Didn't come out of it. Pulse stopped, no vital signs, absolutely moribund. Just a big white dead mackerel. Five minutes later, she fretted back to existence, like a lost explorer with a great scoop of the undiscovered.

MERRICK: She saw heaven?

TREVES: Well. I quote her: it was neither heavenly nor hellish. Rather like perambulating in a London fog. People drifted by, but no one spoke. London, mind you. Hell's probably the provinces. She was shocked it wasn't more exotic. But allowed as how had she stayed, and got used to the familiar, so to speak, it did have hints of becoming a kind of bliss. She fled.

MERRICK: If you do believe–why did you send Mrs. Kendal away?

TREVES: Don't forget. It saved you once. My interference. You know well enough–it was not proper.

MERRICK: How can you tell? If you do not believe?

TREVES: There are still standards we abide by.

MERRICK: They make us happy because they are for our own good.

TREVES: Well. Not always.

MERRICK: Oh.

TREVES: Look, if you are angry, just say so.

MERRICK: Whose standards are they?

TREVES: I am not in the mood for this chipping away at the edges, John.

MERRICK: They do not always make us happy because they are not always for our own good?

TREVES: Everyone's. Well. Mine. Everyone's.

MERRICK: That woman's, that Juliet?

TREVES: Juliet?

MERRICK: Who died, then came back.

TREVES: Oh. I see. Yes. Her standards too.

MERRICK: So.

TREVES: So what?

MERRICK: Did you see her? Naked?

TREVES: When I was operating. Of course—

MERRICK: Oh.

TREVES: Oh what?

MERRICK: Is it okay to see them naked if you cut them up afterwards?

TREVES: Good Lord. I'm a surgeon. That is science.

MERRICK: She died. Mrs. Kendal didn't.

TREVES: Well, she came back too.

MERRICK: And Mrs. Kendal didn't. If you mean that.

TREVES: I am trying to read about anesthetics. There is simply no comparison.

MERRICK: Oh.

TREVES: Science is a different thing. This woman came to me to be. I mean, it is not, well, love, you know.

MERRICK: Is that why you're looking for an anesthetic.

TREVES: It would be a boon to surgery.

MERRICK: Because you don't love them.

TREVES: Love's got nothing to do with surgery.

MERRICK: Do you lose many patients?

TREVES: I—some.

MERRICK: Oh.

TREVES: Oh what? What does it matter? Don't you see? If I love, if any surgeon loves her or any patient or not, what does it matter? And what conceivable difference to you?

MERRICK: Because it is your standards we abide by.

TREVES: For God's sakes. If you are angry, just say it. I won't turn you out. Say it: I am angry. Go on. I am angry. I am angry! I am angry!

MERRICK: I believe in heaven.

TREVES: And it is not okay. If they undress if you cut them up. As you put it. Make me sound like Jack the, Jack the Ripper.

MERRICK: No. You worry about anesthetics.

TREVES: Are you having me on?

MERRICK: You are merciful. I myself am proof. Is it not so? (*Pauses.*)Well? Is it not so?

TREVES: Well. I. About Mrs. Kendal–perhaps I was wrong. I, these days that is, I seem to. Lose my head. Taking too much on perhaps. I do not know–what is in me these days.

MERRICK: Will she come back? Mrs. Kendal?

TREVES: I will talk to her again.

MERRICK: But–will she?

TREVES: No. I don't think so.

MERRICK: Oh.

TREVES: There are other things involved. Very. That is. Other things.

MERRICK: Well. Other things. I want to walk now. Think. Other things. (*Begins to exit. Pauses.*)Why? Why won't she?

Silence. MERRICK *exits.*

TREVES: Because I don't want her here when you die. (*He slumps in chair.*) *Fadeout.*

SCENE XVII

Cruelty Is As Nothing To Kindness

TREVES *asleep in chair dreams the following:* MERRICK *and* GOMM *dressed as* ROSS *in foreground.*

MERRICK: If he is merely papier maché and paint, a swindler and a fake–

GOMM: No, no, a genuine Dorset dreamer in a moral swamp. Look–he has so forgot how to protect himself he's gone to sleep.

MERRICK: I must examine him. I would not keep him for long, Mr. Gomm.

GOMM: It would be inconvenience, Mr. Merrick. He is a mainstay of our institution.

MERRICK: Exactly that brought him to my attention. I am Merrick. Here is
my card. I am with the mutations cross the road.

GOMM: Frederick, stand up. You must understand. He is very very valuable. We have invested a great deal in him. He is personal surgeon to the
Prince of Wales.

MERRICK: But I only wish to examine him. I had not of course dreamed of
changing him.

GOMM: But he is a gentleman and a good man.

MERRICK: Therefore exemplary for study as a cruel or deviant one would
not be.

GOMM: Oh very well. Have him back for breakfast time or you feed him.
Frederick, stand up. Up you bloody donkey, up!

TREVES, *still asleep, stands up. Fadeout.*

SCENE XVIII

We Are Dealing With An Epidemic

TREVES *asleep.* MERRICK *at lecturn.*

MERRICK: The most striking feature about him, note, is the terrifyingly normal head. This allowed him to lie down normally, and therefore to dream in
the exclusive personal manner, without the weight of others' dreams accu-
mulating to break his neck. From the brow projected a normal vision of
benevolent enlightenment, what we believe to be a kind of self-mesmerized
state. The mouth, deformed by satisfaction at being at the hub of the best
of existent worlds, was rendered therefore utterly incapable of self-critical
speech, thus of the ability to change. The heart showed signs of worry at this
unchanging yet untenable state. The back was horribly stiff from being kept
against a wall to face the discontent of a world ordered for his convenience.
The surgeon's hands were well-developed and strong, capable of the most
delicate carvings-up, for other's own good. Due also to the normal head,
the right arm was of enormous power; but, so incapable of the distinction
between the assertion of authority and the charitable act of giving, that it
was often to be found disgustingly beating others–for their own good. The
left arm was slighter and fairer, and may be seen in typical position, hand
covering the genitals which were treated as a sullen colony in constant
need of restriction, governance, punishment. For their own good. To add
a further burden to his trouble, the wretched man when a boy developed
a disabling spiritual duality, therefore was unable to feel what others feel,

nor reach harmony with them. Please. (TREVES *shrugs.*) He would thus be
denied all means of escape from those he had tormented.

PINS *enter.*

FIRST PIN: Mr. Merrick. You have shown a profound and unknown disorder to us. You have said when he leaves here, it is for his prior life again.
I do not think it ought to be permitted. It is a disgrace. It is a pity and a
disgrace. It is an indecency in fact. It may be a danger in ways we do not
know. Something ought to be done about it.

MERRICK: We hope in twenty years we will understand enough to put an
end to this affliction.

FIRST PIN: Twenty years! Sir, that is unacceptable!

MERRICK: Had we caught it early, it might have been different. But his condition has already spread both East and West. The truth is, I am afraid,
we are dealing with an epidemic.

MERRICK *puts another piece on St. Phillip's.* PINS *exit.* TREVES *starts awake.*
Fadeout.

SCENE XIX

They Cannot Make Out What He Is Saying

MERRICK, BISHOP HOW *in the background.* BISHOP *gestures,* MERRICK
on knees. TREVES *foreground. Enter* GOMM.

GOMM: Still beavering away for Christ?

TREVES: Yes.

GOMM: I got your report. He doesn't know, does he?

TREVES: The Bishop?

GOMM: I meant Merrick.

TREVES: No.

GOMM: I shall be sorry when he dies.

TREVES: It will not be unexpected anyway.

GOMM: He's brought the hospital quite a lot of good repute. Quite a lot of
contributions too, for that matter. In fact, I like him; never regretted letting him stay on. Though I didn't imagine he's last this long.

TREVES: His heart won't sustain him much longer. It may even give out
when he gets off his bloody knees with that bloody man.

GOMM: What is it, Freddie? What has gone sour for you?

TREVES: It is just–it is the overarc of things, quite inescapable that as he's
achieved greater and greater normality, his condition's edged him closer to

the grave. So–a parable of growing up? To become more normal is to die? More accepted to worsen? He–it is just a mockery of everything we live by.

GOMM: Sorry, Freddie. didn't catch that one.

TREVES: Nothing has gone sour. I do not know.

GOMM: Cheer up, man. You are knighted. Your clients will be kings. Nothing succeeds my boy like success.

(*Exits.*)

BISHOP *comes from* MERRICK's *room.*

BISHOP: I find my sessions with him utterly moving, Mr. Treves. He struggles so. I suggested he might like to be confirmed; he leaped at it like a man lost in a desert to an oasis.

TREVES: He is very excited to do what others do if he thinks it is what others do.

BISHOP: Do you cast doubt, sir, on his faith?

TREVES: No, sir, I do not. Yet he makes all of us think he is deeply like ourselves. And yet we're not like each other. I conclude that we have polished him like a mirror, and shout hallelujah when he reflects us to the inch. I have grown sorry for it.

BISHOP: I cannot make out what you're saying. Is something troubling you, Mr. Treves?

TREVES: Corsets. How about corsets? Here is a pamphlet I've written due mostly to the grotesque ailments I've seen caused by corsets. Fashion overrules me, of course. My patients do not unstrap themselves of corsets. Some cannot–you know, I have so little time in the week, I spend Sundays in the poor-wards; to keep up with work. Work being twenty-year-old women who look an abused fifty with worn-outedness; young men with appalling industrial conditions I turn out as soon as possible to return to their labors. Happily most of my patients are not poor. They are middle class. They overeat and drink so grossly, they destroy nature in themselves and all around them so fervidly, they will not last. Higher up, sir, above the middle class, I confront these same–deformities–bulged out by unlimited resources and the ruthlessness of privilege into the most scandalous dissipation yoked to the grossest ignorance and constraint. I counsel against it where I can. I am ignored of course. Then, what, sir, could be troubling me? I am an extremely successful Englishman in a successful and respected England which informs me daily by the way it lives that it wants to die. I am in despair in fact. Science, observation, practice, deduction, having led me to these conclusions, can no longer serve as consolation. I apparently see things others don't.

BISHOP: I do wish I understand you better, sir. But as for consolation, there is in Christ's church consolation.

TREVES: I am sure we were not born for mere consolation.

BISHOP: But look at Mr. Merrick's happy example.

TREVES: Oh yes. You'd like my garden too. My dog, my wife, my daughter, pruned, cropped, pollarded and somewhat stupefied. Very happy examples, all of them. Well. Is it all we know how to finally do with–whatever? Nature? Is it? Rob it? No, not really, not nature I mean. Ourselves really. Myself really. Robbed, that is. You do see of course, can't figure out, really, what else to do with them. Can we? (*Laughs.*)

BISHOP: It is not exactly clear, sir.

TREVES: I am an awfully good gardener. Is that clear? By god I take such good care of anything, anything you, we are convinced–are you not convinced, him I mean, is not very dangerously human? I mean how could he be? After what we've given him? What you like, sir, is that he is so grateful for patrons, so greedy to be patronized, and no demands, no rights, no hopes; past perverted, present false, future nil. What better could you ask? He puts up with all of it. Of course I do mean taken when I say given, as in what, what, what we have given him, but. You knew that. I'll bet. Because. I. I. I. I–

BISHOP: Do you mean Charity? I cannot tell what you are saying.

TREVES: Help me. (*Weeps.*)

BISHOP *consoles him.*

MERRICK: (*rises, puts last piece on St. Phillip's*) It is done.

Fadeout.

SCENE XX

The Weight Of Dreams

MERRICK *alone, looking at model. Enter* SNORK *with lunch.*

SNORK: Lunch, Mr. Merrick. I'll set it up. Maybe you'd like a walk after lunch. April's doing wonders for the gardens.

(*A funeral procession passes slowly by.*)

My mate Will, his sister died yesterday. Twenty-eight she was. Imagine that. Wife was sick, his sister nursed her. Was a real bloom that girl. Now wife okay, sister just ups and dies. It's all so–what's that word? Forgot it. It means chance-y. Well. Forgot it. Chance-y'll do. Have a good lunch. (*Exits.*)

MERRICK *eats a little, breathes on model, polishes it, goes to bed, arms on knees, head on arms, the position in which he must sleep.*

MERRICK: Chancey? (*Sleeps.*)

Enter PINHEADS *singing.*

PINS: We are the Queens of the Cosmos
Beautiful darkness' empire
Darkness darkness, light's true flower,
Here is eternity's finest hour
Sleep like others you learn to admire
Be like your mother, be like your sire.

They straighten MERRICK *out to normal sleep position. His head tilts over too far. His arms fly up clawing the air. He dies. As light fades,* SNORK *enters.*

SNORK: I remember it, Mr. Merrick. The word is "arbitrary." Arbitrary. It's all so–oh. Hey! Hey! The Elephant Man is dead!

Fadeout.

SCENE XXI

Final Report To The Investigators

GOMM *reading,* TREVES *listening.*

GOMM: "To the Editors of the *Times*. Sir; In November, 1886, you were kind enough to insert in the *Times* a letter from me drawing attention to the case of Joseph Merrick–"

TREVES: John. John Merrick.

GOMM: Well. "–known as the Elephant Man. It was one of singular and exceptional misfortune" et cetera et cetera " . . . debarred from earning his livelihood in any other way than being exhibited to the gaze of the curious. This having been rightly interfered with by the police . . ." et cetera et cetera, "with great difficulty he succeeded somehow or other in getting to the door of the London Hospital where through the kindness of one of our surgeons he was sheltered for a time." And then . . . and then . . . and . . . ah. "While deterred by common humanity from evict-ing him again into the open street, I wrote to you and from that moment all difficulty vanished; the sympathy of many was aroused, and although no other fitting refuge was offered, a sufficient sum was placed at my disposal, apart from the funds of the hospital, to maintain him for what did not promise to be a prolonged life. As–"

TREVES: I forgot. The coroner said it was death by asphyxiation. The weight of the head crushed the windpipe.

GOMM: Well. I go on to say about how he spent his time here, that all attempted to alleviate his misery, that he was visited by the highest in the land et cetera et cetera, that in general he joined our lives as best he could, and: "In spite of all this indulgence, he was quiet and unassuming, grateful for all that was done for him, and conformed readily to the restrictions which were necessary." Will that do so far, do you think?

TREVES: Should think it would.

GOMM: Wouldn't add anything else, would you?

TREVES: Well. He was highly intelligent. He had an acute sensibility; and worst for him, a romantic imagination. No, no. Never mind. I am really not certain of any of it. (*Exits.*)

GOMM: "I have given these details thinking that those who sent money to use for his support would like to know how their charity was used. Last Friday afternoon, though apparently in his usual health, he quietly passed away in his sleep. I have left in my hands a small balance of the money for his support, and this I now propose, after paying certain gratuities, to hand over to the general funds of the hospital. This course I believe will be consonant with the wishes of the contributors.

"It was the courtesy of the *Times* in inserting my letter in 1886 that procured for this afflicted man a comfortable protection during the last years of a previously wretched existence, and I desire to take this opportunity of thankfully acknowledging it.

> "I am sir, your obedient servant,
> F. C. Carr Gomm
> "House Committee Room, London Hospital."
> 15 April 1890.

TREVES *reenters.*

TREVES: I did think of one small thing.

GOMM: It's too late, I'm afraid. It is done. (*Smiles.*)

Hold before fadeout.

W;t

ℬ

Margaret Edson

INTRODUCTION

W;t, by Margaret Edson, presents an unremitting view of the female body as physiological site, with the main character introducing herself to the audience as a patient who is in the last stages of advanced ovarian cancer. The action takes place during the last two hours of her life, passed in a research hospital where she has been participating in an experimental chemotherapy program. The sentience of pain and physicality are omnipresent in the drama. The spectator is spared little as the woman's treatment and physical decline are graphically represented, nor can there be any escape for the faint of heart since the work is presented without intermission. To complete her self-portrait, the protagonist, Vivian Bearing, also reveals her mind, introducing herself as an academic, a professor of seventeenth-century poetry with a specialization in the work of metaphysical poet John Donne. And should anyone question her credentials, she offers, "I can say with confidence, no one is quite as good as I" (20). We can say that she has her flaws. The intellectual superiority she enjoys over her students often makes her insensitive to their deficiencies to the point where she is frequently unfeeling.

The clinical fellow on her case, Jason Posner, is a former student. Jason is more concerned with research than with patients. Like the poems that Vivian deciphers, patients present challenging puzzles for Jason that demand mental agility and little else. For him, a course he took on bedside manner was "a colossal waste of time for researchers" (55). Apparently the curriculum did succeed in at least one respect: comparing the young doctor to the former undergraduate reveals the outcome of a process undergone in authoritarian institutions such as medical school whereby the novice becomes professionalized to the point where he acquires an exclusive, rigidly defined identity. The exclusion formula that is developed in the training period is open to view in the grand rounds scene, where the senior physician and his fellows are less than grand in their insensitive attitude toward both patients and one another, leading Vivian to characterize the event as "full of subservience, hierarchy, gratuitous displays, sublimated rivalries." She concludes, "It is just like a graduate seminar" (37).

On first meeting Dr. Kelekian, the medical oncology chief, Vivian engages him in an awkward exchange as he bluntly informs her of her malignancy. He proceeds to question her, "You are a professor, Miss Bearing." She replies, "Like yourself, Dr. Kelekian." Embarrassed, he quickly recovers, "Well yes. Now then" (7). It is only on discovering that they both have students with similar failings that the distance between them is reduced. Nonetheless, Vivian's personhood is continually eroded in her encounters with various staff members. To the x-ray technician who asks, "Doctor?" she replies, "Yes, I have a Ph.D." Her response produces an irritated "*Your* doctor." Grasping his meaning, she submits, "Oh, Dr. Harvey Kelekian" (16). Vivian's isolation is complete as even her colleagues at the university fail to show any concern for her. Members of her department confine their interest solely to her position and its imminent availability. Vivian predicts that her colleagues will most likely experience a crisis of conscience on her demise to be eased shortly thereafter by the appearance of a collection of essays on John Donne written by them and dedicated to her memory. Their efforts will gain for her the ultimate distinction—published and perished simultaneously!

The use of a specialized vocabulary links English professors to physicians at the same time that it impedes communication. Vivian's lifelong fascination with words and sounds has resulted in her acquiring a sizable vocabulary that includes the precise language of John Donne as well as words of more common usage. Yet she is confused by medical technology that takes a term such as "insidious" to signify "undetectable" while she understands it to mean "treacherous." Conceding that doctors possess a "potent arsenal" of terminology, Vivian finds it essential to learn the new vocabulary as she undergoes the transformation to research subject. Having acquired many skills during her life and having achieved success in applying her knowledge in intellectual pursuits, she suddenly finds herself in a totally new world where her past training is almost of no account in helping her comprehend and cope with her present reality.

In her current crisis Vivian comes to realize that she has failed to forge any meaningful personal relations of a kind that would sustain her. She must learn the value of feelings. The inhabitants of this new, alien community on whom her life depends are strangers. The procedures to which her body is subjected are as new to her as the IV pole to which that body is attached. The language is foreign, the accommodations are unfamiliar, and her wardrobe is limited to a hospital gown. She must invent herself anew, acquire new knowledge and skills in order to gain familiarity with an existence in which her former identity has been anatomized.

One lesson teaches her the value of kindness. In this she is led by her primary nurse, Susie. In contrast to the insensitive clinical fellow, the nurse is kind and protective of her patient. As such she is representative of many caretakers who are thoroughly attuned to the emotional needs of patients.[1] Compassion is also forthcoming from Vivian's former mentor, E. M. Ashford, who appears in a dreamlike sequence to comfort the dying woman. Instead of discussing the poetry of John Donne, the senior scholar reads from a children's book, *The Runaway Bunny,* and teaches her former student the redeeming power of divine love—the tale being an allegory of the soul. The simple tale contrasts with the complex sonnets of Donne, requiring little wit to decipher it. *The Runaway Bunny* demonstrates the power of feelings over intellect in forging significant human relationships, therapeutic or otherwise. Vivian's error has been to define herself in terms of her mental skills. She learns otherwise, as she admits, "I thought being extremely smart would take care of it. But I see that I have been found out" (70). The last lesson from her former professor teaches Vivian the need to regain the innocence and trust she possessed as a child if she would achieve redemption.

Much of the power of the drama derives from the virtually uninterrupted view that the spectators have of the heroine as she reaches to them across the barrier that separates art from life. Beginning with her initial "Hi" to her last coherent moments, Vivian addresses the audience continually. A series of monologues serve, for one, to narrate the past. Without family or friends, the heroine takes the audience into her confidence, repeatedly defining herself in their eyes. Dominating the action, she compels the spectator to focus on her body, a body in decline. In extreme pain she struggles to convey her bodily experience: "I want to tell you how it feels. I want to explain it, to use *my* words" (70). At times Edson creates variations on the use of monologic speech.[2] In the grand rounds scene, monologue and stage action combine in a contrapuntal tour de force as one element is played against the other. Vivian's observations to the audience on the actions of the medical team that probes her prone body underlines the indignities she must bear. In the earlier scene with Dr. Kelekian, which Anton Chekhov could well appreciate, Vivian half listens to the physician discussing her cancer while she pursues her own thoughts aloud. The speeches in both scenes, spoken simultaneously, reveal the difference in attitudes of the speakers and punctuate the theme of the work, with the personal involvement of the heroine opposing the total detachment of the medical staff.

A further innovative use of monologue occurs as past and present converge in one moment of stage time, most notably when the patient disconnects herself from the IV and stands aside as hospital technicians remove her bed and hand her a pointer. Suddenly powerful once again, Vivian delivers a lecture she has given in the past. Her animated presentation, during which she uses the pointer to "whack" the screen on which a sonnet by Donne is projected, provides a glimpse of a woman the spectator never knew. The empathy of the audience is increased as it views at once the heroine's former self together with her consumed form. Edson makes no radical revisions in the traditional passive role of the audience, though she does increase its involvement in the action. Unable to feel the patient's pain, the spectators can share her most private thoughts and can develop an intimacy with her during the moments of performance that make them one with the heroine as her condition deteriorates and her suffering intensifies.

Only in the final moments of her life does Vivian turn away from the audience. In the last view we have of her, she is seen rising from her bed, discarding all the uses of this world, the last of which is her hospital gown, as she moves slowly—alone—toward a light. Her journey is necessarily solitary; redemption is a singular experience. For company she has only those flights of angels to whom the grieving Horatio consigns the soul of Hamlet and to whom Vivian's mentor now gives over the soul of her student.

Notes

1. For further discussion on this matter, see M. J. Friedrich, "Wit: A Play Raises Issues of Emotional Needs of Patients," JAMA 282.17 (Nov. 3, 1999): 1611–12.

2. For a comprehensive discussion of the use of monologue in the postmodern theater, see Deborah R. Geis, *Postmodern Theatric(k)s: Monologue in Contemporary American Drama* (Ann Arbor: Univ. of Michigan Press, 1993).

Works Cited

Edson, Margaret. *W;t*. New York: Faber and Faber, 1999.

Geis, Deborah R. *Postmodern Theatric(k)s: Monologue in Contemporary American Drama*. Ann Arbor: Univ. of Michigan Press, 1993.

Friedrich, M. J. "Wit: A Play Raises Issues of Emotional Needs of Patients." *JAMA* 282.17 (Nov. 3, 1999): 1611–12.

W;t

By Margaret Edson

CHARACTERS

VIVIAN BEARING, PH.D.   *50; professor of seventeenth-century*
                                poetry at the university
HARVEY KELEKIAN, M.D.   *50; chief of medical oncology, University*
                                Hospital
JASON POSNER, M.D.   *28; clinical fellow, Medical Oncology*
                                Branch
SUSIE MONAHAN, R.N., B.S.N.   *28; primary nurse, Cancer Inpatient Unit*
E.M. ASHFORD, D.PHIL.   *80; professor emerita of English literature*
MR. BEARING   *Vivian's father*
LAB TECHNICIANS
CLINICAL FELLOWS
STUDENTS
CODE TEAM

The play may be performed with a cast of nine: the four TECHNICIANS,
FELLOWS, STUDENTS, *and* CODE TEAM MEMBERS *should double;* DR.
KELEKIAN *and* MR. BEARING *should double.*

NOTES

Most of the action, but not all, takes place in a room of the University Hospital
Comprehensive Cancer Center. The stage is empty, and furniture is rolled on
and off by the technicians.

Jason and Kelekian wear lab coats, but each has a different shirt and tie
every time he enters. Susie wears white jeans, white sneakers, and a different
blouse each entrance.

Scenes are indicated by a line rule in the script; there is no break in the
action between scenes, but there might be a change in lighting. There is no
intermission.

Vivian has a central-venous-access catheter over her left breast, so the IV
tubing goes there, not into her arm. The IV pole, with a Port-a-Pump attached,
rolls easily on wheels. Every time the IV pole reappears, it has a different
configuration of bottles.

(VIVIAN BEARING *walks on the empty stage pushing her IV pole. She is fifty, tall and very thin, barefoot, and completely bald. She wears two hospital gowns–one tied in the front and one tied in the back–a baseball cap, and a hospital ID bracelet. The house lights are at half strength.* VIVIAN *looks out at the audience, sizing them up.*)

VIVIAN: (*In false familiarity, waving and nodding to the audience*) Hi. How are you feeling today? Great. That's just great. (*In her own professorial tone*) This is not my standard greeting, I assure you.

I tend toward something a little more formal, a little less inquisitive, such as, say, "Hello."

But it is the standard greeting here.

There is some debate as to the correct response to this salutation. Should one reply "I feel good," using "feel" as a copulative to link the subject, "I," to its subjective complement, "good"; or "I feel well," modifying with an adverb the subject's state of being?

I don't know. I am a professor of seventeenth century poetry, specializing in the Holy Sonnets of John Donne.

So I just say, "Fine."

Of course it is not very often that I do feel fine.

I have been asked "How are you feeling today?" while I was throwing up into a plastic washbasin. I have been asked as I was emerging from a four-hour operation with a tube in every orifice, "How are you feeling today?"

I am waiting for the moment when someone asks me this question and I am dead.

I'm a little sorry I'll miss that.

It is unfortunate that this remarkable line of inquiry has come to me so late in my career. I could have exploited its feigned solicitude to great advantage: as I was distributing the final examination to the graduate course in seventeenth-century textual criticism–"Hi. How are you feeling today?"

Of course I would not be wearing this costume at the time, so the question's *ironic significance* would not be fully apparent.

As I trust it is now.

Irony is a literary device that will necessarily be deployed to great effect.

I ardently wish this were not so. I would prefer that a play about me be cast in the mythic-heroic-pastoral mode; but the facts, most nobly stage-four metastatic ovarian cancer, conspire against that. *The Faerie Queene* this is not.

And I was dismayed to discover that the play would contain elements of . . . *humor.*

I have been, at best, an *unwitting* accomplice. (*She pauses.*) It is not my intention to give away the plot; but I think I die at the end.

They've given me less than two hours.

If I were poetically inclined, I might employ a threadbare metaphor—the sands of time slipping through the hourglass, the two-hour glass.

Now our sands are almost run;
More a little, and then dumb.

Shakespeare. I trust the name is familiar.
At the moment, however, I am disinclined to poetry.
I've got less than two hours. Then: curtain.

(She disconnects herself from the IV pole and shoves it to a crossing TECHNI-CIAN. *The house lights go out.)*

VIVIAN: I'll never forget the time I found out I had cancer.
(DR. HARVEY KELEKIAN *enters at a big desk piled high with papers.*)
KELEKIAN: You have cancer.
VIVIAN: (*To audience*) See? Unforgettable. It was something of a shock. I had to sit down. (*She plops down.*)
KELEKIAN: Please sit down. Miss Bearing, you have advanced metastatic ovarian cancer.
VIVIAN: Go on.
KELEKIAN: You are a professor, Miss Bearing.
VIVIAN: Like yourself, Dr. Kelekian.
KELEKIAN: Well, yes. Now then. You present with a growth that, unfortunately, went undetected in stages one, two, and three. Now it is an insidious adenocarcinoma, which has spread from the primary adnexal mass–
VIVIAN: "Insidious"?
KELEKIAN: "Insidious" means undetectable at an–
VIVIAN: "Insidious" *means* treacherous.
KELEKIAN: Shall I continue?
VIVIAN: By all means.

KELEKIAN: Good. In invasive epithelial carcinoma, the most effective treatment modality is a chemotherapeutic agent. We are developing an experimental combination of drugs designed for primary-site ovarian, with a target specificity of stage three-and-beyond administration.

Am I going too fast?

Good.

You will be hospitalized as an in-patient for treatment each cycle. You will be on complete intake-and-output measurement for three days after each treatment to monitor kidney function. After the initial eight cycles, you will have another battery of tests.

The antineoplastic will inevitably affect some healthy cells, includ-ing those lining the gastrointes-tinal tract from the lips to the anus, and the hair follicles. We will of course be relying on your resolve to withstand some of the more pernicious side effects.

VIVIAN: Insidious. Hmm. Curious word choice. Cancer. Cancel

"By cancer nature's course untrimmed." No–that's not it.

(*To* KELEKIAN) No.

Must read something about cancer.

Must get some books, articles. Assemble a bibliography.

Is anyone doing research on cancer?

Concentrate.

Antineoplastic. Anti: against. Neo: new. Plastic: to mold. Shap-ing. Antineoplastic. Against new shaping.

Hair follicles. My resolve.

"Pernicious" That doesn't seem–

KELEKIAN: Miss Bearing?
VIVIAN: I beg your pardon?
KELEKIAN: Do you have any questions so far?
VIVIAN: Please, go on.
KELEKIAN: Perhaps some of these terms are new. I realize–
VIVIAN: No, no. Ah. You're being very thorough.

KELEKIAN: I make a point of it. And I always emphasize it with my students–

VIVIAN: So do I. "Thoroughness"–I always tell my students, but they are constitutionally averse to painstaking work.

KELEKIAN: Yours, too.

VIVIAN: Oh, it's worse every year.

KELEKIAN: And this is not dermatology, it's medical oncology, for Chrissake.

VIVIAN: My students read through a text once–*once!*–and think it's time for a break.

KELEKIAN: Mine are blind.

VIVIAN: Well, mine are deaf.

KELEKIAN: *(Resigned, but warmly)* You just have to hope . . .

VIVIAN: *(Not so sure)* I suppose.

(Pause)

KELEKIAN: Where were we, Dr. Bearing?

VIVIAN: I believe I was being thoroughly diagnosed.

KELEKIAN: Right. Now. The tumor is spreading very quickly, and this treatment is very aggressive. So far, so good?

VIVIAN: Yes.

KELEKIAN: Better not teach next semester.

VIVIAN: *(Indignant)* Out of the question.

KELEKIAN: The first week of each cycle you'll be hospitalized for chemotherapy; the next week you may feel a little tired; the next two weeks'll be fine, relatively. This cycle will repeat eight times, as I said before.

VIVIAN: Eight months like that?

KELEKIAN: This treatment is the strongest thing we have to offer you. And, as research, it will make a significant contribution to our knowledge.

VIVIAN: Knowledge, yes.

KELEKIAN: *(Giving her a piece of paper)* Here is the informed-consent form. Should you agree, you sign there, at the bottom. Is there a family member you want me to explain this to?

VIVIAN: *(Signing)* That won't be necessary.

KELEKIAN: *(Taking back the paper)* Good. The important thing is for you to take the full dose of chemotherapy. There may be times when you'll wish for a lesser dose, due to the side effects. But we've got to go full-force. The experimental phase has got to have the maximum dose to be of any use. Dr. Bearing–

VIVIAN: Yes?

KELEKIAN: You must be very tough. Do you think you can be very tough?

VIVIAN: You needn't worry.

KELEKIAN: Good. Excellent.

(KELEKIAN *and the desk exit as* VIVIAN *stands and walks forward.*)

VIVIAN: *(Hesitantly)* I should have asked more questions, because I know there's going to be a test.

I have cancer, insidious cancer, with pernicious side effects–no, the *treatment* has pernicious side effects.

I have stage-four metastatic ovarian cancer. There is no stage five. Oh, and I have to be very tough. It appears to be a matter, as the saying goes, of life and death.

I know all about life and death. I am, after all, a scholar of Donne's Holy Sonnets, which explore mortality in greater depth than any other body of work in the English language.

And I know for a fact that I am tough. A demanding professor. Uncompromising. Never one to turn from a challenge. That is why I chose, while a student of the great E. M. Ashford, to study Donne.

(PROFESSOR E.M. ASHFORD, *fifty-two, enters, seated at the same desk as* KELEKIAN *was. The scene is twenty-eight years ago.* VIVIAN *suddenly turns twenty-two, eager and intimidated.*)

VIVIAN: Professor Ashford?

E.M.: Do it again.

VIVIAN: *(To audience)* It was something of a shock. I had to sit down. *(She plops down.)*

E.M.: Please sit down. Your essay on Holy Sonnet Six, Miss Bearing, is a melodrama, with a veneer of scholarship unworthy of you–to say nothing of Donne. Do it again.

VIVIAN: I, ah . . .

E.M.: You must begin with a text, Miss Bearing, not with a feeling.

Death be not proud, though some have called thee
Mighty and dreadfull, for, thou art not soe.

You have entirely missed the point of the poem, because, I must tell you, you have used an edition of the text that is inauthentically punctuated. In the Gardner edition–

VIVIAN: That edition was checked out of the library–

E.M.: Miss Bearing!

VIVIAN: Sorry.

E.M.: You take this too lightly, Miss Bearing. This is Metaphysical Poetry, not The Modern Novel. The standards of scholarship and critical reading which one would apply to any other text are simply insufficient. The effort must be total for the results to be meaningful. Do you think the punctuation of the last line of this sonnet is merely an insignificant detail?

The sonnet begins with a valiant struggle with death, calling on all the forces of intellect and drama to vanquish the enemy. But it is ultimately about overcoming the seemingly insuperable barriers separating life, death, and eternal life.

In the edition you chose, this profoundly simple meaning is sacrificed to hysterical punctuation:

> And Death–*capital D*–shall be no more–*semicolon!*
> Death–*capital D*–comma–thou shalt die–*exclamation point!*

If you go in for this sort of thing, I suggest you take up Shakespeare.

Gardner's edition of the Holy Sonnets returns to the Westmoreland manuscript source of 1610–not for sentimental reasons, I assure you, but because Helen Gardner is a *scholar.* It reads:

> And death shall be no more, *comma,* Death thou shalt die.

(As she recites this line, she makes a little gesture at the comma.)

Nothing but a breath–a comma–separates life from life everlasting. It is very simple really. With the original punctuation restored, death is no longer something to act out on a stage, with exclamation points. It's a comma, a pause.

This way, the *uncompromising* way, one learns something from this poem, wouldn't you say? Life, death. Soul, God. Past, present. Not insuperable barriers, not semicolons, just a comma.

VIVIAN: Life, death . . . I see. *(Standing)* It's a metaphysical conceit. It's wit! I'll go back to the library and rewrite the paper–

E.M.: *(Standing, emphatically)* It is *not wit,* Miss Bearing. It is truth. *(Walking around the desk to her)* The paper's not the point.

VIVIAN: It isn't?

E.M.: *(Tenderly)* Vivian. You're a bright young woman. Use your intelligence. Don't go back to the library. Go out. Enjoy yourself with your friends. Hmm?

(VIVIAN walks away. E.M. slides off.)

VIVIAN: *(As she gradually returns to the hospital)* I, ah, went outside. The sun was very bright. I, ah, walked around, past the . . . There were students on the lawn, talking about nothing, laughing. The insuperable barrier between one thing and another is . . . just a comma? Simple human truth, uncompromising scholarly standards? They're *connected?* I just couldn't . . .

I went back to the library.

Anyway.

All right. Significant contribution to knowledge.

Eight cycles of chemotherapy. Give me the full dose, the full dose every time.

(In a burst of activity, the hospital scene is created.)

VIVIAN: The attention was flattering. For the first five minutes. Now I know how poems feel.

(SUSIE MONAHAN, VIVIAN's primary nurse, gives VIVIAN her chart, then puts her in a wheelchair and takes her to her first appointment: chest x-ray. This and all other diagnostic tests are suggested by light and sound.)

TECHNICIAN 1: Name.

VIVIAN: My name? Vivian Bearing.

TECHNICIAN 1: Huh?

VIVIAN: Bearing. B-E-A-R-I-N-G. Vivian. V-I-V-I-A-N.

TECHNICIAN 1: Doctor.

VIVIAN: Yes, I have a Ph.D.

TECHNICIAN 1: *Your* doctor.

VIVIAN: Oh. Dr. Harvey Kelekian.

(TECHNICIAN 1 positions her so that she is leaning forward and embracing the metal plate, then steps offstage.)

VIVIAN: I am a doctor of philosophy–

TECHNICIAN 1: *(From offstage)* Take a deep breath, and hold it. *(Pause, with light and sound)* Okay.

VIVIAN:–a scholar of seventeenth-century poetry.

TECHNICIAN 1: *(From offstage)* Turn sideways, arms behind your head, and hold it. (Pause) Okay.

VIVIAN: I have made an immeasurable contribution to the discipline of English literature. (TECHNICIAN 1 *returns and puts her in the wheelchair.)* I am, in short, a force.

(TECHNICIAN 1 rolls her to upper GI series, where TECHNICIAN 2 picks up.)

TECHNICIAN 2: Name.

VIVIAN: Lucy, Countess of Bedford.

TECHNICIAN 2: *(Checking a printout)* I don't see it here.

VIVIAN: My name is Vivian Bearing. B-E-A-R-I-N-G. Dr. Kelekian is my doctor.

TECHNICIAN 2: Okay. Lie down. (*TECHNICIAN 2 positions her on a stretcher and leaves. Light and sound suggest the filming.*)

VIVIAN: After an outstanding undergraduate career, I studied with Professor E.M. Ashford for three years, during which time I learned by instruction and example what it means to be a scholar of distinction.

As her research fellow, my principal task was the alphabetizing of index cards for Ashford's monumental critical edition of Donne's *Devotions upon Emergent Occasions.*

(*During the procedure, another* TECHNICIAN *takes the wheelchair away.*)

I am thanked in the preface: "Miss Vivian Bearing for her able assistance."

My dissertation, "Ejaculations in Seventeenth-Century Manuscript and Printed Editions of the Holy Sonnets: A Comparison," was revised for publication in the *Journal of English Texts,* a very prestigious venue for a first appearance.

TECHNICIAN 2: Where's your wheelchair?

VIVIAN: I do not know. I was busy just now.

TECHNICIAN 2: Well, how are you going to get out of here?

VIVIAN: Well, I do not know. Perhaps you would like me to stay.

TECHNICIAN 2: I guess I got to go find you a chair.

VIVIAN: (*Sarcastically*) Don't inconvenience yourself on my behalf. (*TECHNICIAN 2 leaves to get a wheelchair.*)

My second article, a classic explication of Donne's sonnet "Death be not proud," was published in *Critical Discourse.*

The success of the essay prompted the University Press to solicit a volume on the twelve Holy Sonnets in the 1633 edition, which I produced in the remarkably short span of three years. My book, entitled *Made Cunningly,* remains an immense success, in paper as well as cloth.

In it, I devote one chapter to a thorough examination of each sonnet, discussing every word in extensive detail.

(*TECHNICIAN 2 returns with a wheelchair.*)

TECHNICIAN 2: Here.

VIVIAN: I summarize previous critical interpretations of the text and offer my own analysis. It is exhaustive.

(*TECHNICIAN 2 deposits her at CT scan.*)

Bearing. B-E-A-R-I-N-G. Kelekian.

(*TECHNICIAN 3 has* VIVIAN *lie down on a metal stretcher. Light and sound suggest the procedure.*)

TECHNICIAN 3: Here. Hold still.

VIVIAN: For how long?

TECHNICIAN 3: Just a little while. (TECHNICIAN 3 leaves. *Silence*)

VIVIAN: The scholarly study of poetic texts requires a capacity for scrupu-
lously detailed examination, particularly the poetry of John Donne.

The salient characteristic of the poems is wit: "Itchy outbreaks of far-
fetched wit," as Donne himself said.

To the common reader–that is to say, the undergraduate with a B-plus
or better average–wit provides an invaluable exercise for sharpening the
mental faculties, for stimulating the flash of comprehension that can only
follow hours of exacting and seemingly pointless scrutiny.

(TECHNICIAN 3 *puts* VIVIAN *back in the wheelchair and wheels her toward the
unit. Partway,* TECHNICIAN 3 *gives the chair a shove and* SUSIE MONAHAN,
VIVIAN's *primary nurse, takes over.* SUSIE *rolls* VIVIAN *to the exam room.*)

To the scholar, to the mind comprehensively trained in the subtleties
of seventeenth-century vocabulary, versification, and theological, historical, geographical, political, and mythological allusions, Donne's wit is . . .
a way to see how good you really are.

After twenty years, I can say with confidence, no one is quite as good as I.

(*By now,* SUSIE *has helped* VIVIAN *sit on the exam table.* DR. JASON POSNER,
clinical fellow, stands in the doorway.)

JASON: Ah, Susie?

SUSIE: Oh, hi.

JASON: Ready when you are.

SUSIE: Okay. Go ahead. Ms. Bearing, this is Jason Posner. He's going to do
your history, ask you a bunch of questions. He's Dr. Kelekian's fellow.

(SUSIE *is busy in the room, setting up for the exam.*)

JASON: Hi, Professor Bearing. I'm Dr. Posner, clinical fellow in the medical
oncology branch, working with Dr. Kelekian.

Professor Bearing, I, ah, I was an undergraduate at the U. I took your
course in seventeenth-century poetry.

VIVIAN: You did?

JASON: Yes. I thought it was excellent.

VIVIAN: Thank you. Were you an English major?

JASON: No. Biochemistry. But you can't get into medical school unless
you're well-rounded. And I made a bet with myself that I could get an A
in the three hardest courses on campus.

SUSIE: Howdjya do, Jace?

JASON: Success.

VIVIAN: (*Doubtful*) Really?

JASON: A minus. It was a very tough course. (*To* SUSIE) I'll call you.

SUSIE: Okay. *(She leaves.)*

JASON: I'll just pull this over. *(He gets a little stool on wheels.)* Get the prox-emics right here. There. *(Nervously)* Good. Now. I'm going to be taking your history. It's a medical interview, and then I give you an exam.

VIVIAN: I believe Dr. Kelekian has already done that.

JASON: Well, I know, but Dr. Kelekian wants *me* to do it, too. Now. I'll be taking a few notes as we go along.

VIVIAN: Very well.

JASON: Okay. Let's get started. How are you feeling today?

VIVIAN: Fine, thank you.

JASON: Good. How is your general health?

VIVIAN: Fine.

JASON: Excellent. Okay. We know you are an academic.

VIVIAN: Yes, we've established that.

JASON: So we don't need to talk about your interesting work.

VIVIAN: No.

(The following questions and answers go extremely quickly.)

JASON: How old are you?

VIVIAN: Fifty.

JASON: Are you married?

VIVIAN: No.

JASON: Are your parents living?

VIVIAN: No.

JASON: How and when did they die?

VIVIAN: My father, suddenly, when I was twenty, of a heart attack. My mother, slowly, when I was forty-one and forty-two, of cancer. Breast cancer.

JASON: Cancer?

VIVIAN: Breast cancer.

JASON: I see. Any siblings?

VIVIAN: No.

JASON: Do you have any questions so far?

VIVIAN: Not so far.

JASON: Well, that about does it for your life history.

VIVIAN: Yes, that's all there is to my life history.

JASON: Now I'm going to ask you about your past medical history. Have you ever been hospitalized?

VIVIAN: I had my tonsils out when I was eight.

JASON: Have you ever been pregnant?

VIVIAN: No.

JASON: Ever had heart murmurs? High blood pressure?

VIVIAN: No.

JASON: Stomach, liver, kidney problems?

VIVIAN: No.

JASON: Venereal diseases? Uterine infections?

VIVIAN: No.

JASON: Thyroid, diabetes, cancer?

VIVIAN: No–cancer, yes.

JASON: When?

VIVIAN: Now.

JASON: Well, not including now.

VIVIAN: In that case, no.

JASON: Okay. Clinical depression? Nervous breakdowns? Suicide attempts?

VIVIAN: No.

JASON: Do you smoke?

VIVIAN: No.

JASON: Ethanol?

VIVIAN: I'm sorry?

JASON: Alcohol.

VIVIAN: Oh. Ethanol. Yes, I drink wine.

JASON: How much? How often?

VIVIAN: A glass with dinner occasionally. And perhaps a Scotch every now and then.

JASON: Do you use substances?

VIVIAN: Such as.

JASON: Marijuana, cocaine, crack cocaine. PCP, ecstasy, poppers–

VIVIAN: No.

JASON: Do you drink caffeinated beverages?

VIVIAN: Oh, yes!

JASON: Which ones?

VIVIAN: Coffee. A few cups a day.

JASON: How many?

VIVIAN: Two . . . to six. But I really don't think that's immoderate–

JASON: How often do you undergo routine medical checkups?

VIVIAN: Well, not as often as I should, probably, but I've felt fine, I really have.

JASON: So the answer is?

VIVIAN: Every three to . . . five years.

JASON: What do you do for exercise?

VIVIAN: Pace.

JASON: Are you having sexual relations?

VIVIAN: Not at the moment.

JASON: Are you pre- or post-menopausal?

VIVIAN: Pre.

JASON: When was the first day of your last period?

VIVIAN: Ah, ten days–two weeks ago.

JASON: Okay. When did you first notice your present complaint?

VIVIAN: This time, now?

JASON: Yes.

VIVIAN: Oh, about four months ago. I felt a pain in my stomach, in my abdomen, like a cramp, but not the same.

JASON: How did it feel?

VIVIAN: Like a cramp.

JASON: But not the same?

VIVIAN: No, duller, and stronger. I can't describe it.

JASON: What came next?

VIVIAN: Well, I just, I don't know, I started noticing my body, little things. I would be teaching, and feel a sharp pain.

JASON: What kind of pain?

VIVIAN: Sharp, and sudden. Then it would go away. Or I would be tired. Exhausted. I was working on a major project, the article on John Donne for *The Oxford Encyclopedia of English Literature*. It was a great honor. But I had a very strict deadline.

JASON: So you would say you were under stress?

VIVIAN: It wasn't so much more stress than usual, I just couldn't withstand it this time. I don't know.

JASON: So?

VIVIAN: So I went to Dr. Chin, my gynecologist, after I had turned in the article, and explained all this. She examined me, and sent me to Jefferson the internist, and he sent me to Kelekian because he thought I might have a tumor.

JASON: And that's it?

VIVIAN: Till now.

JASON: Hmmm. Well, that's very interesting.

(Nervous pause)

Well, I guess I'll start the examination. It'll only take a few minutes. Why don't you, um, sort of lie back, and–oh–relax.

(He helps her lie back on the table, raises the stirrups out of the table, raises her legs and puts them in the stirrups, and puts a paper sheet over her.)

Be very relaxed. This won't hurt. Let me get this sheet. Okay. Just stay calm. Okay. Put your feet in these stirrups. Okay. Just. There. Okay? Now.

Oh, I have to go get Susie. Got to have a girl here. Some crazy clinical
rule. Um. I'll be right back. Don't move.

(JASON *leaves. Long pause. He is seen walking quickly back and forth in the
hall, and calling* SUSIE's *name as he goes by.*)

VIVIAN: *(To herself)* I wish I had given him an A. *(Silence)*

Two times one is two.
Two times two is four.
Two times three is six.
Um.
Oh.

> Death be not proud, though some have called thee
> Mighty and dreadfull, for, thou art not soe,
> For, those, whom thou think'st, thou dost overthrow,
> Die not, poore death, nor yet canst thou kill mee . . .

JASON: *(In the hallway)* Has anybody seen Susie?

VIVIAN: *(Losing her place for a second)* Ah.

> Thou' art slave to Fate, chance, kings, and desperate men,
> And dost with poyson, warre, and sicknesse dwell,
> And poppie,' or charmes can make us sleepe as well,
> And better than thy stroake; why swell'st thou then?

JASON: *(In the hallway)* She was here just a minute ago.

VIVIAN:

> One short sleepe past, wee wake eternally,
> And death shall be no more–*comma*–Death thou shalt die.

(JASON *and* SUSIE *return.*)

JASON: Okay. Here's everything. Okay.

SUSIE: What is this? Why did you leave her–

JASON: *(To* SUSIE) I had to find you. Now, come on. *(To* VIVIAN) We're
ready, Professor Bearing. *(To himself, as he puts on exam gloves)* Get these
on. Okay. Just lift this up. Ooh. Okay. *(As much to himself as to her)* Just
relax. *(He begins the pelvic exam, with one hand on her abdomen and the
other inside her, looking blankly at the ceiling as he feels around.)* Okay.
(Silence) Susie, isn't that interesting, that I had Professor Bearing.

SUSIE: Yeah. I wish I had taken some literature. I don't know anything about poetry.

JASON: *(Trying to be casual)* Professor Bearing was very highly regarded on campus. It looked very good on my transcript that I had taken her course. *(Silence)* They even asked me about it in my interview for med school–*(He feels the mass and does a double take.)* Jesus! *(Tense silence. He is amazed and fascinated.)*

SUSIE: What?

VIVIAN: What?

JASON: Um. *(He tries for composure.)* Yeah. I survived Bearing's course. No problem. Heh. *(Silence)* Yeah, John Donne, those metaphysical poets, that metaphysical wit. Hardest poetry in the English department. Like to see *them* try biochemistry. *(Silence)* Okay. We're about done. Okay. That's it. Okay, Professor Bearing. Let's take your feet out, there. *(He takes off his gloves and throws them away.)* Okay. I gotta go. I gotta go.

*(*JASON *quickly leaves.* VIVIAN *slowly gets up from this scene and walks stiffly away.*

SUSIE *cleans up the exam room and exits.)*

VIVIAN: *(Walking downstage to audience)* That . . . was . . . hard. That . . . was . . .

One thing can be said for an eight-month course of cancer treatment: it is highly educational. I am learning to suffer.

Yes, it is mildly uncomfortable to have an electrocardiogram, but the . . . agony . . . of a proctosigmoidoscopy sweeps it from memory. Yes, it was embarrassing to have to wear a nightgown all day long—two nightgowns!—but that seemed like a positive privilege compared to watching myself go bald. Yes, having a former student give me a pelvic exam was thoroughly *degrading*—and I use the term deliberately—but I could not have imagined the depths of humiliation that——

Oh, God—*(*VIVIAN *runs across the stage to her hospital room, dives onto the bed, and throws up into a large plastic washbasin.)* Oh, God. Oh. Oh. *(She lies slumped on the bed, fastened to the IV, which now includes a small bottle with a bright orange label.)* Oh, God. It can't be. *(Silence)* Oh, God. Please. Steady. Steady. (Silence) Oh—Oh, no! *(She throws up again, moans, and retches in agony.)* Oh, God. What's left? I haven't eaten in two days. What's left to puke?

You may remark that my vocabulary has taken a turn for the Anglo-Saxon.

God, I'm going to barf my brains out.

(She begins to relax.) If I actually did barf my brains out, it would be a great loss to my discipline. Of course, not a few of my colleagues would be relieved. To say nothing of my students.

It's not that I'm controversial. Just uncompromising. Ooh–*(She lunges for the basin. Nothing)* Oh. *(Silence)* False alarm. If the word went round that Vivian Bearing had barfed her brains out . . .

Well, first my colleagues, most of whom are my former students, would scramble madly for my position. Then their consciences would flare up, so to honor *my* memory they would put together a collection of *their* essays about John Donne. The volume would begin with a warm introduction, capturing my most endearing qualities. It would be short. But sweet.

Published *and* perished.

Now, watch this. I have to ring the bell *(She presses the button on the bed)* to get someone to come and measure this emesis, and record the amount on a chart of my intake and output. This counts as output.

*(*Susie *enters.)*

Susie: *(Brightly)* How you doing, Ms. Bearing? You having some nausea?

Vivian: *(Weakly)* Uhh, yes.

Susie: Why don't I take that? Here.

Vivian: It's about 300 cc's.

Susie: That all?

Vivian: It was very hard work.

*(*Susie *takes the basin to the bathroom and rinses it.)*

Susie: Yup. Three hundred. Good guess. *(She marks the graph.)* Okay. Anything else I can get for you? Some Jell-O or anything?

Vivian: Thank you, no.

Susie: You okay all by yourself here?

Vivian: Yes.

Susie: You're not having a lot of visitors, are you?

Vivian: *(Correcting)* None, to be precise.

Susie: Yeah, I didn't think so. Is there somebody you want me to call for you?

Vivian: That won't be necessary.

Susie: Well, I'll just pop my head in every once in a while to see how you're coming along. Kelekian and the fellows should be in soon. *(She touches* Vivian's *arm.)* If there's anything you need, you just ring.

Vivian: *(Uncomfortable with kindness)* Thank you.

Susie: Okay. Just call. *(Susie disconnects the IV bottle with the orange label and takes it with her as she leaves.* Vivian *lies still. Silence)*

VIVIAN: In this dramatic structure you will see the most interesting aspects of my tenure as an in-patient receiving experimental chemotherapy for advanced metastatic ovarian cancer.

But as I am a *scholar* before . . . an impresario, I feel obliged to document what it is like here most of the time, between the dramatic climaxes. Between the spectacles.

In truth, it is like this:

(*She ceremoniously lies back and stares at the ceiling.*)

You cannot imagine how time . . . can be . . . so still.

It hangs. It weighs. And yet there is so little of it.

It goes so slowly, and yet it is so scarce.

If I were writing this scene, it would last a full fifteen minutes. I would lie here, and you would sit there.

(*She looks at the audience, daring them.*)

Not to worry. Brevity is the soul of wit.

But if you think eight months of cancer treatment is tedious for the *audience,* consider how it feels to play my part.

All right. All right. It is Friday morning: Grand Rounds. (*Loudly, giving a cue*) Action.

(KELEKIAN *enters, followed by* JASON *and four other* FELLOWS.)

KELEKIAN: Dr. Bearing.

VIVIAN: Dr. Kelekian.

KELEKIAN: Jason.

(JASON *moves to the front of the group.*)

JASON: Professor Bearing. How are you feeling today?

VIVIAN: Fine.

JASON: That's great. That's just great. (*He takes a sheet and carefully covers her legs and groin, then pulls up her gown to reveal her entire abdomen. He is barely audible, but his gestures are clear.*

VIVIAN: "Grand Rounds." The term is theirs. Not "Grand" in the traditional sense of sweeping or magnificent. Not "Rounds" as in a musical canon, or a *round* of applause (though either would be refreshing at this point). Here, "Rounds" seems to signify darting *around* the main issue . . . which I suppose would be the struggle for life . . . *my*

JASON: Very late detection. Staged as a four upon admission. Hexamethophosphacil with Vinplatin to potentiate. Hex at 300 mg. per meter squared, Vin at 100. Today is cycle two, day three. Both cycles at the *full dose.* (The FELLOWS *are impressed.*)

The primary site is–here (*He puts his finger on the spot on her*

life . . . with heated discussions of side effects, other complaints, additional treatments.

Grand Rounds is not Grand Opera. But compared to lying here, it is positively *dramatic.*

Full of subservience, hierarchy, gratuitous displays, sublimated rivalries–I feel right at home. It is just like a graduate seminar.

With one important difference: in Grand Rounds, *they* read *me* like a book. Once I did the teaching, now I am taught.

This is much easier. I just hold still and look cancerous. It requires less acting every time.

Excellent command of details.

abdomen), behind the left ovary. Metastases are suspected in the periotoneal cavity–here. And– here. *(He touches those spots.)*

Full lymphatic involvement. *(He moves his hands over her entire body.)*

At the time of first-look surgery, a significant part of the tumor was de-bulked, mostly in this area–here. *(He points to each organ, poking her abdomen.)* Left, right ovaries. Fallopian tubes. Uterus. All out.

Evidence of primary-site shrinkage. Shrinking in metastatic tumors has not been documented. Primary mass frankly palpable in pelvic exam, frankly, all through here–here. *(Some* FELLOWS *reach and press where he is pointing.)*

KELEKIAN: Excellent command of details.

VIVIAN: *(To herself)* I taught him, you know–

KELEKIAN: Okay. Problem areas with Hex and Vin. *(He addresses all the* FELLOWS, *but* JASON *answers first and they resent him.)*

FELLOW 1: Myelosu–

JASON: *(Interrupting)* Well, first of course is myelosuppression, a lowering of blood-cell counts. It goes without saying. With this combination of agents, nephrotoxicity will be next.

KELEKIAN: Go on.

JASON: The kidneys are designed to filter out impurities in the bloodstream. In trying to filter the chemotherapeutic agent out of the bloodstream, the kidneys shut down.

KELEKIAN: Intervention.

JASON: Hydration.

KELEKIAN: Monitoring

JASON: Full recording of fluid intake and output, as you see here on these graphs, to monitor hydration and kidney function. Totals monitored daily by the clinical fellow, as per the protocol.

KELEKIAN: Anybody else. Side effects.

FELLOW 1: Nausea and vomiting.

KELEKIAN: Jason.

JASON: Routine.

FELLOW 2: Pain while urinating.

JASON: Routine. (*The* FELLOWS *are trying to catch* JASON.)

FELLOW 3: Psychological depression.

JASON: No way.

(*The* FELLOWS *are silent.*)

KELEKIAN: (*Standing by* VIVIAN *at the head of the bed*) Anything else. Other complaints with Hexamethophosphacil and Vinplatin. Come on. (*Silence.* KELEKIAN *and* VIVIAN *wait together for the correct answer.*)

FELLOW 4: Mouth sores.

JASON: Not yet.

FELLOW 2: (*Timidly*) Skin rash?

JASON: Nope.

KELEKIAN: (*Sharing this with* VIVIAN) Why do we waste our time, Dr. Bearing?

VIVIAN: (*Delighted*) I do not know, Dr. Kelekian.

KELEKIAN: (*To the* FELLOWS) Use your eyes. (*All* FELLOWS *look closely at* VIVIAN.) Jesus God. Hair loss.

FELLOWS (*All protesting.* VIVIAN *and* KELEKIAN *are amused.*)

–Come on.

–You can see it.

–It doesn't count.

–No fair.

KELEKIAN: Jason.

JASON: (*Begrudgingly*) Hair loss after first cycle of treatment.

KELEKIAN: That's better. (*To* VIVIAN) Dr. Bearing. Full dose. Excellent. Keep pushing the fluids.

(*The* FELLOWS *leave.* KELEKIAN *stops* JASON.)

KELEKIAN: Jason.

JASON: Huh?

KELEKIAN: Clinical.

JASON: Oh, right. (*To* VIVIAN) Thank you, Professor Bearing. You've been very cooperative. (*They leave her with her stomach uncovered.*)

VIVIAN: Wasn't that . . . Grand? *(She gets up without the IV pole.)* At times, this obsessively detailed examination, this *scrutiny* seems to me to be a nefarious business. On the other hand, what is the alternative? Ignorance? Ignorance may be . . . bliss; but it is not a very noble goal.

So I play my part.

(Pause)

I receive chemotherapy, throw up, am subjected to countless indignities, feel better, go home. Eight cycles. Eight neat little strophes. Oh, there have been the usual variations, subplots, red herrings: hepatotoxicity (liver poison), neuropathy (nerve death).

(Righteously) They are medical terms. I look them up.

It has always been my custom to treat words with respect.

I can recall the time–the very hour of the very day–when I knew words would be my life's work.

(A pile of six little white books appears, with MR. BEARING, VIVIAN's *father, seated behind an open newspaper.)*

It was my fifth birthday.

*(*VIVIAN, *now a child, flops down to the books.)*

I liked that one best.

MR. BEARING: *(Disinterested but tolerant, never distracted from his newspaper)* Read another.

VIVIAN: I think I'll read . . . *(She takes a book from the stack and reads its spine intently)* The Tale of the Flopsy Bunnies. *(Reading the front cover)* The Tale of the Flopsy Bunnies. It has little bunnies on the front.

(Opening to the title page) The Tale of the Flopsy Bunnies *by Beatrix Potter.*
(She turns the page and begins to read.)

It is said that the effect of eating too much lettuce is spoor-sop-or–what is that word?

MR. BEARING: Sound it out.

VIVIAN: Sop-or-fic. Sop-or-i-fic. Soporific. What does that mean?

MR. BEARING: Soporific. Causing sleep.

VIVIAN: Causing sleep.

MR. BEARING: Makes you sleepy.

VIVIAN: "Soporific" means "makes you sleepy"?

MR. BEARING: Correct.

VIVIAN: "Soporific" means "makes you sleepy." Soporific.

MR. BEARING: Now use it in a sentence. What has a soporific effect on *you?*

VIVIAN: A soporific effect on me.

MR. BEARING: What makes you sleepy?

VIVIAN: Aahh–nothing.

MR. BEARING: Correct.

VIVIAN: What about you?

MR. BEARING: What has a soporific effect on me? Let me think: boring conversation, I suppose, after dinner.

VIVIAN: Me too, boring conversation.

MR. BEARING: Carry on.

VIVIAN: It is said that the effect of eating too much lettuce is soporific.

The little bunnies in the picture are asleep! They're sleeping! Like you said, because of *soporific!*

(She stands up, and MR. BEARING *exits.)*

The illustration bore out the meaning of the word, just as he had explained it. At the time, it seemed like magic.

So imagine the effect that the words of John Donne first had on me: ratiocination, concatenation, coruscation, tergiversation.

Medical terms are less evocative. Still, I want to know what the doctors mean when they . . . anatomize me. And I will grant that in this particular field of endeavor they possess a more potent arsenal of terminology than I. My only defense is the acquisition of vocabulary.

---

*(*SUSIE *enters and puts her arm around* VIVIAN's *shoulders to hold her up.* VIVIAN *is shaking, feverish, and weak.)*

VIVIAN: *(All at once)* Fever and neutropenia.

SUSIE: When did it start?

VIVIAN: *(Having difficulty speaking)* I–I was at home–reading–and I–felt so bad. I called. Fever and neutropenia. They said to come in.

SUSIE: You did the right thing to come. Did somebody drive you?

VIVIAN: Cab. I took a taxi.

SUSIE: *(She grabs a wheelchair and helps* VIVIAN *sit. As* SUSIE *speaks, she takes* VIVIAN's *temperature, pulse, and respiration rate.)* Here, why don't you sit? Just sit there a minute. I'll get Jason. He's on call tonight. We'll get him to give you some meds. I'm glad I was here on nights. I'll make sure you get to bed soon, okay? It'll just be a minute. I'll get you some juice, some nice juice with lots of ice.

*(*SUSIE *leaves quickly.* VIVIAN *sits there, agitated, confused, and very sick.* SUSIE *returns with the juice.)*

VIVIAN: Lights. I left all the lights on at my house.

SUSIE: Don't you worry. It'll be all right.

(JASON *enters, roused from his sleep and not fully awake. He wears surgical scrubs and puts on a lab coat as he enters.*)

JASON: *(Without looking at* VIVIAN*)* How are you feeling, Professor Bearing?

VIVIAN: My teeth—are chattering.

JASON: Vitals.

SUSIE: *(Giving* VIVIAN *juice and a straw, without looking at* JASON*)* Temp 39.4. Pulse 120. Respiration 36. Chills and sweating.

JASON: Fever and neutropenia. It's a "shake and bake." Blood cultures and urine, stat. Admit her. Prepare for reverse isolation. Start with acetaminophen. Vitals every four hours. *(He starts to leave.)*

SUSIE: *(Following him)* Jason—I think you need to talk to Kelekian about lowering the dose for the next cycle. It's too much for her like this.

JASON: Lower the dose? No way. Full dose. She's tough. She can take it. Wake me up when the counts come from the lab.

(He pads off. SUSIE *wheels* VIVIAN *to her room.* VIVIAN *collapses on the bed.* SUSIE *connects* VIVIAN'S *IV, then wets a washcloth and rubs her face and neck.* VIVIAN *remains delirious.* SUSIE *checks the IV and leaves with the wheelchair.*

After a while, KELEKIAN *appears in the doorway holding a surgical mask near his face.* JASON *is with him, now dressed and clean-shaven.)*

KELEKIAN: Good morning, Dr. Bearing. Fifth cycle. Full dose. Definite progress. Everything okay.

VIVIAN: *(Weakly)* Yes.

KELEKIAN: You're doing swell. Isolation is no problem. Couple of days. Think of it as a vacation.

VIVIAN: Oh.

(JASON starts to enter, holding a mask near his face, just like KELEKIAN*.)*

KELEKIAN: Jason

JASON: Oh, Jesus. Okay, okay.

(He returns to the doorway, where he puts on a paper gown, mask, and gloves. KELEKIAN *leaves.)*

VIVIAN: *(To audience)* In isolation, I am isolated. For once I can use a term literally. The chemotherapeutic agents eradicating my cancer have also eradicated my immune system. In my present condition, every living thing is a health hazard to me . . .

(JASON comes in to check the intake-and-output.)

JASON: *(Complaining to himself)* I really have not got time for this . . .

VIVIAN: . . . particularly health-care professionals.

JASON: *(Going right to the graph on the wall)* Just to look at the I&O sheets for one minute, and it takes me half an hour to do precautions. Four,

seven, eleven. Two-fifty twice. Okay. *(Remembering)* Oh, Jeez. Clinical.
Professor Bearing. How are you feeling today?

VIVIAN: *(Very sick)* Fine. Just shaking sometimes from the chills.

JASON: IV will kick in anytime now. No problem. Listen, gotta go. Keep
pushing the fluids.

(As he exits, he takes off the gown, mask, and gloves.)

VIVIAN: *(Getting up from bed with her IV pole and resuming her explanation)* I am not in isolation because I have cancer, because I have a tumor
the size of a grapefruit. No. I am in isolation because I am being treated
for cancer. My treatment imperils my health.

Herein lies the paradox. John Donne would revel in it. I would revel in
it, if he wrote a poem about it. My students would flounder in it, because
paradox is too difficult to understand. Think of it as a puzzle, I would tell
them, an intellectual game.

(She is trapped.) Or, I *would have* told them. Were it a game. Which it is not.

(Escaping) If they were here, if I were lecturing: How I would *perplex* them!
I could work my students into a frenzy. Every ambiguity, every shifting
awareness. I could draw so much from the poems.

I could be so powerful.

———————————

*(VIVIAN stands still, as if conjuring a scene. Now at the height of her powers,
she grandly disconnects herself from the IV. TECHNICIANS remove the bed
and hand her a pointer.)*

VIVIAN: The poetry of the early seventeenth century, what has been called
the metaphysical school, considers an intractable mental puzzle by exer-
cising the outstanding human faculty of the era, namely wit.

The greatest wit–the greatest English poet, some would say–was John
Donne. In the Holy Sonnets, Donne applied his capacious, agile wit to
the larger aspects of the human experience: life, death, and God.

In his poems, metaphysical quandaries are addressed, but never
resolved. Ingenuity, virtuosity, and a vigorous intellect that jousts with
the most exalted concepts: these are the tools of wit.

*(The lights dim. A screen lowers, and the sonnet "If poysonous mineralls,
"from the Gardner edition, appears on it. VIVIAN recites.)*

> If poysonous mineralls, and if that tree,
> Whose fruit threw death on else immortall us,
> If lecherous goats, if serpents envious
> Cannot be damn'd; Alas; why should I bee?

Why should intent or reason, borne in mee,
Make sinnes, else equall, in mee, more heinous?
And mercy being easie, 'and glorious
To God, in his sterne wrath, why threatens hee?
But who am I, that dare dispute with thee?
O God, Oh! of thine onely worthy blood,
And my teares, make a heavenly Lethean flood,
And drowne in it my sinnes blacke memorie.
That thou remember them, some claime as debt,
I thinke it mercy, if thou wilt forget.

(VIVIAN *occasionally whacks the screen with a pointer for emphasis. She moves around as she lectures.*)

Aggressive intellect. Pious melodrama. And a final, fearful point. Donne's Holy Sonnet Five, 1609. From the Ashford edition, based on Gardner.

The speaker of the sonnet has a brilliant mind, and he plays the part convincingly; but in the end he finds God's *forgiveness* hard to believe, so he crawls under a rock to *hide.*

If arsenic and serpents are not damned, then why is he? In asking the question, the speaker turns eternal damnation into an intellectual game. Why would God choose to do what is hard, to condemn, rather than what is easy, and also glorious–to show mercy?

(Several scholars have disputed Ashford's third comma in line six, but none convincingly.)

But. Exception. Limitation. Contrast. The argument shifts from cleverness to melodrama, an unconvincing eruption of piety: "O" "God" "Oh!"

A typical prayer would plead "Remember me, O Lord." (This point is nicely explicated in an article by Richard Strier–a former student of mine who once sat where you do now, although I dare say he was awake–in the May 1989 issue of *Modern Philology.*) True believers ask to be *remembered* by God. The speaker of this sonnet asks God to forget. (VIVIAN *moves in front of the screen, and the projection of the poem is cast directly upon her.*) Where is the hyperactive intellect of the first section? Where is the histrionic outpouring of the second? When the speaker considers his own *sins,* and the inevitability of God's *judgment,* he can conceive of but one resolution: to *disappear.* (VIVIAN *moves away from the screen.*) Doctrine assures us that no sinner is denied *forgiveness,* not even one whose sins are overweening *intellect* or overwrought *dramatics.* The speaker does not need to *hide* from God's *judgment,* only to accept God's *forgiveness.* It is very simple. Suspiciously simple.

We want to correct the speaker, to remind him of the assurance of salvation. But it is too late. The poetic encounter is over. We are left to our own consciences. Have we outwitted Donne? Or have we been outwitted?

(SUSIE *comes on.*)

SUSIE: Ms. Bearing?

VIVIAN: *(Continuing)* Will the po–

SUSIE: Ms. Bearing?

VIVIAN: *(Crossly)* What is it?

SUSIE: You have to go down for a test. Jason just called. They want another ultrasound. They're concerned about a bowel obstruction–Is it okay if I come in?

VIVIAN: No. Not now.

SUSIE: I'm sorry, but they want it now.

VIVIAN: Not right now. It's not *supposed* to be now.

SUSIE: Yes, they want to do it now. I've got the chair.

VIVIAN: It should not be now. I am in the middle of–this. I have this planned for now, not ultrasound. No more tests. We've covered that.

SUSIE: I know, I know, but they need for it to be now. It won't take long, and it isn't a bad procedure. Why don't you just come along.

VIVIAN: *I do not want to go now!*

SUSIE: Ms. Bearing.

(Silence. VIVIAN *raises the screen, walks away from the scene, hooks herself to the IV, and gets in the wheelchair* SUSIE *wheels* VIVIAN, *and a* TECH- NICIAN *takes her.*)

TECHNICIAN: Name.

VIVIAN: B-E-A-R-I-N-G. Kelekian.

TECHNICIAN: It'll just be a minute.

VIVIAN: Time for your break.

TECHNICIAN: Yup.

(*The* TECHNICIAN *leaves.*)

VIVIAN: *(Mordantly)* Take a break!

(VIVIAN *sits weakly in the wheelchair*)

VIVIAN:

> This is my playes last scene, here heavens appoint
> My pilgrimages last mile; and my race
> Idly, yet quickly runne, hath this last pace,

My spans last inch, my minutes last point,
And gluttonous death will instantly unjoynt
My body, 'and soule.

John Donne. 1609.

I have always particularly liked that poem. In the abstract. Now I find the image of "my minute's last point" a little too, shall we say, *pointed.*

I don't mean to complain, but I am becoming very sick. Very, very sick. Ultimately sick, as it were.

In everything I have done, I have been steadfast, resolute–some would say in the extreme. Now, as you can see, I am distinguishing myself in illness.

I have survived eight treatments of Hexamethophosphacil and Vin-platin at the *full* dose, ladies and gentlemen. I have broken the record. I have become something of a celebrity. Kelekian and Jason are simply delighted. I think they foresee celebrity status for themselves upon the appearance of the journal article they will no doubt write about me. But I flatter myself. The article will not be about *me*, it will be about my ovaries. It will be about my peritoneal cavity, which, despite their best intentions, is now crawling with cancer. What we have come to think of as *me* is, in fact, just the specimen jar, just the dust jacket, just the white piece of paper that bears the little black marks.

My next line is supposed to be something like this: "It is such a *relief* to get back to my room after those infernal tests."

This is hardly true.

It would be a *relief* to be a cheerleader on her way to Daytona Beach for Spring Break.

To get back to my room after those infernal tests is just the next thing that happens.

(She returns to her bed, which now has a commode next to it. She is very sick.)
  Oh, God. It is such a relief to get back to my goddamn room after those
  goddamn tests.
(JASON enters.)
JASON: Professor Bearing. Just want to check the I&O. Four-fifty, six, five.
  Okay. How are you feeling today? *(He makes notations on his clipboard
  throughout the scene.)*
VIVIAN: Fine.
JASON: That's great. Just great.
VIVIAN: How are my fluids?

JASON: Pretty good. No kidney involvement yet. That's pretty amazing, with Hex and Vin.

VIVIAN: How will you know when the kidneys are involved?

JASON: Lots of in, not much out.

VIVIAN: That simple.

JASON: Oh, no way. Compromised kidney function is a highly complex reaction. I'm simplifying for you.

VIVIAN: Thank you.

JASON: We're supposed to.

VIVIAN: Bedside manner.

JASON: Yeah, there's a whole course on it in med school. It's required. Colossal waste of time for researchers. *(He turns to go.)*

VIVIAN: I can imagine. *(Trying to ask something important)* Jason?

JASON: Huh?

VIVIAN: *(Not sure of herself)* Ah, what . . . *(Quickly)* What were you just saying?

JASON: When?

VIVIAN: Never mind.

JASON: Professor Bearing?

VIVIAN: Yes.

JASON: Are you experiencing confusion? Short-term memory loss?

VIVIAN: No.

JASON: Sure?

VIVIAN: Yes. *(Pause)* I was just wondering: why cancer?

JASON: Why cancer?

VIVIAN: Why not open-heart surgery?

JASON: Oh yeah, why not *plumbing.* Why not run a *lube rack,* for all the surgeons know about *Homo sapiens sapiens.* No way. Cancer's the only thing I ever wanted.

VIVIAN: *(Intrigued)* Huh.

JASON: No, really. Cancer is . . . *(Searching)*

VIVIAN: *(Helping)* Awesome.

JASON: *(Pause)* Yeah. Yeah, that's right. It is. It is awesome. How does it do it? The intercellular regulatory mechanisms–especially for proliferation and differentiation–the malignant neoplasia just don't get it. You grow normal cells in tissue culture in the lab, and they replicate just enough to make a nice, confluent monolayer. They divide twenty times, or fifty times, but eventually they conk out. You grow cancer cells, and they never stop. No contact inhibition whatsoever. They just pile up, just keep replicating forever. *(Pause)* That's got a funny name. Know what it is?

VIVIAN: No. What?

JASON: Immortality in culture.

VIVIAN: Sounds like a symposium.

JASON: It's an error in judgment, in a molecular way. But *why?* Even on the protistic level the normal cell–cell interactions are so subtle they'll take your breath away. Golden-brown algae, for instance, the lowest multi-cellular life form on earth–they're *idiots*–and it's incredible. It's perfect. So what's up with the cancer cells? Smartest guys in the world, with the best labs, funding–they don't know what to make of it.

VIVIAN: What about you?

JASON: Me? Oh, I've got a couple of ideas, things I'm kicking around. Wait till I get a lab of my own. If I can survive this . . . *fellowship.*

VIVIAN: The part with the human beings.

JASON: Everybody's got to go through it. All the great researchers. They want us to be able to converse intelligently with the clinicians. As though *researchers* were the impediments. The clinicians are such troglodytes. So smarmy. Like we have to hold hands to discuss creatinine clearance. Just cut the crap, I say.

VIVIAN: Are you going to be sorry when I–Do you ever miss people?

JASON: Everybody asks that. Especially girls.

VIVIAN: What do you tell them?

JASON: I tell them yes.

VIVIAN: Are they persuaded?

JASON: Some.

VIVIAN: Some. I see. *(With great difficulty)* And what do you say when a patient is . . . apprehensive . . . frightened.

JASON: Of who?

VIVIAN: I just . . . Never mind.

JASON: Professor Bearing, who is the President of the United States?

VIVIAN: I'm fine, really. It's all right.

JASON: You sure? I could order a test–

VIVIAN: No! No, I'm fine. Just a little tired.

JASON: Okay. Look. Gotta go. Keep pushing the fluids. Try for 2,000 a day, okay?

VIVIAN: Okay. To use your word. Okay.

(JASON leaves.)

VIVIAN: *(Getting out of bed, without her IV)* So. The young doctor, like the senior scholar, prefers research to humanity. At the same time the senior scholar, in her pathetic state as a simpering victim, wishes the young doctor would take more interest in personal contact. Now I suppose we shall see, through a series of flashbacks, how the senior scholar ruthlessly denied her simpering students the touch of human kindness she now seeks.

――――――――――

(STUDENTS *appear, sitting at chairs with writing desks attached to the right arm.*)

VIVIAN: *(Commanding attention)* How then would you characterize *(pointing to a student)*–you.

STUDENT 1: Huh?

VIVIAN: How would you characterize the animating force of this sonnet?

STUDENT 1: Huh?

VIVIAN: In this sonnet, what is the principal poetic device? I'll give you a hint. It has nothing to do with football. What propels this sonnet?

STUDENT 1: Um.

VIVIAN: *(Speaking to the audience)* Did I say *(tenderly)* "You are nineteen years old. You are so young. You don't know a sonnet from a steak sandwich." *(Pause)* By no means.

(Sharply, to STUDENT 1*)* You can come to this class prepared, or you can excuse yourself from this class, this department, and this university. Do not think for a moment that I will tolerate anything in between.

(To the audience, defensively) I was teaching him a lesson. *(She walks away from* STUDENT 1, *then turns and addresses the class.)*

So we have another instance of John Donne's agile wit at work: not so much *resolving* the issues of life and God as *reveling* in their complexity.

STUDENT 2: But why?

VIVIAN: Why what?

STUDENT 2: Why does Donne make everything so *complicated?* *(The other* STUDENTS *laugh in agreement.)* No, really, *why?*

VIVIAN: *(To the audience)* You know, someone asked me that every year. And it was always one of the smart ones. What could I say? *(To* STUDENT 2) What do you think?

STUDENT 2: I think it's like he's hiding. I think he's really confused, I don't know, maybe he's scared, so he hides behind all this complicated stuff, hides behind this *wit.*

VIVIAN: *Hides* behind *wit?*

STUDENT 2: I mean, if it's really something he's sure of, he can say it more simple–simply. He doesn't have to be such a brain, or such a performer. It doesn't have to be such a big deal.

(The other STUDENTS *encourage him.)*

VIVIAN: Perhaps he is suspicious of simplicity.

STUDENT 2: Perhaps, but that's pretty stupid.

VIVIAN: *(To the audience)* That observation, despite its infelicitous phrasing, contained the seed of a perspicacious remark. Such an unlikely occurrence left me with two choices. I could draw it out, or I could allow the brain to rest after that heroic effort. If I pursued, there was the chance of great insight, or the risk of undergraduate banality. I could never predict. *(To* STUDENT 2*)* Go on.

STUDENT 2: Well, if he's trying to figure out God, and the meaning of life, and big stuff like that, why does he keep running away, you know?

VIVIAN: *(To the audience, moving closer to* STUDENT 2*)* So far so good, but they can think for themselves only so long before they begin to self-destruct.

STUDENT 2: Um, it's like, the more you hide, the less–no, wait–the more you are getting closer–although you don't know it–and the simple thing is there–you see what I mean?

VIVIAN: *(To the audience, looking at* STUDENT 2, *as suspense collapses)* Lost it.
   (She walks away and speaks to the audience.) I distinctly remember an exchange between two students after my lecture on pronunciation and scansion. I overheard them talking on their way out of class. They were young and bright, gathering their books and laughing at the expense of seventeenth-century poetry, at *my* expense.
   (To the class) To scan the line properly, we must take advantage of the contemporary flexibility in "i-o-n" endings, as in "expansion." The quatrain stands:

> Our two souls therefore, which are one,
> Though I must go, endure not yet
> A breach, but an ex-*pan*-see-on,
> Like gold to airy thinness beat.

Bear this in mind in your reading. That's all for today.

(The STUDENTS *get up in a chaotic burst.* STUDENT 3 *and* STUDENT 4 *pass by* VIVIAN *on their way out.)*

STUDENT 3: I hope I can get used to this pronuncia-see-on.

STUDENT 4: I know. I hope I can survive this course and make it to graduasee-on.

(They laugh. VIVIAN *glowers at them. They fall silent, embarrassed.)*

VIVIAN: *(To the audience)* That was a witty little exchange, I must admit. It showed the mental acuity I would praise in a poetic text. But I admired only the studied application of wit, not its spontaneous eruption.

(STUDENT 1 *interrupts.*)

STUDENT 1: Professor Bearing? Can I talk to you for a minute?

VIVIAN: You May.

STUDENT 1: I need to ask for an extension on my paper. I'm really sorry, and I know your policy, but see–

VIVIAN: Don't tell me. Your grandmother died.

STUDENT 1: You knew.

VIVIAN: It was a guess.

STUDENT 1: I have to go home.

VIVIAN: Do what you will, but the paper is due when it is due.

(*As* STUDENT 1 *leaves and the classroom disappears,* VIVIAN *watches. Pause*)

VIVIAN: I don't know. I feel so much–what is the word? I look back, I see these scenes, and I . . .

(*Long silence.* VIVIAN *walks absently around the stage, trying to think of something. Finally, giving up, she trudges back to bed.*)

VIVIAN: It was late at night, the graveyard shift. Susie was on. I could hear her in the hall.

I wanted her to come and see me. So I had to create a little emergency. Nothing dramatic.

(VIVIAN *pinches the IV tubing. The pump alarm beeps.*)

It worked.

(SUSIE *enters, concerned.*)

SUSIE: Ms. Bearing? Is that you beeping at four in the morning? (*She checks the tubing and presses buttons on the pump. The alarm stops.*) Did that wake you up? I'm sorry. It just gets occluded sometimes.

VIVIAN: I was awake.

SUSIE: You were? What's the trouble, sweetheart?

VIVIAN: (*To the audience, roused*) Do not think for a minute that anyone calls me "Sweetheart." But then . . . I allowed it. (*To* SUSIE) Oh, I don't know.

SUSIE: You can't sleep?

VIVIAN: No. I just keep thinking.

SUSIE: If you do that too much, you can get kind of confused.

VIVIAN: I know. I can't figure things out. I'm in a . . . *quandary,* having these . . . *doubts.*

SUSIE: What you're doing is very hard.

VIVIAN: Hard things are what I like best.

SUSIE: It's not the same. It's like it's out of control, isn't it?

VIVIAN: (*Crying, in spite of herself*) I'm scared.

SUSIE: *(Stroking her)* Oh, honey, of course you are.

VIVIAN: I want . . .

SUSIE: I know. It's hard.

VIVIAN: I don't feel sure of myself anymore.

SUSIE: And you used to feel sure.

VIVIAN: *(Crying)* Oh, yes, I used to feel sure.

SUSIE: Vivian. It's all right. I know. It hurts. I know. It's all right. Do you want a tissue? It's all right. *(Silence)* Vivian, would you like a Popsicle?

VIVIAN: *(Like a child)* Yes, please.

SUSIE: I'll get it for you. I'll be right back.

VIVIAN: Thank you.

(SUSIE leaves.)

VIVIAN: *(Pulling herself together)* The epithelial cells in my GI tract have been killed by the chemo. The cold Popsicle feels good, it's something I can digest, and it helps keep me hydrated. For your information.

(SUSIE returns with an orange two-stick Popsicle. VIVIAN unwraps it and breaks it in half)

VIVIAN: Here.

SUSIE: Sure?

VIVIAN: Yes.

SUSIE: Thanks. (SUSIE *sits on the commode by the bed. Silence)* When I was a kid, we used to get these from a truck. The man would come around and ring his bell and we'd all run over. Then we'd sit on the curb and eat our Popsicles.

Pretty profound, huh?

VIVIAN: It sounds nice.

(Silence)

SUSIE: Vivian, there's something we need to talk about, you need to think about.

(Silence)

VIVIAN: My cancer is not being cured, is it.

SUSIE: Huh-uh.

VIVIAN: They never expected it to be, did they.

SUSIE: Well, they thought the drugs would make the tumor get smaller, and it has gotten a lot smaller. But the problem is that it started in new places too. They've learned a lot for their research. It was the best thing they had to give you, the strongest drugs. There just isn't a good treatment for what you have yet, for advanced ovarian. I'm sorry. They should have explained this–

VIVIAN: I knew.

SUSIE: You did.

VIVIAN: I read between the lines.

SUSIE: What you have to think about is your "code status." What you want them to do if your heart stops.

VIVIAN: Well.

SUSIE: You can be "full code," which means that if your heart stops, they'll call a Code Blue and the code team will come and resuscitate you and take you to Intensive Care until you stabilize again. Or you can be "Do Not Resuscitate," so if your heart stops we'll . . . well, we'll just let it. You'll be "DNR." You can think about it, but I wanted to present both choices before Kelekian and Jason talk to you.

VIVIAN: You don't agree about this?

SUSIE: Well, they like to save lives. So anything's okay, as long as life contin-ues. It doesn't matter if you're hooked up to a million machines. Kelekian is a great researcher and everything. And the fellows, like Jason, they're really smart. It's really an honor for them to work with him. But they always . . . want to know more things.

VIVIAN: I always want to know more things. I'm a scholar. Or I was when I had shoes, when I had eyebrows.

SUSIE: Well, okay then. You'll be full code. That's fine.

(Silence)

VIVIAN: No, don't complicate the matter.

SUSIE: It's okay. It's up to you–

VIVIAN: Let it stop.

SUSIE: Really?

VIVIAN: Yes.

SUSIE: So if your heart stops beating–

VIVIAN: Just let it stop.

SUSIE: Sure?

VIVIAN: Yes.

SUSIE: Okay. I'll get Kelekian to give the order, and then–

VIVIAN: Susie?

SUSIE: Uh-huh?

VIVIAN: You're still going to take care of me, aren't you?

SUSIE: 'Course, sweetheart. Don't you worry.

(As SUSIE *leaves,* VIVIAN *sits upright, full of energy and rage.)*

VIVIAN: That certainly was a *maudlin* display. Popsicles? "Sweetheart"? I can't believe my life has become so . . . *corny.* But it can't be helped. I don't see any other way. We are discussing life and death, and not in the abstract, either; we are discussing *my* life and *my* death, and my brain is dulling, and poor Susie's was never very sharp to begin with, and I can't conceive of any other . . . *tone.*

(*Quickly*) Now is not the time for verbal swordplay, for unlikely flights of imagination and wildly shifting perspectives, for metaphysical conceit, for wit.

And nothing would be worse than a detailed scholarly analysis. Erudition. Interpretation. Complication.

(*Slowly*) Now is a time for simplicity. Now is a time for, dare I say it, kindness.

(*Searchingly*) I thought being extremely smart would take care of it. But I see that I have been found out. Ooohhh.

I'm scared. Oh, God. I want . . . I want . . . No. I want to hide. I just want to curl up in a little ball. (*She dives under the covers.*)

(VIVIAN *wakes in horrible pain. She is tense, agitated, fearful. Slowly she calms down and addresses the audience.*)

VIVIAN: (*Trying extremely hard*) I want to tell you how it feels. I want to explain it, to use *my* words. It's as if . . . I can't . . . There aren't . . . I'm like a student and this is the final exam and I don't know what to put down because I don't understand the question and I'm *running out of time.*

The time for extreme measures has come. I am in terrible pain. Susie says that I need to begin aggressive pain management if I am going to stand it.

"It": such a little word. In this case, I think "it" signifies "being alive."

I apologize in advance for what this palliative treatment modality does to the dramatic coherence of my play's last scene. It can't be helped. They have to do something. I'm in terrible pain.

Say it, Vivian. *It hurts like hell. It really does.*

(SUSIE *enters.* VIVIAN *is writhing in pain.*)

Oh, God. Oh, God.

SUSIE: Sshh. It's okay. Sshh. I paged Kelekian up here, and we'll get you some meds.

VIVIAN: Oh, God, it is so painful. So painful. So much pain. So much pain.

SUSIE: I know, I know, it's okay. Sshh. Just try and clear your mind. It's all right. We'll get you a Patient-Controlled Analgesic. It's a little pump, and you push a little button, and you decide how much medication you want. (*Importantly*) It's very simple, and it's up to you.

(KELEKIAN *storms in;* JASON *follows with chart.*)

KELEKIAN: Dr. Bearing. Susie.

SUSIE: Time for Patient-Controlled Analgesic. The pain is killing her.

KELEKIAN: Dr. Bearing, are you in pain? (KELEKIAN *holds out his hand for chart;* JASON *hands it to him. They read.*)

VIVIAN: *(Sitting up, unnoticed by the staff)* Am I in pain? I don't believe this. Yes, I'm in goddamn pain. *(Furious)* I have a fever of 101 spiking to 104. And I have bone metastases in my pelvis and both femurs. *(Screaming)* There is cancer eating away at my goddamn bones, and I did not know there could be such pain on this earth.

(She flops back on the bed and cries audibly to them.) Oh, God.

KELEKIAN: *(Looking at* VIVIAN *intently)* I want a morphine drip.

SUSIE: What about Patient-Controlled? She could be more alert–

KELEKIAN: *(Teaching)* Ordinarily, yes. But in her case, no.

SUSIE: But–

KELEKIAN: *(To* SUSIE) She's earned a rest. *(To* JASON) Morphine, ten push now, then start at ten an hour. *(To* VIVIAN) Dr. Bearing, try to relax. We're going to help you through this, don't worry. Dr. Bearing? Excellent. *(He squeezes* VIVIAN's *shoulder. They all leave.)*

VIVIAN: *(Weakly, painfully, leaning on her IV pole, she moves to address the audience.)* Hi. How are you feeling today?

(Silence)

These are my last coherent lines. I'll have to leave the action to the professionals.

It came so quickly, after taking so long. Not even time for a proper conclusion.

*(*VIVIAN *concentrates with all her might, and she attempts a grand summation, as if trying to conjure her own ending.)*

And Death–*capital* D–shall be no more–semicolon.
Death–*capital* D–thou shalt die–*ex-cla-mation point!*

(She looks down at herself, looks out at the audience, and sees that the line doesn't work. She shakes her head and exhales with resignation.)
I'm sorry.

———————

(She gets back into bed as SUSIE *injects morphine into the IV tubing.* VIVIAN *lies down and, in a final melodramatic gesture, shuts the lids of her own eyes and folds her arms over her chest.)*

VIVIAN: I trust this will have a soporific effect.

SUSIE: Well, I don't know about that, but it sure makes you sleepy.

(This strikes VIVIAN *as delightfully funny. She starts to giggle, then laughs out loud.* SUSIE *doesn't get it.)*

SUSIE: What's so funny? *(*VIVIAN *keeps laughing.)* What?

VIVIAN: Oh! It's that–"Soporific" *means* "makes you sleepy."

SUSIE: It does?

VIVIAN: Yes. *(Another fit of laughter)*

SUSIE: *(Giggling)* Well, that was pretty dumb–

VIVIAN: No! No, no! It was *funny!*

SUSIE: *(Starting to catch on)* Yeah, I guess so. *(Laughing)* In a dumb sort of way. *(This sets them both off laughing again)* I never would have gotten it. I'm glad you explained it.

VIVIAN: *(Simply)* I'm a teacher.

(They laugh a little together Slowly the morphine kicks in, and VIVIAN's *laughs become long sighs. Finally she falls asleep.* SUSIE *checks everything out, then leaves. Long silence)*

---

*(*JASON *and* SUSIE *chat as they enter to insert a catheter.)*

JASON: Oh, yeah. She was a great scholar. Wrote tons of books, articles, was the head of everything. *(He checks the I&O sheet.)* Two hundred. Seventy-five. Five-twenty. Let's up the hydration. She won't be drinking anymore. See if we can keep her kidneys from fading. Yeah, I had a lot of respect for her, which is more than I can say for the *entire* biochemistry department.

SUSIE: What do you want? Dextrose?

JASON: Give her saline.

SUSIE: Okay.

JASON: She gave a hell of a lecture. No notes, not a word out of place. It was pretty impressive. A lot of students hated her, though.

SUSIE: Why?

JASON: Well, she wasn't exactly a cupcake.

SUSIE: *(Laughing, fondly)* Well, she hasn't exactly been a cupcake here, either. *(Leaning over* VIVIAN *and talking loudly and slowly in her ear)* Now, Ms. Bearing, Jason and I are here, and we're going to insert a catheter to collect your urine. It's not going to hurt, don't you worry. *(During the conversation she inserts the catheter.)*

JASON: Like she can hear you.

SUSIE: It's just nice to do.

JASON: Eight cycles of Hex and Vin at the full dose. Kelekian didn't think it was possible. I wish they could all get through it at full throttle. Then we could really have some data.

SUSIE: She's not what I imagined. I thought somebody who studied poetry would be sort of dreamy, you know?

JASON: Oh, not the way she did it. It felt more like boot camp than English class. This guy John Donne was incredibly intense. Like your whole brain had to be in knots before you could get it.

SUSIE: He made it hard on purpose?

JASON: Well, it has to do with the subject. The Holy Sonnets we worked on most, they were mostly about Salvation Anxiety. That's a term I made up in one of my papers, but I think it fits pretty well. Salvation Anxiety. You're this brilliant guy, I mean, brilliant–this guy makes Shakespeare sound like a Hallmark card. And you know you're a sinner. And there's this promise of salvation, the whole religious thing. But you just can't deal with it.

SUSIE: How come?

JASON: It just doesn't stand up to scrutiny. But you can't face life without it either. So you write these screwed-up sonnets. Everything is brilliantly convoluted. Really tricky stuff. Bouncing off the walls. Like a game, to make the puzzle so complicated.

(The catheter is inserted. SUSIE puts things away.)

SUSIE: But what happens in the end?

JASON: End of what?

SUSIE: To John Donne. Does he ever get it?

JASON: Get what?

SUSIE: His Salvation Anxiety. Does he ever understand?

JASON: Oh, no way. The puzzle takes over. You're not even trying to solve it anymore. Fascinating, really. Great training for lab research. Looking at things in increasing levels of complexity.

SUSIE: Until what?

JASON: What do you mean?

SUSIE: Where does it end? Don't you get to solve the puzzle?

JASON: Nah. When it comes right down to it, research is just trying to quantify the complications of the puzzle.

SUSIE: But you *help* people! You save lives and stuff.

JASON: Oh, yeah, I save some guy's life, and then the poor slob gets hit by a bus!

SUSIE: (Confused) Yeah, I guess so. I just don't think of it that way. Guess you can tell I never took a class in poetry.

JASON: Listen, if there's one thing we learned in Seventeenth-Century Poetry, it's that you can forget about that sentimental stuff. *Enzyme Kinetics* was more poetic than Bearing's class. Besides, you can't think about that *meaning-of-life* garbage all the time or you'd go nuts.

SUSIE: Do you believe in it?

JASON: In what?

SUSIE: Umm. I don't know, the meaning-of-life garbage. *(She laughs a little.)*

JASON: What do they *teach* you in nursing school? *(Checking* VIVIAN'S *pulse)* She's out of it. Shouldn't be too long. You done here?

SUSIE: Yeah, I'll just . . . tidy up.

JASON: See ya. *(He leaves.)*

SUSIE: Bye, Jace. *(She thinks for a minute, then carefully rubs baby oil on* VIVIAN's *hands. She checks the catheter, then leaves.)*

(Professor E.M. ASHFORD, *now eighty, enters.)*

E.M.: Vivian? Vivian? It's Evelyn. Vivian?

VIVIAN: *(Waking, slurred)* Oh, God. *(Surprised)* Professor Ashford. Oh, God.

E.M.: I'm in town visiting my great-grandson, who is celebrating his fifth birthday. I went to see you at your office, and they directed me here. *(She lays her jacket, scarf, and parcel on the bed.)* I have been walking all over town. I had forgotten how early it gets chilly here.

VIVIAN: *(Weakly)* I feel so bad.

E.M.: I know you do. I can see. (VIVIAN *cries.)* Oh, dear, there, there. There, there. (VIVIAN *cries more, letting the tears flow.)* Vivian, Vivian. (E.M. *looks toward the hall, then furtively slips off her shoes and swings up on the bed. She puts her arm around* VIVIAN.) There, there. There, there, Vivian. *(Silence)*

It's a windy day. *(Silence)*

Don't worry, dear. *(Silence)*

Let's see. Shall I recite to you? Would you like that? I'll recite something by Donne.

VIVIAN: *(Moaning)* Nooooooo.

E.M.: Very well. *(Silence)* Hmmm. *(Silence)* Little Jeffrey is very sweet. Gets into everything.

(Silence. E.M. *takes a children's book out of the paper bag and begins reading.* VIVIAN *nestles in, drifting in and out of sleep.)*

Let's see. *The Runaway Bunny.* By Margaret Wise Brown. Pictures by Clement Hurd. Copyright 1942. First Harper Trophy Edition, 1972. Now then.

Once there was a little bunny who wanted to run away.

So he said to his mother, "I am running away."

> "If you run away," said his mother, "I will run after you. For you are my little bunny."
>
> "If you run after me," said the little bunny, "I will become a fish in a trout stream and I will swim away from you."
>
> "If you become a fish in a trout stream," said his mother, "I will become a fisherman and I will fish for you."

(Thinking out loud) Look at that. A little allegory of the soul. No matter where it hides, God will find it. See, Vivian?

VIVIAN: *(Moaning)* Uhhhhhh.

E.M.:

> "If you become a fisherman," said the little bunny, "I will be a bird and fly away from you."
>
> "If you become a bird and fly away from me," said his mother, "I will be a tree that you come home to."

(To herself) Very clever.

> "Shucks," said the little bunny, "I might just as well stay where I am and be your little bunny."
>
> And so he did.
>
> "Have a carrot," said the mother bunny.

(To herself) Wonderful.

*(*VIVIAN *is now fast asleep.* E.M. *slowly gets down and gathers her things. She leans over and kisses her.)*

It's time to go. And flights of angels sing thee to thy rest. *(She leaves.)*

*(*JASON *strides in and goes directly to the I&O sheet without looking at* VIVIAN.*)*

JASON: Professor Bearing. How are you feeling today? Three p.m. IV hydration totals. Two thousand in. Thirty out. Uh-oh. That's it. Kidneys gone.

(He looks at VIVIAN.*)* Professor Bearing? Highly unresponsive. Wait a second–*(Puts his head down to her mouth and chest to listen for heartbeat and breathing)* Wait a sec–Jesus Christ! *(Yelling)* CALL A CODE!

*(*JASON *throws down the chart, dives over the bed, and lies on top of her body as he reaches for the phone and punches in the numbers.)*

(To himself) Code: 4-5-7-5. *(To operator)* Code Blue, room 707. Code Blue, room 707. Dr. Posner–P-O-S-N-E-R. Hurry up!

(He throws down the phone and lowers the head of the bed.)

Come on, come on, COME ON.

(He begins CPR, kneeling over VIVIAN, *alternately pounding frantically and giving mouth-to-mouth resuscitation. Over the loudspeaker in the hall, a droning voice repeats "Code Blue, room 707. Code Blue, room 707.")*
    One! Two! Three! Four! Five! *(He breathes in her mouth.)*
*(*SUSIE, *hearing the announcement, runs into the room.)*
SUSIE: WHAT ARE YOU DOING?
JASON: A GODDAMN CODE. GET OVER HERE!
SUSIE: She's DNR! *(She grabs him.)*
JASON: *(He pushes her away.)* She's Research!
SUSIE: She's NO CODE!
*(*SUSIE *grabs* JASON *and hurls him off the bed.)*
JASON: Ooowww! Goddamnit, Susie!
SUSIE: She's no code!
JASON: Aaargh!
SUSIE: Kelekian put the order in—you saw it! You were right there, Jason!
    Oh, God, the code! *(She runs to the phone. He struggles to stand.)* 4-5-7-5.
(The CODE TEAM *swoops in. Everything changes. Frenzy takes over. They knock* SUSIE *out of the way with their equipment.)*
SUSIE: *(At the phone)* Cancel code, room 707. Sue Monahan, primary nurse.
    Cancel code. Dr. Posner is here.
JASON: *(In agony)* Oh, God.
CODE TEAM:
    –Get out of the way!
    –Unit staff out!
    –Get the board!
    –Over here!
(They throw VIVIAN's *body up at the waist and stick a board underneath for CPR. In a whirlwind of sterile packaging and barked commands, one team member attaches a respirator, one begins CPR, and one prepares the defibrillator.* SUSIE *and* JASON *try to stop them but are pushed away. The loudspeaker in the hall announces "Cancel code, room 707. Cancel code, room 707.")*
CODE TEAM:
    –Bicarb amp!
    –I got it! *(To* SUSIE*)* Get out!
    –One, two, three, four, five!
    –Get ready to shock! *(To* JASON*)* Move it!
SUSIE: *(Running to each person, yelling)* STOP! Patient is DNR!
JASON: *(At the same time, to the* CODE TEAM*)* No, no! Stop doing this.
    STOP!

CODE TEAM:
- −Keep it going!
- −What do you get?
- −Bicarb amp!
- −No pulse!

SUSIE: She's NO CODE! Order was given−*(She dives for the chart and holds it up as she cries out)* Look! Look at this! DO NOT RESUSCITATE. KELEKIAN.

CODE TEAM: *(As they administer electric shock,* VIVIAN's *body arches and bounces back down.)*
- −Almost ready!
- −Hit her!
- −CLEAR!
- −Pulse? Pulse?

JASON: *(Howling)* I MADE A MISTAKE!

(Pause. The CODE TEAM *looks at him. He collapses on the floor.)*

SUSIE: No code! Patient is no code.

CODE TEAM HEAD: Who the hell are you?

SUSIE: Sue Monahan, primary nurse.

CODE TEAM HEAD: Let me see the goddamn chart. CHART!

CODE TEAM: *(Slowing down)*
- −What's going on?
- −Should we stop?
- −What's it say?

SUSIE: *(Pushing them away from the bed)* Patient is no code. Get away from her!

*(*SUSIE *lifts the blanket.* VIVIAN *steps out of the bed.*

She walks away from the scene, towards a little light.

She is now attentive and eager, moving slowly toward the light.

She takes off her cap and lets it drop.

She slips off her bracelet

CODE TEAM HEAD: *(Reading)* Do Not Resuscitate. Kelekian. Shit.

(The CODE TEAM *stops working.)*

JASON: *(Whispering)* Oh, God.

CODE TEAM HEAD: Order was put in yesterday.

CODE TEAM:
- −It's a doctor fuck-up.
- −What is he, a resident?

She loosens the ties and the top gown slides to the floor. She lets the second gown fall.

The instant she is naked, and beautiful, reaching for the light–

Lights out.)

–Got us up here on a DNR
–Called a code on a no-code.

JASON: Oh, God.

(The bedside scene fades.)

HEAVEN?

Wings

ℬ

Arthur Kopit

INTRODUCTION

Wings, by Arthur Kopit, depicts the experience of a woman who suffers a cerebral stroke. The play leads the audience through the various stages of the event as the victim struggles to define her fragmented self in what she perceives to be an alien world. In an informative preface to his play, the dramatist reveals the inspiration for his work in a similar crisis suffered by his father some months earlier. Additional stimuli resulted from his subsequent meetings with patients and staff at the Burke Rehabilitation Center in New York where his father was cared for. Besides his personal observations at Burke, Kopit made a serious study of brain damage in order to ground his work in clinical accuracy. Specifically, he acknowledged two sources that informed him. The first, *The Shattered Mind,* by neuropsychologist Howard Gardner, appeared a year before the play and deals with the result of brain injury. The second is A. R. Luria's *The Man with a Shattered World,* first published in 1972. The latter, written by one of the major neurologists of the twentieth-century, includes a narrative of brain damage in the language of the patient.[1]

In being scrupulous about accuracy in dramatic situations, Kopit was following the recommendations of Anton Chekhov. He also followed the Russian author's advice regarding limits on the depiction of medical situations on stage. Chekhov had noted, for example, that one cannot show death by poisoning on the stage as it actually occurs. Kopit, similarly, felt that his father's case was "too severe, too grim" for the audience. In addition, he could not use his father as a model for the protagonist since he lacked the necessary objectivity. Yet he felt compelled to interpret what was going on inside the elder Kopit, to comprehend his intolerable isolation, and to transmit his father's recognition of his own condition as revealed by the terror in his eyes. As he strained to overcome the barrier that illness had erected between them, Kopit was haunted by one question: "What was it like inside?" (180). He was convinced that despite his impairment, the afflicted man was essentially the same person he had always been. The dramatist also knew that to arrive at an understanding of his father's interior life and to recreate that life for an audience, he would have to work by analogy. He decided to focus on two patients and a therapist he had met at the Burke Center with the intention of creating a composite figure for his main character. The figure who ultimately emerged from his imagination was a woman named Emily Stilson. While the facts of her illness are accurate, the play is neither a case study nor a documentary. The audience comes to know the character's world through her own consciousness. Kopit offers a note of caution: any attempt to render a person's consciousness through words must be speculative. His goal was to convey emotional truth informed by fact.

The patient on whom the protagonist is based was an elderly woman who, in her youth during the post–World War I era, had been, to the playwright's astonishment, a barnstorming aviatrix. She thrilled crowds with breathtaking stunts performed on the wings of planes. An old photograph, pinned on the wall in her room, shows her dressed in pilot's garb as she stands on the wing of an old Curtiss Jenny about to take off. In comparing the youthful, imperious face in the photograph with that of the aged woman he had met earlier, Kopit detected a feature that gave evidence of the same essential being at the core of both forms, a noble and slightly quizzical smile. He grasped the bravery and spirit that was part of her nature and knew that her courage prevailed as she withstood the challenge of her illness. Kopit sensed that his father tolerated his condition with a similar muted strength.

Wings is constructed of four sections corresponding to the character's experience from the moment she is stricken: "Prelude," "Catastrophe," "Awakening," and "Explorations." During the course of the drama, she moves from isolation to frustrated attempts at communication with her doctors, on to tentative mingling with other patients, and through a final relationship with her therapist. To render his character's state intelligible, the playwright had to reproduce her universe where language, time, and space had become suddenly and horrifically disjointed. And then he had to place his audience within her damaged consciousness. In keeping with his emphasis on language disorder and its implications, the playwright proceeded first to create a rich stage language for the impaired woman that combined the speech patterns of other patients suffering varying forms of aphasia. He then added strains of the language created by expressionist dramatist August Strindberg as well as that of James Joyce and Samuel Beckett to express inner experience. One recalls Beckett's character Lucky and his mention of aphasia in his long, disordered monologue in *Waiting For Godot*. In *Wings,* as with other postmodern dramas, the realist aesthetic gives ground as action is suspended and attention is deflected to verbal imagery and spatial and temporal rearrangements while a new theatrical discourse takes precedence.

In a fortuitous blending of structure and theme, the apparent disorder of the stage world occasioned by the displacement of traditional stage conventions—most notably linear progression—magnifies the disordered inner world of the protagonist. Mrs. Stilson delivers what is virtually a dramatic monologue, interspersed with occasional passages of dialogue, throughout the play. Addressing the audience directly, she draws them into her consciousness. In such a manner the character's worldview becomes that of the audience who witnesses her confusion and fear. Her words lead us to shape her splintered visual and aural perceptions as we participate in her painful struggle to communicate. Yet, as monolgic language can at times be deceptive, given an unreliable narrator, Mrs. Stilson's speech can be equally misleading, though not intentionally so. A question exists regarding the extent to which the recollections of a mind that has been damaged may be regarded as truth. And given Mrs. Stilson's severe language deficit, how much can her verbal recollections be trusted? (187). Hence the playwright strives for emotional validity. As the woman begins to show signs of recovery and her world becomes more integrated, the audience is shifted to its traditional position of observer. Doctors, nurses, and hospital equipment appear as discernible images. Another view prevails as doctors attempt to communicate with their patient. Trying to evaluate the damage, they put simple questions to her: "Name something that grows on trees" "Who fixes teeth?" "What is Jim short for?" "Point to your shoulder" "No, your shoulder" (222). The questions are understandable to the audience that now confronts the patient's confusion from a distance. The distance widens when Mrs. Stilson assesses her situation in a later monologue. Evoking the time and place of another realm, she imagines that her plane has crashed, that she is being held prisoner in a farmhouse disguised as a hospital, and that she is being interrogated by an enemy that puts foolish questions to her. In his vivid simulation of the mental state of the stroke victim, Kopit indicates the way in which her aphasia has caused her cognitive damage as well as linguistic impairment. Nevertheless, despite its grim subject, the play is not without humor, transmitting the heroine's good cheer as she comes to terms with her inverted world. At one point she confides, "Yesterday my children came to see me. Or at least I was told they were my children. Never saw them before in my life" (231).

Realism asserts itself intermittently. One instance occurs with the visual rendition of the hospital environment in a scene depicting a group therapy session; another is achieved with an aural effect as the patient listens to a tape recorder as a doctor lectures on stroke. Alternately, when the landscape blurs, bits of dialogue remind us of the presence of professionals in the background. Conflicting theories regarding the patient's mental abilities reach the audience as one doctor, failing to support his opinion with scientific fact, is accused of "flying blind." The image is especially apt for the former aviatrix and her healers who frequently fail to understand one another. Clearly, each acts in good faith. The warmest relationship of the play is that between the patient and her therapist. Mrs. Stilson's interaction with Amy is tender and loving. While science may fail at curing her, the heroine discovers the healing power of—dare one admit it?—a kiss. It is in Amy's company, too, that Emily Stilson is finally able to find the word to describe what she is experiencing at the moment. Naming the "something wet" on her cheeks, she finds the word for tears and knows that she is sad.

Kopit spares his audience little in his powerfully accurate depiction of the devastation caused by a stroke, obliging them to remain fixed in their seats without benefit of an intermission as he reveals the grueling facts. Remaining true to his commitment to tell his story with clinical accuracy, Kopit nonetheless makes it possible for a lay audience to gain insight into a serious health crisis likely to occur commonly. Scientific truth retains its validity as the dramatist answers the question "What was it like inside?" But his response is that of an artist creating a stage illusion that conveys truth by means of its own discourse. Probing the patient's mind, Kopit discovers one person's courage and resiliency that time and illness cannot diminish. While science can determine the essential elements of the body, it cannot decipher the human spirit. For the latter, we applaud the artist.

NOTES

1. A study contextualizing *Wings* against these two specific sources has been made by James Hurt in his fine study "Arthur Kopit's *Wings* and the Languages of the Theater," *American Drama* 8.1 (Fall 1998): 75–94.

WORKS CITED

Hurt, James. "Arthur Kopit's *Wings* and the Languages of the Theater." *American Drama* 8.1 (Fall 1998): 75–94.
Kopit, Arthur. *Wings: Three Plays*. New York: Hill and Wang, 1997.

WINGS
Arthur Kopit

To George Kopit, my father
1913–1977

CHARACTERS

EMILY STILSON
AMY
DOCTORS
NURSES
BILLY
MR. BROWNSTEIN
MRS. TIMMONS

The play takes place over a period of two years; it should be performed without an intermission.

NOTES ON THE PRODUCTION OF THIS PLAY

The stage as a void.

System of black scrim panels that can move silently and easily, creating the impression of featureless, labyrinthine corridors.

Some panels mirrored so they can fracture light, create the impression of endlessness, even airiness, multiply and confuse images, confound one's sense of space.

Sound both live and pre-recorded, amplified; speakers all around the theater.

No attempt should be made to create a literal representation of Mrs. Stilson's world, especially since Mrs. Stilson's world is no longer in any way literal.

The scenes should blend. No clear boundaries or domains in time or space for Mrs. Stilson any more.

It is posited by this play that the woman we see in the center of the void is the intact inner self of Mrs. Stilson. This inner self does not need to move physically when her external body (which we cannot see) moves. Thus, we infer movement from the context; from whatever clues we can obtain. It is the same for her, of course. She learns as best she can.

And yet, sometimes, the conditions change; then the woman we observe is Mrs. Stilson as others see her. We thus infer who it is we are seeing from the context, too. Sometimes we see both the inner and outer self at once.

Nothing about her world is predictable or consistent. This fact is its essence. The progression of the play is from fragmentation to integration. By the end, boundaries have become somewhat clearer. But she remains always in another realm from us.

PRELUDE

As audience enters, a cozy armchair visible downstage in a pool of light, darkness surrounding it.
A clock heard ticking in the dark.
Lights to black.
Hold.
When the lights come back, EMILY STILSON, *a woman well into her seventies, is sitting in the armchair reading a book. Some distance away, a floor lamp glows dimly. On the other side of her chair, also some distance away, a small table with a clock. The chair, the lamp, and the table with the clock all sit isolated in narrow pools of light, darkness between and around them.*
The clock seems to be ticking a trifle louder than normal.
MRS. STILSON, *enjoying her book and the pleasant evening, reads on serenely.*
And then she looks up.
The lamp disappears into the darkness.
But she turns back to her book as if nothing odd has happened; resumes reading.
And then, a moment later, she looks up again, an expression of slight perplexity on her face. For no discernible reason, she turns toward the clock.
The clock and the table it is sitting on disappear into the darkness.
She turns front. Stares out into space.
Then she turns back to her book. Resumes reading. But the reading seems an effort; her mind is on other things.
The clock skips a beat.
Only after the clock has resumed its normal rhythm does she look up. It is as if the skipped beat has only just then registered. For the first time, she displays what one might call concern.
And then the clock stops again. This time the interval lasts longer.
The book slips out of MRS. STILSON's *hands; she stares out in terror.*
Blackout.
Noise.

The moment of a stroke, even a relatively minor one, and its immediate after-math, are an experience in chaos. Nothing at all makes sense. Nothing except perhaps this overwhelming disorientation will be remembered by the victim. The stroke usually happens suddenly. It is a catastrophe.

It is my intention that the audience recognize that some real event is occur-ring; that real information is being received by the victim, but that it is coming in too scrambled and too fast to be properly decoded. Systems overload.

And so this section must not seem like utter "noise," though certainly it must be more noisy than intelligible. I do not believe there is any way to be true to this material if it is not finally "composed" in rehearsal, on stage, by "feel." Theoretically, any sound or image herein described can occur anywhere in this section. The victim cannot process. Her familiar world has been rear-ranged. The puzzle is in pieces. All at once, and with no time to prepare, she has been picked up and dropped into another realm.

In order that this section may be put together in rehearsal (there being no one true "final order" to the images and sounds she perceives), I have divided this section into three discrete parts with the understanding that in perfor-mance these parts will blend together to form one cohesive whole.

The first group consists of the visual images MRS. STILSON perceives.

The second group consists of those sounds emanating outside herself. Since these sounds are all filtered by her mind, and since her mind has been drastically altered, the question of whether we in the audience are hearing what is actually occurring or only hearing what she believes is occurring is unanswerable.

The third group contains MRS. STILSON's words: the words she thinks and the words she speaks. Since we are perceiving the world through MRS. STILSON's senses, there is no sure way for us to know whether she is actually saying any of these words aloud.

Since the experience we are exploring is not one of logic but its opposite, there is no logical reason for these groupings to occur in the order in which I have presented them. These are but components, building blocks, and can therefore be repeated, spliced, reversed, filtered, speeded up or slowed down. What should determine their final sequence and juxtaposition, tempi, intensity, is the "musical" sense of this section as a whole; it must pulse and build. An explosion quite literally is occurring in her brain, or rather, a series of explo-sions: the victim's mind, her sense of time and place, her sense of self, all are being shattered if not annihilated. Fortunately, finally, she will pass out. Were her head a pinball game it would register TILT—game over—stop. Silence. And resume again. Only now the victim is in yet another realm. The Catastrophe section is the journey or the fall into this strange and dreadful realm.

In the world into which MRS. STILSON has been so violently and suddenly transposed, time and place are without definition. The distance from her old familiar world is immense. For all she knows, she could as well be on another planet.

In this new world, she moves from one space or thought or concept to another without willing or sometimes even knowing it. Indeed, when she moves in this maze-like place, it is as if the world around her and not she were doing all the moving. To her, there is nothing any more that is commonplace or predictable. Nothing is as it was. Everything comes as a surprise. Something has relieved her of command. Something beyond her comprehension has her in its grip.

In the staging of this play, the sense should therefore be conveyed of physical and emotional separation (by the use, for example, of the dark transparent screens through which her surrounding world can be only dimly and partly seen, or by alteration of external sound) and of total immersion in strangeness.

Because our focus is on MRS. STILSON's inner self, it is important that she exhibit no particular overt physical disabilities. Furthermore, we should never see her in a wheelchair, even though, were we able to observe her through the doctors' eyes, a wheelchair is probably what she would, more often than not, be in.

One further note: because MRS. STILSON now processes information at a different rate from us, there is no reason that what we see going on around her has to be the visual equivalent of what we hear.

CATASTROPHE

IMAGES	SOUNDS OUTSIDE HERSELF
	(Sounds live or on tape, altered or unadorned)
	Of wind.
Mostly it is whiteness. Dazzling, blinding.	Of someone breathing with effort, unevenly.
	Of something ripping, like a sheet.

MRS. STILSON'S VOICE

(Voice live or on tape, altered or
unadorned)

Oh my God oh my God oh my
God—

—trees clouds houses mostly planes
flashing past, images without words,
utter disarray disbelief, never seen
this kind of thing before!

Where am I? How'd I get here?

My leg (What's my leg?) feels wet
arms . . . wet too, belly same chin
nose everything (Where are they
taking me?) something sticky (What
has happened to my plane?) feel
something sticky.

Doors! Too many doors!

Must have . . . fallen cannot . . . move
at all sky . . . (Gliding!) dark cannot
. . . talk (Feel as if I'm gliding!).

Yes, feels cool, nice . . . Yes, this is
the life all right!

My plane! What has happened to
my plane!

Help . . .

IMAGES	SOUNDS OUTSIDE HERSELF
Occasionally, there are brief rhombs of color, explosions of color, the color red being dominant.	Of something flapping, the sound suggestive of an old screen door perhaps, or a sheet or sail in the wind. It is a rapid fibrillation. And it is used mostly to mark transitions. It can seem ominous or not.
The mirrors, of course, reflect endlessly. Sense of endless space, endless corridors.	Of a woman's scream (though this sound should be altered by filters so it resembles other things, such as sirens).
	Of random noises recorded in a busy city hospital, then altered so to be only minimally recognizable.
Nothing seen that is not a fragment. Every aspect of her world has been shattered.	Of a car's engine at full speed.
	Of a siren (altered to resemble a woman screaming).
	Of an airplane coming closer, thundering overhead, then zooming off into silence.
Utter isolation.	
In this vast whiteness, like apparitions, partial glimpses of doctors and NURSES *can be seen. They appear and disappear like a pulse. They are never in one place for long. The mirrors multiply their incomprehensibility.*	Of random crowd noises, the crowd greatly agitated. In the crowd, people can be heard calling for help, a doctor, an ambulance. But all the sounds are garbled.
	Of people whispering.
	Of many people asking questions simultaneously, no question comprehensible.

MRS. STILSON'S VOICE

—all around faces of which nothing known no sense ever all wiped
out blank like ice I think saw it once
flying over something some place
all was white sky and sea clouds
ice almost crashed couldn't tell
where I was heading right side up
topsy-turvy under over I was flying
actually if I can I do yes do recall
was upside down can you believe
it almost scraped my head on the
ice caps couldn't tell which way was
up wasn't even dizzy strange things
happen to me that they do!

What's my name? I don't know my
name!

Where's my arm? I don't have an
arm!

What's an arm?

AB-ABC-ABC123DEF451212 what?
123—12345678972357 better yes no
problem I'm okay soon be out be
over storm . . . will pass I'm sure.
Always has.

IMAGES	SOUNDS OUTSIDE HERSELF
Sometimes the dark panels are opaque, sometimes transparent. Always, they convey a sense of layers, multiplicity, separation. Sense constant of doors opening, closing, opening, closing.	Of doors opening, closing, opening, closing.
	Of someone breathing oxygen through a mask.
	VOICES (garbled): Just relax. / No one's going to hurt you. / Can you hear us? / Be careful! / You're hurting her! / No, we're not. / Don't lift her, leave her where she is! / Someone call an ambulance! / I don't think she can hear.
Fragments of hospital equipment appear out of nowhere and disappear just as suddenly. Glimpse always too brief to enable us to identify what this equipment is, or what its purpose.	MALE VOICE: Have you any idea—
	Other Voices (garbled): Do you know your name? / Do you know where you are? / What year is this? / If I say the tiger has been killed by the lion, which animal is dead?
MRS. STILSON's movements seem random. She is a person wandering through space, lost.	A hospital paging system is heard.
Finally, MRS. STILSON is led by attendants downstage, to a chair. Then left alone.	Equipment being moved through stone corridors, vast vaulting space. Endless echoing.

AWAKENING

In performance, the end of the Catastrophe section should blend, without interruption, into the beginning of this.

MRS. STILSON *downstage on a chair in a pool of light, darkness all around*
  her. In the distance behind her, muffled sounds of a hospital. Vague images
  of doctors, nurses attending to someone we cannot see. One of the doctors
  calls MRS. STILSON's *name. Downstage,* MRS. STILSON *shows no trace*
  of recognition. The doctor calls her name again. Again no response. One of
  the doctors says, "it's possible she may hear us but be unable to respond."
One of the nurses tries calling out her name. Still no response. The doctor
  leaves. The remaining doctors and nurses fade into the darkness:
Only MRS. STILSON *can be seen.*
Pause.

MRS. STILSON: Still . . . sun moon too or . . . three times happened maybe
  globbidged rubbidged uff and firded-forded me to nothing there try
  again *[we hear a window being raised somewhere behind her]* window! up
  and heard *[sounds of birds]* known them know I know them once upon a
  birds! that's it better getting better soon be out of this.
Pause.

  Out of . . . what?
Pause.

  Dark . . . space vast of . . . in I am or so it seems feels no real clues to speak
  of. *[Behind her, brief image of a doctor passing]* Something tells me I am
  not alone. Once! Lost it. No here back thanks work fast now, yes empty
  vast reach of space desert think they call it I'll come back to that anyhow
  down I . . . something what *[brief image of a nurse]* it's SOMETHING ELSE
  IS ENTERING MY!—no wait got it crashing OH MY GOD! CRASH-
  ING! deadstick dead-of-night thought the stars were airport lights upside
  down was I what a way to land glad no one there to see it, anyhow tubbish
  blaxed and vinkled I commenshed to uh-oh where's it gone to somewhere
  flubbished what? with *[brief images of hospital staff on the move]* images are
  SOMETHING ODD IS! . . . yes, then there I thank you crawling sands and
  knees still can feel it hear the wind all alone somehow wasn't scared why a
  mystery, vast dark track of space, we've all got to die that I know, anyhow
  then day came light came with it so with this you'd think you'd hope just
  hold on they will find me I am . . . still intact.
Pause.

  In here.

Long silence.

Seem to be the word removed.

Long silence.

How long have I been here? . . . And wrapped in dark.

Pause.

Can remember nothing.

*Outside sounds begin to impinge; same for images. In the distance, an atten-
dant dimly seen pushing a floor polisher. Its noise resembles an animal's
growl.*

[Trying hard to be cheery]: No, definitely I am not alone!

*The sound of the polisher grows louder, seems more bestial, voracious; it over-
whelms everything. Explosion! She gasps.*

*[Rapidly and in panic, sense of great commotion behind her. A crisis has
occurred]:* There I go there I go hallway now it's screaming crowded
pokes me then the coolbreeze needle scent of sweetness can see palms
flowers flummers couldn't fix the leaking sprouting everywhere to save
me help me CUTS UP THROUGH to something movement I am something moving without movement!

*Sound of a woman's muffled scream from behind her. The scream grows
louder.*

[With delight]: What a strange adventure I am having!

Lights to black on everything.

In the dark, a pause.

*When her voice is heard again, it is heard first from all the speakers. Her voice
sounds groggy, slurred. No longer any sense of panic discernible. A few
moments after her voice is heard, the lights come up slowly on her. Soon,
only she is speaking; the voice from the speakers has disappeared.*

Hapst aporkshop fleetish yes of course it's yes the good ol' times when we
would mollis I mean collis all around still what my son's name is cannot
for the life of me yet face gleams smiles as he tells them what I did but
what his name is cannot see it pleasant anyway yes palms now ocean
sea breeze wafting floating up and lifting holding weightless and goes
swooooping down with me least I . . . think it's me.

Sound of something flapping rapidly open and closed, open and closed.

Sound of wind.

Lights change into a cool and airy blue. Sense of weightlessness, serenity.

In another realm now.

Yes, out there walking not holding even danger ever-present how I loved
it love it still no doubt will again hear them cheering wisht or waltz away
to some place like Rumania . . .

The wind disappears.

Nothing . . .

The serene blue light begins to fade away. Some place else now that she is going.
    Of course beyond that yet 1, 2 came before the yeast rose bubbled and
    MY CHUTE DIDN'T OPEN PROPERLY! Still for a girl did wonders
    getting down and it was Charles! no Charlie, who is Charlie? see him
    smiling as they tell him what I—

Outside world begins to impinge. Lights are changing, growing brighter, some-
    thing odd is happening. Sense of imminence. She notices.

[Breathless with excitement]: Stop hold cut stop wait stop come-out-break-
    out light can see it ready heart can yes can feel it pounding something
    underway here light is getting brighter lids I think the word is that's it
    lifting of their own but slowly knew I should be patient should be what?
    wait hold on steady now it's spreading no no question something under-
    way here spreading brighter rising lifting light almost yes can almost
    there a little more now yes can almost see this . . . place I'm . . . in and . . .

Look of horror.

Oh my God! Now I understand! THEY'VE GOT ME!

For first time doctors, nurses, hospital equipment all clearly visible behind her.
    All are gathered around someone we cannot see. From the way they are all
    bending over, we surmise this person we cannot see is lying in a bed.

Lights drop on MRS. STILSON, *downstage.*

NURSE: *[talking to the person upstage we cannot see]:* Mrs. Stilson, can you
    open up your eyes?

Pause.

MRS. STILSON *[separated from her questioners by great distance]:* Don't
    know how.

DOCTOR: Mrs. Stilson, you just opened up your eyes. We saw you. Can you
    open them again?

No response.

Mrs. Stilson . . . ?

MRS. STILSON *[proudly, triumphantly]:* My name then—Mrs. Stilson!

VOICE ON P.A. SYSTEM: Mrs. Howard, call on three! Mrs. Howard . . . !

MRS. STILSON: My name then—Mrs. Howard?

Lights fade to black on hospital staff.

Sound of wind, sense of time passing.

Lights come up on MRS. STILSON. *The wind disappears.*

The room that I am in is large, square. What does large mean?

Pause.

The way I'm turned I can see a window. When I'm on my back the win-
    dow isn't there.

DOCTOR *[in the distance, at best only dimly seen]:* Mrs. Stilson, can you
  hear me?

MRS. STILSON: Yes.

SECOND DOCTOR: Mrs. Stilson, can you hear me?

MRS. STILSON: Yes! I said yes! What's wrong with you?

FIRST DOCTOR: Mrs. Stilson, CAN YOU HEAR ME!

MRS. STILSON: Don't believe this—I've been put in with the deaf.

SECOND DOCTOR: Mrs. Stilson, if you can hear us, nod your head.

MRS. STILSON: All right, fine, that's how you want to play it—there!

She nods.

The doctors exchange glances.

FIRST DOCTOR: Mrs. Stilson, if you can hear us, NOD YOUR HEAD!

MRS. STILSON: Oh my God, this is grotesque!

Cacophony of sounds heard from all around, both live and from the speak-
  ers. Images suggesting sensation of assault as well. Implication of all these
  sounds and images is that MRS. STILSON is being moved through the
  hospital for purposes of examination, perhaps even torture. The informa-
  tion we receive comes in too fast and distorted for rational comprehension.
  The realm she is in is terrifying. Fortunately, she is not in it long.

As long as she is, however, the sense should be conveyed that her world moves
  around her more than she through it.

WHAT WE HEAR (the components): Are we moving you too fast? / Mus-
  tlian pottid or blastigrate, no not that way this, that's fletchit gottit careful
  now. / Now put your nose here on this line, would you? That's it, thank
  you, well done, well done. / How are the wickets today? / *[sound of a*
  cough] / Now close your—/ Is my finger going up or—/ Can you feel
  this? / Can you feel this? / Name something that grows on trees. / Who
  fixes teeth? / What room do you cook in? / What year is this? / How long
  have you been here? / Are we being too rippled shotgun? / Would you
  like a cup of tea? / What is Jim short for? / Point to your shoulder. / No,
  your shoulder. / What do you do with a book? / Don't worry, the water's
  warm. We're holding you, don't worry. In we go, that's a girl!

And then, as suddenly as the assault began, it is over.

Once again, MRS. STILSON all alone on stage, darkness all around her, no
  sense of walls or furniture. Utter isolation.

MRS. STILSON *[trying hard to keep smiling]:* Yes, all in all I'd say while
  things could be better could be worse, far worse, how? Not quite sure.
  Just a sense I have. The sort of sense that only great experience can
  mallees or rake, plake I mean, flake . . . Drake! That's it.

She stares into space.

Silence.

In the distance behind her, two DOCTORS *appear.*

FIRST DOCTOR: Mrs. Stilson, who was the first President of the United States?

MRS. STILSON: Washington.

Pause.

SECOND DOCTOR *[speaking more slowly than the* FIRST DOCTOR *did; perhaps she simply didn't hear the question]*: Mrs. Stilson, who was the first President of the United States?

MRS. STILSON: Washington!

SECOND DOCTOR *[to* FIRST*]*: I don't think she hears herself.

FIRST DOCTOR: No, I don't think she hears herself.

The two DOCTORS *emerge from the shadows, approach* MRS. STILSON. *She looks up in terror. This should be the first time that the woman on stage has been directly faced or confronted by the hospital staff. Her inner and outer worlds are beginning to come together.*

FIRST DOCTOR: Mrs. Stilson, makey your naming powers?

MRS. STILSON: What?

SECOND DOCTOR: Canju spokeme?

MRS. STILSON: Can I what?

FIRST DOCTOR: Can do peeperear?

MRS. STILSON: Don't believe what's going on!

SECOND DOCTOR: Ahwill.

FIRST DOCTOR: Pollycadjis.

SECOND DOCTOR: Sewyladda?

First Doctor *[with a nod]*: Hm-hm.

Exit doctors.

MRS. STILSON *[alone again]*: How it came to pass that I was captured! *[She ponders]* Hard to say really. I'll come back to that.

Pause.

The room that I've been put in this time is quite small, square, what does square mean? . . . Means . . .

Sense of time passing. The lights shift. The space she is in begins to change its shape.

Of course morning comes I think . . . *[She ponders]* Yes, and night of course comes . . . *[Ponders more]* Though sometimes . . .

MRS. STILSON *some place else now. And she is aware of it.*

Yes, the way the walls choose to move around me . . . Yes, I've noticed that, I'm no fool!

A NURSE *appears carrying a dazzling bouquet of flowers. This bouquet is the first real color we have seen.*

NURSE: Good morning! Look what somebody's just sent you! *[She sets them on a table]* Wish I had as many admirers as you.

Exit NURSE, smiling warmly.

MRS. STILSON's *eyes are drawn to the flowers. And something about them apparently renders it impossible for her to shift her gaze away. Something about these flowers has her in their thrall.*

What it is is their color.

It is as if she has never experienced color before. And the experience is so overwhelming, both physiologically and psychologically, that her brain cannot process all the information. Her circuitry is overloaded. It is too much sensory input for her to handle. An explosion is imminent. If something does not intervene to divert her attention, MRS. STILSON *will very likely faint, perhaps even suffer a seizure.*

A narrow beam of light, growing steadily in intensity, falls upon the bouquet of flowers, causing their colors to take on an intensity themselves that they otherwise would lack. At the same time, a single musical tone is heard, volume increasing.

A NURSE *enters the room.*

NURSE: May I get you something?

MRS. STILSON *[abstracted, eyes remaining on the flowers]*: Yes, a sweater.

NURSE: Yes, of course. Think we have one here. *[The NURSE opens a drawer, takes out a pillow, hands the pillow to* MRS. STILSON*]* Here.

MRS. STILSON *accepts the pillow unquestioningly, eyes never leaving the flowers. She lays the pillow on her lap, promptly forgets about it. The musical tone and the beam of light continue relentlessly toward their peak.*

The NURSE, *oblivious of any crisis, exits.*

The single tone and the beam of light crest together.

Silence follows. The beam disappears. The flowers seem normal. The lights around MRS. STILSON *return to the way they were before the gift of flowers was brought in.*

MRS. STILSON *[shaken]*: This is not a hospital of course, and I know it! What it is is a farmhouse made up to look like a hospital. Why? I'll come back to that.

Enter another NURSE.

NURSE: Hi! Haven't seen you in a while. Have you missed me?

MRS. STILSON *[no hint of recognition visible]*: What?

Nurse *[warmly]*: They say you didn't touch your dinner. Would you like some pudding?

MRS. STILSON: No.

NURSE: Good, I'll go get you some.

Exit NURSE, very cheerfully.

MRS. STILSON: Yes no question they have got me I've been what that word was captured is it? No it's—Yes, it's captured how? Near as it can figure. I was in my prane and crashed, not unusual, still in all not too common. Neither is it very grub. Plexit rather or I'd say propopic. Well that's that, jungdaball! Anyhow to resume, what I had for lunch? That's not it, good books I have read, good what, done what? Whaaaaat? Do the busy here! Get inside this, rubbidge all around let the vontul do some yes off or it of above semilacrum pwooosh! what with noddygobbit nip-n-crashing inside outside witsit watchit funnel vortex sucking into backlash watchit get-out caught-in spinning ring-grab grobbit help woooosh! cannot stoppit on its own has me where it wants *[and suddenly she is in another realm. Lights transformed into weightless blue. Sense of ease and serenity]* Plane! See it thanks, okay, onto back we were and here it is. Slow down easy now. Captured. After crashing, that is what we said or was about to, think it so, cannot tell for sure, slow it slow it, okay here we go . . . *[Speaking slower now]* captured after crashing by the enemy and brought here to this farm masquerading as a hospital. Why? For I would say offhand information. Of what sort though hard to tell. For example, questions such as can I raise my fingers, what's an overcoat, how many nickels in a rhyme, questions such as these. To what use can they be to the enemy? Hard to tell from here. Nonetheless, I would say must be certain information I possess that they want well I won't give it I'll escape! Strange things happen to me that they do! Good thing I'm all right! Must be in Rumania. Just a hunch of course. *[The serene blue light starts to fade]* Ssssh, someone's coming.

A NURSE has entered. The NURSE guides MRS. STILSON to a DOCTOR. The blue light is gone. The NURSE leaves.

The space MRS. STILSON now is in appears much more "real" and less fragmentary than what we have so far been observing. We see MRS. STILSON here as others see her.

DOCTOR: Mrs. Stilson, if you don't mind, I'd like to ask you some questions. Some will be easy, some will be hard. Is that all right?

MRS. STILSON: Oh yes I'd say oh well yes that's the twither of it.

DOCTOR: Good. Okay. Where were you born?

MRS. STILSON: Never. Not at all. Here the match wundles up you know and drats flames fires I keep careful always—

DOCTOR: Right . . . *[Speaking very slowly, precise enunciation]* Where were you born?

MRS. STILSON: Well now well now that's a good thing knowing yushof course wouldn't call it such as I did andinjurations or aplovia could it?

No I wouldn't think so. Next?

Pause.

DOCTOR: Mrs. Stilson, are there seven days in a week?

MRS. STILSON: ... Seven ... Yes.

DOCTOR: Are there five days in a week?

Pause.

Mrs. Stilson *[after much pondering]:* No.

DOCTOR: Can a stone float on water?

Long pause.

MRS. STILSON: No.

DOCTOR: Mrs. Stilson, can you cough?

MRS. STILSON: Somewhat.

DOCTOR: Well, would you show me how you cough?

MRS. STILSON: Well now well now not so easy what you cromplie is to put
   these bushes open and—

DOCTOR: No no, Mrs. Stilson, I'm sorry—I would like to hear you cough.

MRS. STILSON: Well I'm not bort you know with plajits or we'd see it
   wencherday she brings its pillow with the fistils-opening I'd say outward
   always outward never stopping it.

Long silence.

DOCTOR: Mrs. Stilson, I have some objects here. *[He takes a comb, a toothbrush, a pack of matches, and a key from his pocket, sets them down where
   she can see]* Could you point to the object you would use for cleaning
   your teeth?

Very long silence.

*Finally she picks up the comb and shows it to him. Then she puts it down.
   Waits.*

Mrs. Stilson, here, take this object in your hand. *[He hands her the tooth-
   brush]* Do you know what this object is called?

MRS. STILSON *[with great difficulty]:* Toooooooovvvv ... bbbrum?

DOCTOR: Very good. Now put it down.

She puts it down.

Now, pretend you have it in your hand. Show me what you'd do with it.

She does nothing.

What does one do with an object such as that, Mrs. Stilson?

No response.

Mrs. Stilson, what is the name of the object you are looking at?

MRS. STILSON: Well it's ... wombly and not at all ... rigged or tuned like
   we might twunter or toring to work the clambness out of it or—

DOCTOR: Pick it up.

Mrs. Stilson [*as soon as she's picked it up*]: Tooovebram, tooove-brach bratch brush bridge, two-bridge.

DOCTOR: Show me what you do with it.

For several moments she does nothing.

Then she puts it to her lips, holds it there motionless.

Very good. Thank you.

She sighs heavily, puts it down.

The doctor gathers up his objects, leaves.

Once again MRS. STILSON *all alone.*

She stares into space.

Then her voice is heard coming from all around; she herself does not speak.

Her Voice: Dark now again out the window on my side lying here all alone . . .

Very long silence.

MRS. STILSON: Yesterday my children came to see me.

Pause.

Or at least, I was told they were my children. Never saw them before in my life.

She stares out, motionless. No expression.

Then after a while she looks around. Studies the dark for clues.

Time has become peculiar.

And she continues this scrutiny of the dark.

But if this activity stems from curiosity, it is a mild curiosity at most. No longer does she convey or probably even experience the extreme, disoriented dread we saw earlier when she first arrived in this new realm. Her sense of urgency is gone. Indeed, were we able to observe MRS. STILSON *constantly, we would inevitably conclude that her curiosity is now only minimally purposeful; that, in fact, more likely her investigations are the actions, possibly merely the reflex actions, of someone with little or nothing else to do.*

This is not to deny that she is desperately trying to piece her shattered world together. Undoubtedly, it is the dominant motif in her mind. But it is a motif probably more absent from her consciousness than present, and the quest it inspires is intermittent at best. Her mental abilities have not only been severely altered, they have been diminished: that is the terrible fact one cannot deny.

And then suddenly she is agitated.

Mother! . . . didn't say as she usually . . .

Pause.

And I thought late enough or early rather first light coming so when didn't move I poked her then with shoving but she didn't even eyes or giggle when I tickled.

Pause.

What it was was not a trick as I at first had—

Pause.

Well I couldn't figure, he had never lied, tried to get her hold me couldn't it was useless. Then his face was, I had never known a face could . . . It was like a mask then like sirens it was bursting open it was him then I too joining it was useless. Can still feel what it was like when she held me.

Pause.

So then well I was on my own. He was all destroyed, had I think they say no strength for this.

Then she's silent. No expression. Stares into space.

Enter a DOCTOR and a NURSE.

DOCTOR *[warmly]*: Hello, Mrs. Stilson.

He comes over next to her. We cannot tell if she notices him or not. The NURSE, chart in hand, stands a slight distance away.

You're looking much, much better. *[He smiles and sits down next to her. He watches her for several moments, searching for signs of recognition]*

Mrs. Stilson, do you know why you're here?

MRS. STILSON: Well now well now . . .

She gives it up.

Silence.

DOCTOR: You have had an accident—

MRS. STILSON *[her words overpowering his]*:	DOCTOR *[to all intents and purposes, what he says is lost]*:
I don't trust anyone. Must get word out, send a message where I am. Like a wall between me and others. No one ever gets it right even though I tell them right. They are playing tricks on me, two sides, both not my friends, goes in goes out too fast too fast hurts do the busy I'm all right I talk right why acting all these others like I don't, what's he marking, what's he writing?	At home. Not in an airplane. It's called a stroke. This means that your brain has been injured and brain tissue destroyed, though we are not certain of the cause. You could get better, and you're certainly making progress. But it's still too soon to give any sort of exact prognosis. *[He studies her. Then he rises and marks something on his on his clipboard]*

Exit DOCTOR *and* NURSE.

MRS. STILSON: I am doing well of course!

Pause.

> [*Secretive tone*]: They still pretend they do not understand me. I believe they may be mad.

Pause.

> No they're not mad, I am mad. Today I heard it. Everything I speak is wronged. SOMETHING HAS BEEN DONE TO ME!

DOCTOR [*barely visible in the distance*]: Mrs. Stilson, can you repeat this phrase: "We live across the street from the school."

She ponders.

MRS. STILSON: "Malacats on the forturay are the kesterfats of the romancers."

Look of horror comes across her face; the doctor vanishes.

Through the screens, upstage, we see a NURSE *bringing on a tray of food.*

NURSE [*brightly*]: Okay ups-a-girl, ups-a-baby, dinnertime! Open wide now, mustn't go dribble-dribble-at's-a-way!

MRS. STILSON *screams, swings her arms in fury. In the distance, upstage, the tray of food goes flying.*

MRS. STILSON [*screaming*]: Out! Get out! Take this shit away, I don't want it! Someone get me out of here!

NURSE [*while* MRS. STILSON *continues shouting*]: Help, someone, come quick! She's talking! Good as you or me! It's a miracle! Help! Somebody! Come quick!

While MRS. STILSON *continues to scream and flail her arms,* NURSES *and* DOCTORS *rush on upstage and surround the patient we never see.*

And although MRS. STILSON *continues to scream coherently, in fact she isn't any better, no miracle has occurred. Her ability to articulate with apparent normalcy has been brought on by extreme agitation and in no way implies that she could produce these sounds again "if she only wanted"; will power has nothing to do with what we hear.*

Her language, as it must, soon slips back into jargon. She continues to flail her arms. In the background, we can see a NURSE *preparing a hypodermic.*

MRS. STILSON [*struggling*]: —flubdgy please no-mommy-callming hold-meplease to sleeEEEEP SHOOOOP shop shnoper CRROOOOOCK SNANNNNG wuduitcoldly should I gobbin flutter truly HELP ME yessis-nofun, snofun, wishes awhin dahd killminsilf if . . . could [*in the distance, we see the needle given*] OW! . . . would I but . . . [*She's becoming drowsy*] . . . awful to me him as well moas of all no cantduit . . . jusscantduit . . .

Head drops.

Into sleep she goes.

Exit DOCTORS, NURSES.

Sound of a gentle wind is heard. Lights fade to black on MRS. STILSON.

Darkness everywhere; the sound of the wind fades away.

Silence.

Lights up on AMY, *downstage right.*

Then lights up on MRS. STILSON *staring into space.*

AMY: Mrs. Stilson?

MRS. STILSON *turns toward the sound, sees* AMY.

You have had what's called a stroke.

Change of lights and panels open. Sense of terrible enclosure gone. Birds heard. We are outside now. AMY *puts a shawl around* MRS. STILSON'S *shoulders.*

AMY: Are you sure that will be enough?

MRS. STILSON: Oh yes . . . thhhankyou.

She tucks the shawl around herself.

Then AMY *guides her through the panels as if through corridors; no rush, slow gentle stroll.*

They emerge other side of stage. Warm light. AMY *takes in the view.* MRS. STILSON *appears indifferent.*

AMY: Nice to be outside, isn't it? . . . Nice view.

MRS. STILSON *[still with indifference]:* Yes indeed.

There are two chairs nearby, and they sit.

Silence for a time.

AMY: Are you feeling any better today?

But she gets no response.

Then, a moment later, MRS. STILSON *turns to* AMY; *it is as if* AMY'S *question has not even been heard.*

MRS. STILSON: The thing is . . .

But the statement trails off into nothingness.

She stares out, no expression.

AMY: Yes? What?

Long silence.

MRS. STILSON: I can't make it do it like it used to.

AMY: Yes, I know. That's because of the accident.

MRS. STILSON *[seemingly oblivious of* AMY'S *words]:* The words, they go in somelimes then out they go, I can't stop them here inside or make maybe globbidge to the tubberway or—

AMY: Emily. Emily!

MRS. STILSON *[shaken out of herself]:* . . . What?

AMY: Did you hear what you just said?

MRS. STILSON: . . . Why?

AMY *[speaking slowly]:* You must listen to what you're saying.

MRS. STILSON: Did I . . . do . . .

AMY *[nodding, smiling; clearly no reproach intended]:* Slow down. Listen to what you're saying.

Silence.

MRS. STILSON *[slower]:* The thing is . . . doing all this busy in here gets, you know with the talking it's like . . . sometimes when I hear here *[she touches her head]* . . . but when I start to . . . kind more what kind of voice should . . . it's like pfffft! *[She makes a gesture with her hand of something flying away]*

AMY *[smiling]:* Yes, I know. It's hard to find the words for what you're thinking of.

MRS. STILSON: Well yes.

Long pause.

And then these people, they keep waiting . . . And I see they're smiling and . . . they keep . . . waiting . . . *[Faint smile, helpless gesture. She stares off]*

Long silence.

AMY: Emily.

MRS. STILSON looks up.

Can you remember anything about your life . . . before the accident?

MRS. STILSON: Not sometimes, some days it goes better if I see a thing or smell . . . it . . . remembers me back, you see? And I see things that maybe they were me and maybe they were just some things you know that happens in the night when you . . . *[Struggling visibly]* have your things closed, eyes.

AMY: A dream you mean.

MRS. STILSON *[with relief]:* Yes. So I don't know for sure.

Pause.

If it was really me.

Long silence.

AMY: Your son is bringing a picture of you when you were younger. We thought you might like that.

No visible response. Long silence.

You used to fly, didn't you?

MRS. STILSON *[brightly]:* Oh yes indeed! Very much! I walked . . . out . . .

Pause.

[Softly, proudly]: I walked out on wings.

Lights fade on AMY. MRS. STILSON alone again.

Sitting here on my bed I can close my eyes shut out all that I can't do with, hearing my own talking, others, names that used to well just be

there when I wanted now all somewhere else. No control. Close my eyes
then, go to—

Sound of something flapping rapidly.

A fibrillation.

Lights become blue. Sense of weightlessness, serenity.

Here I go. No one talks here. Images coming I seem feel it feels better
this way here is how it goes: this time I am still in the middle Stilson in
the middle going out walking out wind feels good hold the wires feel
the hum down below far there they are now turn it bank it now we spin!
Looks more bad than really is, still needs good balance and those nerves
and that thing that courage thing don't fall off! . . . And now I'm out . . .
and back and . . . *[With surprise]* there's the window.

Lights have returned to normal. She is back where she started.

Amy enters.

Amy: Hello, Emily.

Mrs. Stilson: Oh, Amy! . . . Didn't hear what you was . . . coming here to
. . . Oh!

Amy: What is it?

Mrs. Stilson: Something . . . wet.

Amy: Do you know what it is?

Mrs. Stilson: Don't . . . can't say find it word.

Amy: Try. You can find it.

Mrs. Stilson: Wet . . . thing, many, both sides yes.

Amy: Can you name them? What they are? You do know what they are.

Pause.

Mrs. Stilson: . . . Tears?

Amy: That's right, very good. Those are tears. And do you know what that
means?

Mrs. Stilson: . . . Sad?

Amy: Yes, right, well done, it means . . . that you are sad.

EXPLORATIONS

Stage dark.

*In the dark, a piano heard: someone fooling around on the keyboard, brief
halting snatches of old songs emerging as the product; would constitute a
medley were the segments only longer, more cohesive. As it is, suspicion
aroused that what we hear is all the pianist can remember.*

Sound of general laughter, hubbub.

Lights rise.

What we see is a rec room, in some places clearly, in others not (the room being observed partly through the dark scrim panels).

Upstage right, an upright piano, players and friends gathered round. Doctors, therapists, nurses, attendants, patients, visitors certainly are not all seen, but those we do see come from such a group. We are in the rec room of a rehabilitation center. Some patients in wheelchairs.

The room itself has bright comfortable chairs, perhaps a card table, magazine rack, certainly a TV set. Someone now turns on the TV.

What emerges is the sound of Ella Fitzgerald in live performance. She sings scat: mellow, upbeat.

The patients and staff persuade the pianist to cease. Ella's riffs of scat cast something like a spell.

MRS. STILSON wanders through the space.

The rec room, it should be stressed, shows more detail and color than any space we've so far seen. Perhaps a vase of flowers helps to signal that MRS. STILSON's world is becoming fuller, more integrated.

Movements too seem normal, same for conversations that go on during all of this, though too softly for us to comprehend.

The music of course sets the tone. All who listen are in its thrall.

New time sense here, a languor almost. The dread MRS. STILSON felt has been replaced by an acknowledgment of her condition, though not an understanding.

In this time before she speaks, and in fact during, we observe the life of the rec room behind and around her. This is not a hospital any more, and a kind of normalcy prevails.

The sense should be conveyed of corridors leading to and from this room.

Then the music and the rec room sounds grow dim; MRS. STILSON comes forward, lost in the drifts of a thought.

MRS. STILSON *[relaxed, mellow]*: Wonder . . . what's inside of it . . . ?

Pause.

I mean, how does it work? What's inside that . . . makes it work?

Long pause. She ponders.

I mean when you . . . think about it all . . .

Pause.

And when you think that it could . . . ever have been . . . possible to . . . be another way . . .

She ponders.

But it's hard for her to keep in mind what she's been thinking of, and she has to fight the noise of the rec room, its intrusive presence. Like a novice juggler, MRS. STILSON is unable to keep outside images and inner thoughts going

simultaneously. When she's with her thoughts, the outside world fades away.
When the outside world is with her, her thoughts fade away.

But she fights her way through it, and keeps the thought in mind.

The rec room, whose noise has just increased, grows quiet.

Maybe . . . if somehow I could—*[she searches for the words that match her concept]*—get inside . . .

Pause.

Sounds of the rec room pulse louder. She fights against it. The rec room sounds diminish.

Prob'ly . . . very dark inside . . . *[She ponders; tries to picture what she's thinking]* Yes . . . twisting kind of place I bet . . . *[Ponders more]* With lots of . . . *[She searches for the proper word; finds it]* . . . passageways that . . . lead to . . . *[again, she searches for the word]*

The outside world rushes in.

PATIENT IN A WHEELCHAIR *[only barely audible]*: My foot feels sour.

An attendant puts a lap rug over the patient's limbs. Then the rec room, once again, fades away.

MRS. STILSON *[fighting on]*: . . . lead to . . . something . . . Door! Yes . . . closed off now I . . . guess possib . . . ly for good I mean . . . forever, what does that mean? *[She ponders]*

ATTENDANT: Would you like some candy?

MRS. STILSON: No.

ATTENDANT: Billy made it.

MRS. STILSON: No!

The attendant moves back into the shadows.

Where was I? *[She looks around]* Why can't they just . . . let me . . . be when I'm . . .

Lights start to change. Her world suddenly in flux. The rec room fades from view. Sounds of birds heard, dimly at first.

[aware of the change as it is occurring] . . . okay. Slipping out of . . . it and . . .

MRS. *STILSON in a different place.*

Outside now! How . . . did l do that?

AMY *[emerging from the shadows]*: Do you like this new place better?

MRS. STILSON: Oh well oh well yes, much, all . . . nice flowers here, people seem . . . more like me. Thank you.

AMY *moves back toward the shadows.*

And then I see it happen once again . . .

AMY *gone from sight.*

Amy kisses me. Puts her—what thing is it, arm! yes, arm, puts her arm around my . . .

Pause.

. . . shoulder, turns her head away so I can't . . .
Pause.
Well, it knows what she's doing. May not get much better even though
I'm here. No, I know that. I know that. No real need for her to . . .
Long pause.
Then she kisses me again.
Pause.
Walks away . . .
Pause.
Lights change again, world again in flux. Noises of the building's interior can
be heard like a Babel, only fleetingly coherent. The rec room seen dissolving.
MRS. STILSON: Where am I?
She begins to wander through a maze of passageways. The mirrors multiply
her image, create a sense of endlessness.

[Note. The following blocks of sound, which accompany her expedition, are
meant to blend and overlap in performance and, to that end, can be used in
any order and combined in any way desired, except for the last five blocks,
numbers 12–16, which must be performed in their given sequence and in a way
that is comprehensible. The sounds themselves may be live or pre-recorded;
those which are pre-recorded should emanate from all parts of the theater and
in no predictable pattern. The effect should be exhilarating and disorienting.
An adventure. With terrifying aspects to be sure. But the sense of mystery and
adventure must never be so overwhelmed by the terror that it is either lost
altogether or submerged to the point of insignificance.

Mrs. Stilson may be frightened here, but the fear does not prevent her from
exploring.

She wanders through the labyrinth of dark panels as if they were so many
doors, each door leading into yet another realm.]

BLOCK 1: It was but a few years later that Fritsch and Hitzig stimulated the
cortex of a dog with an electric current. Here at last was dramatic and
indisputable evidence that—
BLOCK 2: Would you like me to change the channel?
BLOCK 3: . . . presented, I would say, essentially similar conclusions on the
behavioral correlates of each cerebral convolution.
BLOCK 4 *[being the deep male voice, speaking slowly, enunciating carefully,*
that one hears on the speech-therapy machine known as "the language
master"]: Mother led Bud to the bed.
BLOCK 5: . . . In the laboratory then, through electrical stimulation of neu-

ral centers or excisions of areas of the brain, scientists acquired information about the organization of mental activities in the monkey, the dog, the cat, and the rat. The discovery of certain peculiar clinical pictures, reminiscent of bizarre human syndromes, proved of special interest.

BLOCK 6: Can you tell me what this object's called?

BLOCK 7: *Ella's riffs of scat, as if we were still in the rec room after all.*

BLOCK 8: One has only to glance through the writings of this period to sense the heightened excitement attendant upon these discoveries!

BLOCK 9: Possibly some diaschisis, which would of course help account for the apparent mirroring. And then, of course, we must not overlook the fact that she's left-handed.

BLOCK 10: Of course, you understand, these theories may all be wrong! *[Sound of laughter from an audience]* Any other questions? Yes, over there, in the corner.

BLOCK 11: Mrs. Stilson, this is Dr. Rogans. Dr. Rogans, this is Emily Stilson.

BLOCK 12: MALE VOICE: —definite possibility I would say of a tiny subclinical infarct in Penfield's area. Yes? Female Voice: Are you sure there is a Penfield's area? Male voice: No. *[Laughter from his audience]* Male Voice Again *[itself on the verge of laughter]*: But *something* is wrong with her! *[Raucous laughter from his audience]*

[Note. Emerging out of the laughter in Block 12, a single musical TONE. This tone increases in intensity. It should carry through Block 16 and into Mrs. Stilson's emergence from the maze of panels, helping to propel her into the realm and the memory to which this expedition has been leading.]

BLOCK 13: The controversy, of course, is that some feel it's language without thought, and others, thought without language . . .

Block 14: What it is, of course, is the symbol system. Their symbol system's shot. They can't make analogies.

Block 15: You see, it's all so unpredictable. There are no fixed posts, no clear boundaries. The victim, you could say, has been cut adrift . . .

Block 16: Ah, now you're really flying blind there!

MRS. STILSON *emerges from the maze of corridors. Sound perhaps of wind, or bells. Lights blue, sense again of weightlessness, airiness.*

MRS. STILSON *[in awe and ecstasy]*: As I see it now, the plane was flying BACKWARDS! Really, wind that strong, didn't know it could be! Yet the sky was clear, not a cloud, crystal blue, gorgeous, angels could've lived in sky like that . . . I think the cyclone must've blown in on the Andes from the sea . . .

Blue light fades. Wind gone, bells gone, musical tone is gone.

[Coming out of it] Yes . . . *[She looks around; gets her bearings]* Yes, no question, this . . . place better. *[And now she's landed]* All these people just . . . like me, I guess.

She takes in where she is, seems slightly stunned to be back where she started. Sense of wonderment apparent.

An attendant approaches.

ATTENDANT: Mrs. Stilson?

MRS. STILSON *[startled]*: Oh!

ATTENDANT: Sorry to—

MRS. STILSON: Is it . . . ?

ATTENDANT: Yes.

MRS. STILSON: Did I . . . ?

ATTENDANT: No, no need to worry. Here, I'll take you.

The ATTENDANT *guides* MRS. STILSON *to a therapy room, though, in fact, more likely (on the stage) the room assembles around her. In the room are* AMY, BILLY *(a man in his middle thirties),* MRS. TIMMINS *(elderly, in a wheelchair), and* MR. BROWNSTEIN *(also elderly and in a wheelchair).*

The attendant leaves.

AMY: Well! Now that we're all here on this lovely afternoon, I thought that maybe—

BILLY: She looks really good.

AMY: What?

BILLY: This new lady here, can't remember what her name is, no bother, anyhow, she looks really nice all dressed like this, an' I jus' wanna extent a nice welcome here on behalf o' all of us.

The other patients mumble their assent.

AMY: Well, that is very nice, Billy, very nice. Can any of the rest of you remember this woman's name?

BILLY: I seen her I think when it is, yesterday, how's that?

AMY: Very good, that's right, you met her for the first time yesterday. Now, can any of you remember her name?

BILLY: Dolores.

AMY *[laughing slightly]*: No, not Dolores.

MR. BROWNSTEIN: She vas, I caught sight ya know, jussaminute, flahtied or vhat, vhere, midda *[he hums a note]*

AMY: Music.

MR. BROWNSTEIN: Yeah right goodgirlie right she vas lissning, I caught slight, saw her vooding bockstond tipping-n-topping de foot vas jussnow like dis. *[He starts to stamp his foot]*

AMY: Mrs. Stilson, were you inside listening to some music just now?

MRS. STILSON: Well . . .

Pause.

[Very fast]: Well now I was yes in the what in-the-in-the where the—

AMY *[cheerfully]:* Sssssllllow dowwwwwn.

The other patients laugh; MRS. TIMMINS softly echoes the phrase "slow down."

[Speaking very slowly]: Listen to yourself talking.

MRS. STILSON *[speaking slowly]:* Well yes, I was . . . listening and it was it was going in . . . good I think, I'd say, very good yes I liked it very nice it made it very nice inside.

AMY: Well, good.

MRS. TIMMINS: Applawdgia!

AMY: Ah, Mrs. Timmins! You heard the music, too?

MRS. TIMMINS *[with a laugh]:* Ohshorrrrrrn. Yossssso, TV.

AMY: Well, good for you! Anyway, I'd like you all to know that this new person in our group is named Mrs. Stilson.

MR. BROWNSTEIN: Sssssstaa-illllllssssim.

AMY: Right! Well done, Mr. Brownstein!

MR. BROWNSTEIN *[laughing proudly]:* It's vurktiddiDINGobitch!

AMY: That's right it's working, I told you it would.

BILLY: Hey! Wait, hold on here-jus' remembered!

AMY: What's that, Billy?

BILLY: You've been holdin' out pay up where is it?

AMY: Where . . . is what?

BILLY: Where is for all what I did all that time labor which you—don't kid me, I see you grinning back there ate up *[he makes munching sounds]* so where is it, where's the loot?

AMY: For the cheesecake.

BILLY: That's right you know it for the cheesecape, own recipe, extra-special, pay up.

AMY *[to MRS. STILSON]:* Billy is a terrific cook.

MRS. STILSON *[delighted]:* Oh!

BILLY: Well used t' be, not now much what they say, anyhow, hah-hah! see? look, laughing, giggles, tries t' hide it, she knows she knows, scoundrel, thief, can't sleep nights can you, people give their arms whatnots recipe like that one is. Cheapskate. Come on fork over hand it over, don't be chief.

AMY: . . . What?

BILLY: Don't be chief.

Pause.

You know, when someone don' pay, you say he's chief.

AMY [*warmly, nearly laughing*]: Billy, you're not listening.

BILLY: Okay not the word not the right word what's the word? I'll take any help you can give me. [*He laughs*]

AMY: Cheap.

BILLY: That's it that's the word that's what you are, from now on I'm gonna sell my recipes somewheres else.

AMY: Billy, say cheap.

He sighs mightily.

BILLY: . . . Chief.

Her expression tells him everything.

Not right okay, try again this thing we can, what's its, lessee okay here we go CHARF! Nope. Not right. Ya know really, this could take all day.

AMY: Well then, the sooner you do it, the sooner we can go on to what I've planned.

BILLY: You've got somethin' planned? You've never got somethin' planned.

AMY: I've *always* got something planned.

BILLY: Oh come on don' gimme that, you're jus' tryin' to impress this new lady, really nice new lady, Mrs. . . .

AMY: Stilson.

BILLY: Yeah her, you're jus' tryin'—what's that word again?

AMY: Cheap.

BILLY: Cheap right okay lessee now—

AMY: Billy! You just said it!

BILLY: Did I? Good. Then maybe we can go on to somethin' else, such as when you're gonna fork over for the cheesecake, I could be a rich man now.

AMY: Billy, I never made the cheesecake.

BILLY: I'll bet you've gone sold the recipe to all the stores the whatnot everywhere fancy bigdeal places made a fortune, gonna retire any day t' your farm in New Jersey.

AMY: I don't have a farm in New Jersey, you have a farm in New Jersey!

BILLY: Oh? Then what were you doin' on my farm then?

AMY: I wasn't on your farm, Billy, I've been here!

[BILLY *starts arguing about something incomprehensible and seemingly unrelated to farm life, the argument consisting mostly of the recitation of a convoluted string of numbers;* AMY *cuts him short before he goes too far astray*]: Billy, cheap, say cheap!

Long silence.

BILLY [*simply and without effort*]: Cheap.

AMY *cheers.*

[*Overjoyed*]: Cheap!—Cheap-cheap-cheap-cheap-cheap!

MR. BROWNSTEIN: I vas hoping you could polsya and git vid mustard all
    dis out of dis you gottit right good I say hutchit and congratulupsy!
AMY: Congratulations.
MR. BROWNSTEIN: Yeah right dassit goodgirlie, phhhhew! fin'lly!
Lights fade to black all around MRS. STILSON. *Nothing seen but her.*
Silence for a time.
MRS. STILSON: What it was . . . how I heard it how I said it not the same,
    you would think so but it's not. Sometimes . . . well it just goes in so fast,
    in-and-out all the sounds. I know they mean
Pause.

> I mean I know they're . . . well like with me, helping, as their at their in
> their best way knowing how I guess they practice all the time so I'd say
> must be good or even better, helps me get the dark out just by going you
> know sssslowww and thinking smiling . . . it's not easy.

Pause.

> Sometimes . . . how can . . . well it's just I think these death things, end
> it, stuff like sort of may be better not to listen anything no more at all or
> trying even talking cause what good's it, I'm so far away! Well it's crazy
> I don't mean it I don't think, still it's just like clouds that you can't push
> through. Still you do it, still you try to. I can't hear things same as others
> say them.

Pause.

> So the death thing, it comes in, I don't ask it, it just comes in, plays
> around in there, I can't get it out till it's ready, goes out on its own. Same I
> guess for coming. I don't open up the door.

Silence.
Lights up on a chair, small table. On the table, a cassette recorder.
MRS. STILSON *goes to the chair. Sits. Stares at the recorder.*
A few moments later, BILLY *and a* DOCTOR *enter.*
BILLY: Oh, I'm sorry, I didn't know you was in . . . here or . . .
MRS. STILSON: Dr. Freedman said I could . . . use room and his . . . this . . .
    [She gestures toward the recorder]
DOCTOR: No problem, we'll use another room.
He smiles. Exit BILLY *and* DOCTOR.
MRS. STILSON *turns back to the machine. Stares at it. Then she reaches out,*
    presses a button.
DOCTOR'S VOICE *[from cassette recorder]:* All right, essentially, a stroke
    occurs when there's a stoppage . . . When blood flow ceases in one part
    of the brain . . . And that brain can no longer get oxygen . . . And sub-
    sequently dies. Okay? Now, depending upon which part of the brain

is affected by the stroke, you'll see differences in symptoms. Now what you've had is a left cerebral infarction. Oh, by the way, you're doing much, much better. We were very worried when you first arrived . . .

Silence.

She clicks off the recording machine. Does nothing, stares at nothing. Then she reaches out and pushes the rewind button. The machine rewinds to start of tape. Stops automatically. She stares at the machine. Deep breath. Reaches out again. Presses the playback button.

DOCTOR'S VOICE: All right, essentially, a stroke occurs when there's a stoppage . . . When blood flow ceases in one part of the brain . . . And that brain can no long—

She shuts it off.

Stares into space.

Silence.

MRS. STILSON *with* AMY *sitting next to her on another chair.*

MRS. STILSON *[still staring into space]:* "Memory" . . .

Pause.

AMY: Yes, come on, "memory"

No response.

   Anything.

Still no response.

   [Warmly]: Oh, come on, I bet there are lots of things you can talk about . . . You've been going out a lot lately . . . With your son . . . With your niece . . .

Pause.

   What about Rhinebeck? Tell me about Rhinebeck.

Pause.

MRS. STILSON: On . . . Saturday . . . *[She ponders]* On . . . Sunday my . . . son . . . *[Ponders again]* On Saturday my son . . . took me to see them out at Rhinebeck.

AMY: See what?

MRS. STILSON: What I used to . . . fly in.

AMY: Can you think of the word?

MRS. STILSON: . . . What word?

AMY: For what you used to fly in.

Long pause.

MRS. STILSON: Planes!

AMY: Very good!

MRS. STILSON: Old . . . planes.

AMY: That is very good. Really!

MRS. STILSON: I sat . . . inside one of them. He said it was like the kind I used to . . . fly in and walk . . . out on wings in. I couldn't believe I could have ever done this.

Pause.

But he said I did, I had. He was very . . . proud.

Pause.

Then . . . I saw my hand was pushing on this . . . stick . . . Then my hand was . . . pulling. Well I hadn't you know asked my hand to do this, it just went and did it on its own. So I said okay Emily, if this is how it wants to do it you just sit back here and watch . . . But . . . my head, it was really . . . hurting bad. And I was up here both . . . sides, you know . . .

AMY: Crying.

MRS. STILSON [*with effort*]: Yeah.

Long pause.

And then all at once—it remembered everything!

Long pause.

But now it doesn't.

Silence.

Faint sound of wind. Hint of bells.

The screens open.

We are outside. Sense of distance, openness. All feeling of constraint is gone.

AMY helps MRS. STILSON into an overcoat; AMY is in an overcoat already.

AMY: Are you sure you'll be warm enough?

MRS. STILSON: Oh yes . . .

And they start to walk—a leisurely stroll through a park or meadow, sense of whiteness everywhere. They head toward a bench with snow on its slats. The sound of wind grows stronger.

Faint sound of an airplane overhead, the sound quickly disappearing.

MRS. STILSON: This is winter, isn't it?

AMY: Yes.

MRS. STILSON: That was just a guess, you know.

AMY [*with a warm, easy laugh*]: Well, it was a good one, keep it up!

MRS. STILSON laughs.

AMY stops by the bench.

Do you know what this is called?

MRS. STILSON: Bench!

AMY: Very good! No, I mean what's on top of it.

No response.

What I'm brushing off . . .
Still no response.
　　What's falling from the sky . . .
Long silence.
MRS. STILSON: Where do you get names from?
AMY: I? From in here, same as you.
MRS. STILSON: Do you know how you do it?
AMY: No.
MRS. STILSON: Then how am I supposed . . . to learn?
AMY *[softly]:* I don't really know.
MRS. STILSON stares at AMY. Then she points at her and laughs.
At first, AMY doesn't understand. Then she does.
And then both of them are laughing.
MRS. STILSON: Look. You see? *[She scoops some snow off the bench]* If I
　　pick this . . . stuff up in my hand, then . . . I know its name. I didn't have
　　to pick it up to know . . . what it *was.*
AMY: No . . .
MRS. STILSON: But to find its name . . . *[She stares at what is in her hand]* I
　　had to pick it up.
AMY: What's its name?
MRS. STILSON: Snow. It's really nuts, isn't it!
AMY: It's peculiar!
They laugh.
Then, laughter gone, they sit; stare out.
Silence for a time.
MRS. STILSON: A strange thing happened to me . . .
Pause.
　　I think last night.
AMY: Can you remember it?
MRS. STILSON: Perfectly.
AMY: Ah!
MRS. STILSON: I think it may have been . . . you know, when you sleep . . .
AMY: A dream.
MRS. STILSON: Yes, one of those, but I'm not . . . sure that it was . . . that.
Pause. Then she notices the snow in her hand.
　　Is it all right if I . . . eat this?
AMY: Yes! We used to make a ball of it, then pour maple syrup on top. Did
　　you ever do that?
MRS. STILSON: I don't know.
Pause.

No, I remember—I did!

She tastes the snow. Smiles.

After a time, the smile vanishes.

She turns back to AMY.

Who was that man yesterday?

AMY: What man?

MRS. STILSON: In our group. He seemed all right.

AMY: Oh, that was last week.

MRS. STILSON: I thought for sure he was all right! I thought he was maybe, you know, a doctor.

AMY: Yes, I know.

MRS. STILSON *[searching her memory]:* And you asked him to show you where his . . . hand was.

AMY: And he knew.

MRS. STILSON: That's right, he raised his hand, he knew. So I thought, why is Amy joking?

She ponders.

Then you asked him . . . *[She tries to remember]* . . . where . . . *[She turns to AMY]*

AMY: His elbow was.

MRS. STILSON: Yes! And he . . . *[she struggles to find the word]*

AMY *[helping]:* Pointed

MRS. STILSON *[at the same time]:* Pointed! to . . . *[But the struggle's getting harder]*

AMY: The corner of the room.

MRS. STILSON: Yes.

Pause.

[Softly]: That was very . . . scary.

AMY: Yes.

MRS. STILSON stares into space.

Silence.

What is it that happened to you last night?

MRS. STILSON: Oh yes! Well, this . . . *person* . . . came into my room. I couldn't tell if it was a man or woman or . . . young or old. I was in my bed and it came. Didn't seem to have to walk just . . . came over to my . . . bed and . . . smiled at where I was.

Pause.

And then it said . . . *[In a whisper]* "Emily . . . we're glad you changed your mind."

Pause.

And then . . . it turned and left.

AMY: Was it a doctor? [MRS. STILSON *shakes her head*] One of the staff?
[MRS. STILSON *shakes her head*] How do you know?

MRS. STILSON: I just know.

Pause.

Then . . . I left my body.

AMY: *What?*

MRS. STILSON [*with great excitement*]: I was on the . . . what's the name
over me—

AMY: Ceiling?

MRS. STILSON: Yes! I was floating like a . . .

AMY: Cloud?

MRS. STILSON *shakes her head.*

Bird?

MRS. STILSON: Yes, up there at the—[*she searches for the word; finds it*]—
ceiling, and I looked down and I was still there in my bed! Wasn't even
scared, which you'd think I would be . . . And I thought, wow! this is the
life isn't it?

Sound of wind.

Lights begin to change.

AMY *recedes into the darkness.*

It comes now without my asking . . . Amy is still beside me but I am
somewhere else. I'm not scared. It has taken me, and it's clear again.
Something is about to happen.

Pause.

AMY *now completely gone.*

MRS. STILSON *in a narrow spot of light, darkness all around.*

I am in a plane, a Curtiss Jenny, and it's night. Winter. Snow is falling.
Feel the tremble of the wings! How I used to walk out on them! Could I
have really done—. . . Yes. What I'd do, I'd strap myself with a tether to
the stays, couldn't see the tether from below, then out I'd climb! Oh my,
but it was wonderful! I could feel the wind! shut my eyes, all alone—
FEEL THE SOARING!

The wind grows stronger. Then the wind dies away. Silence.

She notices the change.

MRS. STILSON: But this is in another time. Where I've been also . . . It is
night and no one else is in the plane. Is it . . . remembering?

Pause.

No . . . No, I'm simply there again!

Pause.

And I'm lost . . . I am lost, completely lost, have to get to . . . somewhere, Omaha I think. The radio is out, or rather for some reason picks up only Bucharest. Clouds all around, no stars only snow, don't possess a clue to where I am, flying blind, soon be out of gas . . . And then the clouds open up a bit, just a bit, and lights appear below, faint, a hint, like torches. Down I drop! heart pounding with relief, with joy, hoping for a landing place, I'll take anything—a field, a street, and down I drop! No place to land . . . It's a town but the smallest—one tiny street is all, three street lamps, no one on the street, all deserted . . . just a street and some faint light in the middle of darkness. Nothing. Still, down I go! Maybe I can find a name on a railroad station, find out where I am! . . . But I see nothing I can read . . . So I begin to circle, though I know I'm wasting fuel and I'll crash if I keep this up! But somehow, I just can't tear myself away! Though I know I should pull back on the stick, get the nose up, head north into darkness—Omaha must be north! But no, I keep circling this one small silly street in this one small town . . . I'm scared to leave it, that's what, as if I guess once away from it I'll be inside something empty, black, and endless . . .

Pause.

So I keep circling—madness! but I love it, what I see below! And I just can't bring myself to give it up, it's that simple—just can't bring myself to give it up!

Pause.

Then I know I have to. It's a luxury I can't afford. Fuel is running low, almost gone, may be too late anyway, so—

I pull the nose up, kick the rudder, bank, and head out into darkness all in terror! GOD, BUT IT TAKES EFFORT! JUST DON'T WANT TO DO IT! . . . But I do.

Pause.

[Suddenly calm]: Actually, odd thing, once I did, broke free, got into the dark, found I wasn't even scared . . . Or was I? *[Slight laugh]* Can't remember . . . Wonder where that town was . . . ?

Pause.

Got to Omaha all right.

Pause.

Was it Omaha . . . ?

Pause.

Yes, I think so . . . Yes, Topeka, that was it!

Pause.

God, but it was wonderful! *[Slight laugh]* Awful scary sometimes, though!

AMY *seen in the distance.*

AMY: Emily! Emily, are you all right!

Sudden, sharp, terrifying flapping sound.

MRS. STILSON *gasps.*

AMY *disappears.*

MRS. STILSON *[rapidly]:* Around! There here spins saw it rumple chumps and jumps outgoes inside up and . . . takes it, gives it, okay . . .

Pause.

[Easier]: Touch her for me, would you?

Pause.

[Even easier]: Oh my, yes, and here it goes then out . . . there I think on . . . wings? Yes . . .

Pause.

[Softly, faint smile]: Thank you.

No trace of terror.

Music. Hint of bells.

Lights to black.

Silence.

The Sandbox

℘

Edward Albee

INTRODUCTION

Edward Albee's *The Sandbox* is a remarkable work for its concise and intense exploration of a vital issue, aging. Foreshadowing a longer work, *The American Dream,* the short piece details a broad canvas that reveals a satirical view of American society with its substitution of artificial values for real ones, especially regarding the corruption of relationships within the family. Dissecting marriage and parent-child interactions, Albee lays bare once more the conflict that intrigued Shakespeare centuries before. *King Lear* presents the tragic consequences of the clash through the incantation of verse, captivating its audience and drawing it into its circumscribed world. With all due respect to the science of gerontology, the drama transmits the truth of aging with a force and totality that cannot be duplicated. Albee creates a variation on the theme by focusing on a married couple, Mommy and Daddy, as the errant younger generation. And he makes of the couple a loveless, hypocritical duo maintaining a union simply to satisfy selfish interests. In *The Sandbox* their sole act is to keep a final watch over Grandma, Mommy's eighty-six-year-old mother, whom they regard as a nuisance and long to be rid of. In the process, they trade vacuous remarks that expose the fiction of their marriage. The emasculated head of the family is clearly under his wife's domination as he declines to offer any opinions, repeating, "Whatever you say, Mommy" (10). Hesitantly, he makes an attempt at communication, "Shall we talk to each other?" and is instantly rebuffed with, "Well, you can talk, if you want to . . . if you can think of anything to say . . . if you can think of anything new"(12). Daddy retreats. The painful exchanges indicate the couple's lack of esteem for one another. As their marriage is a sham, their love counterfeit, so too is their grief for Grandma as they celebrate the social rituals associated with dying and burial. In conclusion, Mommy echoes the usual comment on how well the corpse looks and departs with Daddy, who expresses no compassion for Grandma since, as he has told Mommy, "She's *your* mother, not mine" (10).

And it is precisely that mother in an aged body that takes center stage in *The Sandbox*. Despite the attention paid to the relationship between Mommy and Daddy, Grandma is the focal point of the play. Distanced from one another, the couple abandons Grandma as well. They convey the action in a single visual image, carrying the aged woman's taut frame across the bare stage—the set represents a lonely beach—and depositing her in a child's sandbox, a symbolic grave. The action satirizes the practice of transferring the elderly from their home to an institution to live out their final years. The sight of Grandma as she is borne aloft is startling. Rigid in body, with legs drawn up, feet off the ground, she appears as some subhuman oddity. Only an expression of puzzlement and fear on her face gives evidence of a living being. Apparently incapable of speech, she cries unintelligibly. The image sets the tone for the play's duration. We approach the realm of the absurd, at least in mood, as Albee dispenses with linear plot, creates a language charged with irony, and works with visual and aural effects enhanced by background music and lights.

The most striking theatrical device is that of the monologue as Grandma, mute before her daughter and son-in-law, suddenly finds her voice as well as a confidant in the audience, whom she addresses virtually without interruption. She proceeds to reconstruct her past in a narration that, for all its brevity, is a brilliant bit of stagecraft: it establishes the character of Grandma in word and in action and, perhaps more significantly, it functions to point up a major problem in aging—the question of changing identity likely to occur with changes in social roles.[1] From Grandma the audience learns that she was a farmer's bride at seventeen, a widow and single mother at thirty. In each capacity she was a vital force in the lives of those who depended on her. In her later years, when she no longer filled the needs of husband and child, she experienced a reversal of roles that left her dependent on her daughter who had become the wife of Daddy for no other reason, as Grandma tells it, than for "money, money, money" (14). The couple took Grandma off the farm and relocated her under the stove of their big townhouse, providing her with an old army blanket, her very own dish, and a new identity—that of a dog. One may dismiss her account as a touch of the bitter humor with which absurdist dramatists frequently infuse their work. Even so, the underlying seriousness of her language demands our attention. The audience is made vividly aware of the degree to which the aged woman has been discarded. Her depressed condition brings to mind the plight of the impoverished elderly who often rely for sustenance on dog food.

The character of Grandma is drawn with infinite warmth and depth. In her interaction with her daughter and son-in-law, she assumes the type of a spoiled child; she wails and tosses sand at them. Her behavior suits the stereotype of the aged who revert to childhood. Yet the hostility that prompts Grandma's actions arises from singular experience. She repeatedly punctures the negative images with which aging is fixed and proves that the perception reflects a cultural view as much as a personal and psychological one. As with disability, aging is given a value consonant with the attributes that society attaches to it. Where the notion prevails that helplessness and dependency are synonymous with old age, many elderly themselves succumb to the stereotype and doubt their own abilities, adding credence to the distorted view.

Society's signification of the aged often results in limited contact between the generations. Grandma's vitality leads her to form the one significant contact in the piece, with the Young Man, a character who assumes a dual role. He is at once a fledgling actor and the Angel of Death. In his human identity, he could be any young person in need of support from an elder with whom he establishes a sincere bond. As a good-looking specimen in a swimsuit, he performs calisthenics on the beach under Grandma's admiring gaze. He similarly gains her approval for his developing acting skills. That Grandma is attracted to him as a sexual being demonstrates the truth that, contrary to the popular conviction, aging individuals maintain romantic and sexual interests. Grandma's reaction to the Young Man is best expressed in a line from *The American Dream* where she responds to the same character, "Yup . . . yup. You know, if I were about a hundred and fifty years younger I could go for you" (106). In her tender moments, Grandma offers the young man pure affection, addressing him in endearing terms. Her love and approval at such instances is that of a nurturing parent, and she strikes a responsive chord in him, catalyzing his transfiguration into the Angel of Death. Soothing her with a kiss and placing his hands on hers, he eases her way toward eternity.

In envisioning the character of Grandma and foregrounding her conflict with Mommy and Daddy, Albee magnifies the deleterious consequences of false values as they tear asunder all meaningful human contact, jolting the audience with a piercing vision, all the more powerful for its condensation. Albee exposes the ugliness of hypocrisy and pretence in nullifying loving relationships. And he illustrates the brutality with which man abandons those with whom he shares a common humanity. Certainly there is ample evidence of such desertion in the fourteen minutes of stage time to leave the audience chilled. Nevertheless, the figure of Grandma carries the seed of redemption. As her life ebbs with the receding tide, she affirms the authenticity that destroys falseness and embodies the love that defeats rejection. For all the ugliness that has emerged from the playwright's dissection of spurious contacts, the final moments of union between the aged woman and the youth at her side are filled with beauty and peace that surpasses all. On a tranquil beach, edged by life-giving waters, mankind is renewed yet again. The dramatist has given new life to the woman, recreating her in the brief moments of stage time. The spectator that never knew the living being becomes familiar with her spirited, endearing nature. When the moment of death comes, abruptly as often in life, the audience that has been taken unawares by Grandma's magnetism suddenly knows the pain of loss. Written a long time ago in Edward Albee's career, *The Sandbox* remains a miniature gem, conveying as forcefully as ever the truth of its vision and the worth and dignity of the human spirit that inspired it.

Notes

1. For a discussion of changing identities and their significance among an aging population, see the Introduction to *Literature and Aging: An Anthology,* ed. Martin Kohn, Carol Donley, and Delese Wear (Kent, Ohio: Kent State Univ. Press, 1992).

Works Cited

Albee, Edward. *An American Dream: Two Plays by Edward Albee.* New York: Penguin, 1961.
———. *The Sandbox: Two Plays by Edward Albee.* New York: New American Library, 1960.
Kohn, Martin, Carol Donley, and Delease Wear. Introduction. *Literature and Aging: An Anthology.* Kent, Ohio: Kent State Univ. Press, 1992. 3–4.

THE SANDBOX

By Edward Albee

A Brief Play, in Memory of My Grandmother (1876–1959)

The Players:

The Young Man	25	A good-looking, well-built boy in a bathing suit
Mommy	55	A well-dressed, imposing woman.
Daddy	60	A small man; gray, thin.
Grandma	86	A tiny wizened woman with bright eyes

| THE MUSICIAN | No particular age, but young would be nice |

NOTE:

When, in the course of the play, MOMMY and DADDY call each other by these names, there should be no suggestion of regionalism. These names are of empty affection and point up the pre-senility and vacuity of their characters.

THE SCENE:

A bare stage, with only the following: Near the footlights, far stage-right, two simple chairs set side by side facing the audience; near the footlights, far stage-left, a chair facing stage-right with a music stand before it; farther back, and stage-center, slightly elevated and raked, a large child's sandbox with a toy pail and shovel; the background is the sky, which alters from brightest day to deepest night.

At the beginning, it is brightest day; the YOUNG MAN is alone on stage, to the rear of the sandbox, and to one side. He is doing calisthenics; he does calisthenics until quite at the very end of the play. These calisthenics, employing the arms only, should suggest the beating and fluttering of wings. The YOUNG MAN is, after all, the Angel of Death.

MOMMY *and* DADDY *enter from stage-left,* MOMMY *first.*
MOMMY: *(Motioning to* DADDY*)* Well, here we are; this is the beach.
DADDY: *(Whining)* I'm cold.
MOMMY: *(Dismissing him with a little laugh)* Don't be silly; it's as warm as toast. Look at that nice young man over there: *he* doesn't think it's cold. *(Waves to the* YOUNG MAN*)* Hello.
YOUNG MAN: *(With an endearing smile)* Hi!
MOMMY: *(Looking about)* This will do perfectly . . . don't you think so, Daddy? There's sand there . . . and the water beyond. What do you think, Daddy?
DADDY: *(Vaguely)* Whatever you say, Mommy.
MOMMY: *(With the same little laugh)* Well, of course . . . whatever I say. Then, it's settled, is it?
DADDY: *(Shrugs)* She's *your* mother, not mine.
MOMMY: I know she's my mother. What do you take me for? *(A pause)* All right, now; let's get on with it. *(She shouts into the wings, stage-left)* You! Out there! You can come in now.

(The MUSICIAN *enters, seats himself in the chair, stage-left. places music on the music stand, is ready to play.* MOMMY *nods approvingly)*

MOMMY: Very nice; very nice. Are you ready, Daddy? Let's go get Grandma.

DADDY: Whatever you say, Mommy.

MOMMY: *(Leading the way out, stage-left)* Of course, whatever I say. *(To the* MUSICIAN*)* You can begin now.

(The MUSICIAN *begins playing;* MOMMY *and* DADDY *exit; the* MUSICIAN, *all the while playing, nods to the* YOUNG MAN*)*

YOUNG MAN: *(With the same endearing smile)* Hi!

(After a moment, MOMMY *and* DADDY *re-enter, carrying* GRANDMA. *She is borne in by their hands under her armpits; she is quite rigid; her legs are drawn up; her feet do not touch the ground; the expression on her ancient face is that of puzzlement and fear)*

DADDY: Where do we put her?

MOMMY: *(The same little laugh)* Wherever I say, of course. Let me see . . . well . . . all right, over there . . . in the sandbox. *(Pause)* Well, what are you waiting for, Daddy? . . . The sandbox!

(Together they carry GRANDMA *over to the sandbox and more or less dump her in)*

GRANDMA: *(Righting herself to a sitting position; her voice a cross between a baby's laugh and cry)* Ahhhhhh! Graaaaa!

DADDY: *(Dusting himself)* What do we do now?

MOMMY: *(To the* MUSICIAN*)* You can stop now.

(The MUSICIAN *Stops)*

(Back to DADDY*)* What do you mean, what do we do now? We go over there and sit down, of course. *(To the* YOUNG MAN*)* Hello there.

YOUNG MAN: *(Again smiling)* Hi!

*(*MOMMY *and* DADDY *move to the chairs, stage-right, and sit down. A pause)*

GRANDMA: *(Same as before)* Ahhhhhh! Ah-haaaaaa! Graaaaaa!

DADDY: Do you think . . . do you think she's . . . comfortable?

MOMMY: *(Impatiently)* How would I know?

DADDY: *(Pause)* What do we do now?

MOMMY: *(As if remembering)* We . . . wait. We . . . sit here . . . and we wait . . . that's what we do.

DADDY: *(After a pause)* Shall we talk to each other?

MOMMY: *(With that little laugh; picking something off her dress)* Well, *you* can talk, if you want to . . . if you can think of anything to *say* . . . if you can think of anything *new*.

DADDY: *(Thinks)* No . . . I suppose not.

MOMMY: *(With a triumphant laugh)* Of course not!

GRANDMA: *(Banging a toy shovel against the pail)* Haaaaaa! Ah-haaaaaa!

MOMMY: *(Out over the audience)* Be quiet, Grandma . . . just be quiet, and wait.

(GRANDMA *throws a shovelful of sand at* MOMMY)

MOMMY: *(Still out over the audience)* She's throwing sand at me! You stop that, Grandma; you stop throwing sand at Mommy! *(To* DADDY) She's throwing sand at me.

(DADDY *looks around at* GRANDMA, *who screams at him*)

GRANDMA: GRAAAAAA!

MOMMY: Don't look at her. Just . . . sit here . . . be very still . . . and wait. *(To the* MUSICIAN) You . . . uh . . . you go ahead and do whatever it is you do.

(The MUSICIAN *plays)*

(MOMMY *and* DADDY *are fixed, staring out beyond the audience.* GRANDMA *looks at them, looks at the* MUSICIAN, *looks at the sand box, throws down the shovel)*

GRANDMA: Ah-haaaaaa! Graaaaaa! *(Looks for reaction; gets none. Now . . . directly to the audience)* Honestly! What a way to treat an old woman! Drag her out of the house . . . stick her in a car . . . bring her out here from the city . . . dump her in a pile of sand . . . and leave her here to set. I'm eighty-six years old! I was married when I was seventeen. To a farmer. He died when I was thirty. *(To the* MUSICIAN) Will you stop that, please?

(The MUSICIAN *stops playing)*

I'm a feeble old woman . . . how do you expect anybody to hear me over that peep! peep! peep! *(To herself)* There's no respect around here. *(To the* YOUNG MAN) There's no respect around here!

YOUNG MAN: *(Same smile)* Hi!

GRANDMA: *(After a pause, a mild double-take, continues, to the audience)* My husband died when I was thirty *(indicates* MOMMY) , and I had to raise that big cow over there all by my lonesome. You can imagine what *that was like.* Lordy! *(To the* YOUNG MAN) Where'd they get *you?*

YOUNG MAN: Oh . . . I've been around for a while.

GRANDMA: I'll bet you have! Heh, heh, heh. Will you look at you!

YOUNG MAN: *(Flexing his muscles)* Isn't that something? *(Continues his calisthenics)*

GRANDMA: Boy, oh boy; I'll say. Pretty good.

YOUNG MAN: *(Sweetly)* I'll say.

GRANDMA: Where ya from?

YOUNG MAN: Southern California.

GRANDMA: *(Nodding)* Figgers; figgers. What's your name, honey?

YOUNG MAN: I don't know. . . .

GRANDMA: *(To the audience)* Bright, too!

YOUNG MAN: I mean . . . I mean, they haven't given me one yet . . . the studio. . . .

GRANDMA: *(Giving him the once-over)* You don't say . . . you don't say. Well . . . uh, I've got to talk some more . . . don't you go 'way.

YOUNG MAN: Oh, no.

GRANDMA: *(Turning her attention back to the audience)* Fine; fine. *(Then, once more, back to the* YOUNG MAN*)* You're . . . you're an actor, hunh?

YOUNG MAN: *(Beaming)* Yes. I am.

GRANDMA: *(To the audience again; shrugs)* I'm smart that way. *Anyhow,* I had to raise . . . *that* over there all by my lonesome; and what's next to her there . . . that's what she married. Rich? I tell you . . . money, money, money. They took me off the *farm* . . . which was real decent of them . . . and they moved me into the big town house with *them* . . . fixed a nice place for me under the stove . . . gave me an army blanket . . . and my own dish . . . my very own dish! So, what have I got to complain about? Nothing of course. I'm not complaining. *(She looks up at the sky, shouts to someone off stage)* Shouldn't it be getting dark now, dear?

(The lights dim; night comes on. The MUSICIAN *begins to play; it becomes deepest night. There are spots on all the players, including the* YOUNG MAN *who is, of course, continuing his calisthenics)*

DADDY: *(Stirring)* It's nighttime

MOMMY: Shhh. Be still . . . wait.

DADDY: *(Whining)* It's so hot.

MOMMY: Shhhhhh. Be still . . . wait.

GRANDMA: *(To herself)* That's better. Night. *(To the* MUSICIAN*)* Honey, do you play all through this part?

(The MUSICIAN *nods)*

Well, keep it nice and soft; that's a good boy.

(The MUSICIAN *nods again; plays softly)*

That's nice.

(There is an off-stage rumble)

DADDY: *(Starting)* What was that?

MOMMY: *(Beginning to weep)* It was nothing.

DADDY: It was . . . it was . . . thunder . . . or a wave breaking . . . or something.

MOMMY: *(Whispering, through her tears)* It was an off-stage rumble . . . and you know what *that* means. . . .

DADDY: I forget. . . .

MOMMY: *(Barely able to talk)* It means the time has come for poor
     Grandma . . . and I can't bear it!
DADDY: *(Vacantly)* I . . . I suppose you've got to be brave.
GRANDMA: *(Mocking)* That's right, kid; be brave. You'll bear up; you'll get
     over it.
(Another off-stage rumble . . . louder)
MOMMY: Ohhhhhhhhhh . . . poor Grandma . . . poor Grandma. . . .
GRANDMA: *(To* MOMMY*)* I'm fine! I'm all right! It hasn't happened yet!
(A violent off-stage rumble. All the lights go out, save the spot on the YOUNG
     MAN; *the* MUSICIAN *stops playing)*
MOMMY: Ohhhhhhhhhh. . . . Ohhhhhhhhhh. . . .
(Silence)
GRANDMA: Don't put the lights up yet . . . I'm not ready; I'm not quite
     ready. *(Silence)*
All right, dear . . . I'm about done.
(The lights come up again, to brightest day; the MUSICIAN *begins to play.*
     GRANDMA *is discovered, still in the sandbox, lying on her side propped up*
     on an elbow, half covered, busily shoveling sand over herself)
GRANDMA: *(Muttering)* I don't know how I'm supposed to do anything
     with this goddam toy shovel. . . .
DADDY: Mommy! It's daylight!
MOMMY: *(Brightly)* So it is! Well! Our long night is over. We must put away
     our tears, take off our mourning . . . and face the future. It's our duty.
GRANDMA: *(Still shoveling; mimicking)* . . . take off our mourning . . . face
     the future. . . . Lordy!
*(*MOMMY *and* DADDY *rise, stretch.* MOMMY *waves to the* YOUNG MAN*)*
YOUNG MAN: *(With that smile)* Hi!
*(*GRANDMA *plays dead. (!)* MOMMY *and* DADDY *go over to look at her; she*
     is a little more than half buried in the sand; the toy shovel is in her hands,
     which are crossed on her breast)
MOMMY: *(Before the sandbox; shaking her head)* Lovely! It's . . . it's hard to
     be sad . . . she looks . . . so happy. *(With pride and conviction)* It pays to
     do things well. *(To the* MUSICIAN*)* All right, you can stop now, if you
     want to. I mean, stay around for a swim, or something; it's all right with
     us. *(She sighs heavily)* Well, Daddy . . . off we go.
DADDY: Brave Mommy!
MOMMY: Brave Daddy!
(They exit stage-left)
GRANDMA: *(After they leave; lying quite still)* It pays to do things well. . . .
     Boy, oh Boy! *(She tries to sit up)* . . . well, kids . . . *(but she finds she can't)*
     . . . I . . . I can't get up. I . . . I can't move. . . .

(*The* YOUNG MAN *stops his calisthenics, nods to the* MUSICIAN, *walks over to* GRANDMA, *kneels down by the sandbox*)

GRANDMA: I . . . I can't move. . . .

YOUNG MAN: Shhhhh . . . be very still. . . .

GRANDMA: I . . . I can't move

YOUNG MAN: Uh . . . ma'am; I . . . I have a line here.

GRANDMA: Oh, I'm sorry, sweetie; you go right ahead.

YOUNG MAN: I am . . . uh . . .

GRANDMA: Take your time, dear.

YOUNG MAN: (*Prepares; delivers the line like a real amateur*) I am the Angel of Death. I am . . . uh . . . I am come for you.

GRANDMA: What . . . wha . . . (*Then, with resignation*) . . . ohhhh . . . ohhhh, I see.

(*The* YOUNG MAN *bends over, kisses* GRANDMA *gently on the forehead*)

GRANDMA:

(*Her eyes closed, her hands folded on her breast again, the shovel between her hands, a sweet smile on her face*)

Well . . . that was very nice, dear. . . .

YOUNG MAN: (*Still kneeling*) Shhhhhh . . . be still. . . .

GRANDMA: What I meant was . . . you did that very well, dear . . .

YOUNG MAN: (*Blushing*) . . . oh . . .

GRANDMA: No; I mean it. You've got that . . . you've got a quality.

YOUNG MAN: (*With his endearing smile*) Oh . . . thank you; thank you very much . . . ma'am.

GRANDMA:

(*Slowly; softly—as the* YOUNG MAN *puts his hands on top of* GRANDMA'S)

You're . . . you're welcome . . . dear.

(*Tableau. The* MUSICIAN *continues to play as the curtain slowly comes down*)

The Shadow Box

ℰ๑

Michael Cristofer

INTRODUCTION

In *The Shadow Box* Michael Cristofer presents an unvarnished view of terminally ill patients who are living out their lives in a hospice. The facility is composed of three cottages on the grounds of a large hospital. In 1975, when the play first appeared, hospice was a new concept in health care in America, the first facility having been opened in Connecticut the previous year followed shortly by an inpatient hospice program at Yale Medical Center. One may well speculate on the influence of Cristofer's play in introducing the concept of hospice care and dramatizing its dynamics to an audience largely unaware of the movement's mission. By the early 1980s Congress had created legislation establishing Medicare coverage for hospice services, and the movement spread quickly across the country.

The Shadow Box tells the story of three individuals suffering the identical experience of coming to terms with their approaching death. Their separate dramas are played out in the cottage each occupies. All the action occurs on the same set within a twenty-four-hour period. Stage space is compressed as the three narratives are presented in turn, each seemingly independent of the other with strikingly disparate characters as their subjects. Linear development is replaced by the simultaneous unfolding of the three tales. The past is reconstructed through memory as each character recalls time gone by while attempting to order the present. As the audience is witness to the physical and emotional state of each of the trio, it discovers that the accounts inform one another as they interact and resonate with equal intensity in affirming the same truth. The unity of the three-in-one structure is supported in the coda that concludes the piece as all the characters come together simultaneously and proclaim as one their acceptance of both death and life.

The three patients—Joe, a middle-aged, hardworking nonprofessional; Brian, an unsuccessful author; and Felicity, an elderly woman—become

increasingly cut off from others in their social interactions as their deteriora-
tion progresses. Each case is presented on a personal level through dialogue
between patient and family or friends. Formal exchanges occur between
each patient and a clinician known as the Interviewer, who never appears on
stage but whose disembodied voice is heard over a loudspeaker as he draws
the patients out and encourages them to express their feelings. While such
exchanges are limited, the contact ensures that the patient is not isolated for
the time he is cared for, as occurs in instances where the dying are set apart in
a clinical unit, heavily sedated or made dependent on life-sustaining technology. Cristofer's drama reflects the philosophy of hospice care, revealing how
the quality of life may be maintained and respect for human dignity upheld
even when invasive means are no longer beneficial and all treatment options
have been exhausted.

The Shadow Box records a significant development in medicine, the shift
to alternative approaches to end-of-life care. Situating the patients within the
cottages is a strategy meant to meet their needs as well as those of their loved
ones as the focus comes to rest on helping people live with catastrophic illness
and approaching death. A social construct is developed as family and friends
are admitted to the patient's living space. Joe is joined by his wife, Maggie, and
young son; Brian welcomes his domestic partner, Mark, and ex-wife, Beverly;
Felicity admits her daughter, Agnes. One of the virtues of hospice care is its
conception of the ill person as part of a larger whole, acknowledging his inter-
relatedness to others. Since what happens to the patient impacts the family, and
vice versa, the struggle of the family to come to terms with death is foregrounded
in the drama. The audience observes the extent to which those who witness
the patient's decline similarly share feelings of helplessness and abandonment
experienced by the dying. In agreeing to live together and support each other,
they renew their commitment to one another and lose their sense of isolation,
which is felt as much by the family as the patient due to the latter's sense of
helplessness in preventing the inevitable. Joe's plea is made on behalf of all as he
tells his wife, "I'm going to die, Maggie. . . . Don't make me do it alone" (94).

Characteristic of those approaching the end of life is the tendency to ponder
the past and reflect on previous successes and failures. Cristofer's characters
are never as affective as when, in their misery, they recall fleeting moments
of happiness and feel regret for injudicious choices. Such recollections can
be shattering. Consider an early treatment of the experience in medieval literature, the moment in *The Divine Comedy* when Dante meets Francesca da
Rimini in the *Inferno*. Pausing to listen to Francesca's account of how love led
her to adultery, Dante hears her cry, "There is no greater pain than happiness
recalled in misery."[1] Unable to bear the sight of the woman's suffering, the
poet collapses, falling senseless to the floor, an action to recur on two other

extraordinary moments within the poem. In *The Shadow Box* the characters are able to bear the reality of their lives by interacting with those who listen to them, encouraging them to express their thoughts and aiding them to put their past into perspective. The absence of linear plot allows for the revelation of the characters' histories as they reminisce and reveal the details of their emotional lives. In contrast to actual patients whose reality is limited to standard case histories, Cristofer's fictional characters have the vitality of whole beings who chronicle their lives in their own voices. They reveal intense inner lives that help personalize them. The audience is not spared any of the clinical details while it is permitted access to the private worlds of the patients.

Cristofer is also adept at creating monologic speech that enables family members to add depth to the initial depiction of the patients. The stunning recollections by Agnes in Act II provide sufficient details of her mother's emotional history to complete the portrait of the elderly woman who first appears as a medical curiosity. The playwright has grasped the vulnerability of individuals in circumstances similar to those he creates, and he points a direction in endurance. Illustrating the hospice philosophy that the patient is a living person who should be encouraged to seize each moment, the playwright draws the figure of Brian as a man with a passion for life that is awakened upon learning that his time on earth is soon to end. Although he has been an unsuccessful writer, he proceeds to turn out volumes of work. He becomes increasingly active and even goes to the extraordinary length of visiting Passaic, New Jersey, just to confirm his suspicion that he has absolutely no desire to go there. (In consideration of the citizens of Passaic, Cristofer is simply injecting a bit of comic relief, as he does regularly throughout the play.) And contemplating his limited expectations, Brian concludes that he'd best close out his charge account at Bloomingdale's. The effect of such levity is to underline the reality that dying is a natural part of living and that the quality of life is enhanced by humor, which functions as a coping mechanism.

Quoting his agent, Brian passes on another wry joke, "There's a huge market for dying people just now" (44). The contemporary scene had just witnessed the publication of Elizabeth Kübler-Ross's *On Death and Dying* only a few years before, and death as a subject had taken on an added dimension in America. Kübler-Ross traveled widely promoting the fledgling hospice movement with its sensitivity to the psychological needs of dying people, especially as expressed in the now familiar stages of grief as she identified them—denial, anger, bargaining, depression, and acceptance. One of the achievements of the drama is the characters' passage through the different stages, a progression they relate in their own words, making the dramatic account sufficiently real to impact the audience substantially. Not the most articulate of the characters, Joe nonetheless is forceful in describing his passage through fear to anger: "You get scared at first. Plenty. And then you get pissed off" (6). Family members experience similar transitions. Joe's wife denies her husband's approaching death, repeating, "You look fine. I can see it" (91). She stops short at the door of the cottage, refusing to enter, for to do so would be to acknowledge the truth. Instead, she pleads with her husband to return with her to the home they have left. Since *The Shadow Box* is a work for the theater and not a study in contemporary medical practice, Cristofer concentrates less on the clinical significance of each stage for the individual than on the dramatic conflict occurring when characters fail to meet on the same level.[2] Where Maggie is in denial, Joe has moved on to acceptance.

At the conclusion of the drama, all characters come to accept the finite nature of life as they overcome fear and acquire the strength to endure. Reaching deep within themselves, they find the love and compassion that enable them to support each other while reaffirming life and upholding the dignity of those who live it with grace.

NOTES

1. The lines in the original read "Nessun maggior dolore / che ricordarsi del tempo felice / ne la miseria." Dante Alighieri, *The Divine Comedy: The Inferno.* (ll. 121–23, Canto V). Translated by the author.

2. For a fine discussion of the changes occurring in societal perceptions of death, see Donald F. Duclow, "Dying on Broadway: Contemporary Drama and Mortality," *Soundings: An Interdisciplinary Journal* 64:2 (Summer 1981): 197–216.

WORKS CITED

Cristofer, Michael. *The Shadow Box*. New York: Drama Book Specialists, 1977.
Duclow, Donald F. "Dying on Broadway: Contemporary Drama and Mortality." *Soundings: An Interdisciplinary Journal* 64:2 (Summer 1981): 197–216.

THE SHADOW BOX
By Michael Cristofer

For my mother and father,
Mary and Joseph Procaccino

CHARACTERS

THE INTERVIEWER
Cottage One
   JOE
   STEVE
   MAGGIE
Cottage Two
   BRIAN
   MARK
   BEVERLY
Cottage Three
   AGNES
   FELICITY

The play takes place in three cottages on the grounds of a large hospital.

ACT ONE

Morning
A small cottage that looks like a vacation house, set in the trees, secluded. A front porch, a living room area and a large kitchen area.
The lights come up first on a small area downstage and away from the cottage. A stool is there. We will call this area the "Interview Area."
JOE *is surprised by the light. He is a strong, thick-set man, a little bit clumsy with moving and talking, but full of energy.*
He steps into the light and looks out toward the back of the theatre. A MIKED VOICE *speaks to him.*
VOICE OF INTERVIEWER: Joe? Joe, can you hear me?
JOE: Huh? *(Looking around)* What ... uh ... ?
VOICE OF INTERVIEWER: Can you hear me?
JOE: Oh, yeah. Sure. I can hear you real good.
VOICE OF INTERVIEWER: Good. Have a seat, Joe.
JOE: *(Still looking around, a little amused)* What? Hey, where ... uh ... I can't see ...
VOICE OF INTERVIEWER: We're out here.
JOE: What? Oh, yeah. I get it.
VOICE OF INTERVIEWER: Yes.
JOE: You can see me. Right?
VOICE OF INTERVIEWER: Yes. That's correct.

JOE: You can see me, but I . . .

VOICE OF INTERVIEWER: Yes.

JOE: . . . can't see you. Yeah. *(He laughs)* I get it now. You can see me, huh?

VOICE OF INTERVIEWER: Yes, we can.

JOE: Far out.

VOICE OF INTERVIEWER: What?

JOE: *(Smiling)* Nothing. Nothing. Well, how do I look?

VOICE OF INTERVIEWER: Have a seat, Joe.

JOE: That bad, huh? I *feel* all right. Lost a little weight, but outside of that . . .

VOICE OF INTERVIEWER: Have a seat, Joe.

JOE: Sure. Sure. *(He sits)* Okay. What?

VOICE OF INTERVIEWER: Nothing special. We just wanted to talk. Give you a chance to see how we do this.

JOE: Sure.

VOICE OF INTERVIEWER: There's nothing very complicated about it. It's just a way for us to stay in touch.

JOE: Yeah. It's like being on TV.

VOICE OF INTERVIEWER: Just relax.

JOE: Right. Fire away.

VOICE OF INTERVIEWER: You seem to be in very good spirits.

JOE: Never better. Like I said, I feel great.

VOICE OF INTERVIEWER: Good.

(There is a pause. JOE *looks out into the lights)*

JOE: My family is coming today.

VOICE OF INTERVIEWER: Yes. We know.

JOE: It's been a long time. Almost six months. They would have come sooner, but we couldn't afford it. Not after all these goddamn bills. And then I always figured I'd be going home. I always figured I'd get myself back into shape and . . . *(Pause)*

VOICE OF INTERVIEWER: Have you seen the cottage?

JOE: Yeah. Yeah, it's real nice. It's beautiful. They're going to love it.

VOICE OF INTERVIEWER: Good.

JOE: Maggie always wanted a place in the mountains. But I'm an ocean man. So, every summer, we always ended up at the beach. She liked it all right. It just takes her a while to get used to things. She'll love it here, though. She will. It's real nice.

VOICE OF INTERVIEWER: Good.

JOE: It just takes her a little time.

(The lights slowly start to come up on the cottage area. MAGGIE'S *and* STEVE'S *voices are heard off stage)*

STEVE: Here. Over here.

MAGGIE: Stephen!

VOICE OF INTERVIEWER: *(To* JOE*)* Then everything is settled, right?

JOE: What? Oh, yeah. Maggie knows the whole setup. I wrote to her.

VOICE OF INTERVIEWER: And your son?

JOE: Steve? Yeah. I told Maggie to tell him. I figured he should know before he got here.

VOICE OF INTERVIEWER: Good.

JOE: It's not an easy thing.

STEVE: *(Still off stage–overlapping)* Come on, Mom.

JOE: I guess you know that.

MAGGIE: *(Still offstage)* Give me a chance to catch my breath.

JOE: You get used to the idea, but it's not easy.

VOICE OF INTERVIEWER: You seem fine.

JOE: Oh, Me. Yeah, Sure. But Maggie . . .

MAGGIE: *(Overlapping)* What number did you say it was?

VOICE OF INTERVIEWER: *(Overlapping)* What number cottage are you in?

JOE: Uh . . . one. Number one.

STEVE: *(Overlapping)* Number one. One, they said.

JOE: You get scared at first. Plenty. And then you get pissed off. Oh, is that all right to say?

VOICE OF INTERVIEWER: Yes, Joe. That's all right. It's all right for you to be angry or depressed or even happy . . . if that's how you feel. We want to hear as much as you want to tell us.

STEVE: *(Still off stage)* Look at all these goddamn trees!

MAGGIE: *(Still off)* Watch your mouth.

JOE: Yeah, 'cause I was. Plenty pissed off. I don't mind telling you that. In fact, I'm glad just to say it. You get tired of keeping it all inside. But it's like, nobody wants to hear about it. You know what I mean? Even the doctors . . . they shove a thermometer in your mouth and a stethoscope in their ears . . . How the hell are you supposed to say anything? But then, like I said, you get used to it . . . I guess . . .

STEVE: Come on, Mom!

JOE: There's still a few things . . .

MAGGIE: You're going to give me a heart attack.

JOE: I could talk to you about them . . . maybe later.

VOICE OF INTERVIEWER: Even if it's just to listen. That's what we're here for, Joe.

JOE: I mean, it happens to everybody, right? I ain't special.

VOICE OF INTERVIEWER: I guess not Joe.

JOE: I mean, that's the way I figure it. We could talk about that, too.

VOICE OF INTERVIEWER: Yes, we can.

JOE: But maybe tomorrow.

VOICE OF INTERVIEWER: All right, Joe. We won't keep you now.

JOE: I'm a little nervous today.

VOICE OF INTERVIEWER: But if you need anything . . .

JOE: Huh . . . What . . . ?

VOICE OF INTERVIEWER: If you need anything . . .

JOE: Oh, sure. Thanks. We'll be all right.

VOICE OF INTERVIEWER: You know where to find us.

JOE: Is that it?

VOICE OF INTERVIEWER: That's it. Unless *you* have something . . .

JOE: Oh . . . yeah. One thing . . . I . . . uh . . .

STEVE: (STEVE *is a young boy, about fourteen years old.*) Dad? *(He rushes onto the stage, runs around the cottage.)*

MAGGIE: *(Still off stage)* Stephen?

STEVE: Here! Over here!

JOE: I . . . uh . . . no. No. I guess not.

VOICE OF INTERVIEWER: All right, then. Thank you, Joe.

JOE: Sure. Any time.

STEVE: *(Rushing into the cottage)* Number one. This is it! Jesus!

JOE: Oh, yeah. I want to thank you for making all this possible. *(He looks out into the lights. There is no answer.)* Hello?

STEVE: He's not there.

JOE: You still there? *(Still no answer)* Well, I'd better be getting back.

(Still no answer. The lights fade on the Interview Area and come up full on the cottage.)

STEVE: *(Running out of the cottage)* Mom? Where the . . .

JOE: *(Turning toward the cottage)* Stephen! Hey, dad!

STEVE: Holy shit! Holy . . . ! *(He does a little dance, runs to his father and embraces him)* Where the hell . . .

JOE: There you are . . . I been waiting all day.

STEVE: . . . have you been? We been traipsing around the whole goddamn place . . .

JOE: *(Laughing)* I been here. Waiting. Where's your mother?

STEVE: One cottage after another. Is this it? Is this it?

MAGGIE: *(Still off)* Joe? Stephen, is that your father?

STEVE: Far out! I brought my guitar. Wait till you hear . . .

(Calling off) Mom! Over here, for Christ's sake.

(To JOE) So many goddamn trees . . .

JOE: What do you think? Huh?

STEVE: So many . . .

JOE: There's a bunk in there.

MAGGIE: *(Off)* Joe?

JOE: Hey, Maggie. Get the lead out!

STEVE: Yeah. I saw. Bunk beds and a fireplace . . . we got any wood?

JOE: You can take the top one night and the bottom the next.

STEVE: Uh-uh. I'll take the bottom. I fall off, I'll break my fucking head.

JOE: I'll break your fucking head, if you don't watch your fucking mouth.

STEVE: Holy, holy shit!

(STEVE hugs his father again.

   JOE *holds him at arms length for a second, to catch his breath)*

STEVE: You okay?

JOE: *(Quickly recovers and returns to his previous level of energy)* Yeah, yeah, I'm great.

STEVE: You look terrific. I was worried. I missed you. Hey! How long can we stay? Huh?

JOE: I don't know. A couple of weeks . . . I don't know how long it . . .

STEVE: Great. *(He drags* JOE *into the cottage)* Come on. I'll show you the guitar. It was pretty cheap. I ripped off the case, so that didn't cost anything. It's got a little compartment on the inside for picks and capos and dope and shit like that . . .

(They go in to the cottage. MAGGIE *struggles onto the stage, a mass of bundles, shopping bags and suitcases. She's dressed up–high heels, bright yellow print dress–but she looks a mess. She's been walking too long, carrying too big a load. Finally, she stops near the cottage.)*

MAGGIE: End of the line. Everybody off.

(And she lets all the shopping bags, packages, and suitcases crash to the ground around her. She straightens her back with a groan and looks around her.)

   Steve? Joe? The jackass is here! Come and get your luggage?

(No answer. She walks up to the porch of the cabin, and takes one step up. But the cottage seems to frighten her. She stops, looks at it and then backs away from it.)

   You leave me alone out here for one more minute and I'm taking the next plane back to Newark.

(She gives out a long, loud whistle through her teeth.)

   Stephen, are you in there or not?

STEVE: *(From inside the cottage)* Hey, Mom, come on in if you're coming.

MAGGIE: I'm not coming in. You're coming out. And don't give me . . .

JOE: *(Coming out of the cottage and saying her line with her)* . . . and don't give me any smart back talk or I'll split your lip.

(Surprised by JOE'S *sudden appearance, she doesn't move for a second. Then, very carefully, she takes a few slow steps toward him.* JOE *walks down to meet her. All* MAGGIE *can manage to do is reach out one hand and touch him, just to see if he's really there. When she is sure that he's not an illusion, she takes a deep breath, goes back to her bundles, and starts talking very quickly, trying to keep control of herself.)*

MAGGIE: Well . . . I brought you some things . . . I didn't know what, what for sure you'd want, but I thought it was better to be sure, safe . . . so . . .

JOE: We'll take them inside . . .

MAGGIE: No . . . Steve'll get them. I been dragging them all . . .

JOE: Let me look at you, huh?

MAGGIE: *(Continues to fumble nervously with her hair, her dress, the packages)* I didn't know what you'd need. There's some jelly and some peppers I put up . . . *(She starts pulling jars out of one of the bags.)* I thought it was forty pounds on the plane, but they let you have extra. You can put things under the seat. A lot of people didn't *have* anything, so I put stuff under *their* seats, too.

JOE: How are you, Maggie?

MAGGIE: Oh, fine, I brought the newspapers. *(She pulls more jars out.)* Some cookies, and some pumpkin flowers. The airplane made me sick. There was a man sitting next to me. He kept talking and talking. All those clouds. It looked like you could walk on them. I wanted to throw up, but the man next to me made me so nervous I couldn't. Where did I put . . .

JOE: Come on inside. You want some coffee?

MAGGIE: *(Reaching into another bag)* I brought some coffee. You've got everything here already. You should've told me.

JOE: I did. I told you over the phone.

MAGGIE: I don't remember. I'll clean up tomorrow. First thing. Straighten everything out.

JOE: It's already clean.

MAGGIE: You want to live in somebody else's dirt?

JOE: Maggie, it isn't the Poconos. It's clean. It's clean.

MAGGIE: Well, you can't be too sure. Mom sent some bread . . .

JOE: How is she?

MAGGIE: Oh, good. Yeah. She fell down and hurt her leg. I don't know. It's not healing so good. She's getting old. What can you do. But she made the bread anyway. I told her not to, but she said she wanted to. So . . .

And Fanny says hello. She gave me . . . uh, something . . . where is it? Oh, yeah. Here . . . *(She pulls out a wrapped package.)*

JOE: I can see it later.

MAGGIE: I don't know what it is. You know Fanny. It could be anything . . . and some clam broth. Oh, Pop and Josie, they went crabbing, they took the kids. Steve went with them. They gave me almost a whole bushel. So I made some sauce. *(Another jar emerges.)* We can . . . do you have a stove in there?

JOE: Sure. Come on inside. I'll show you. It's real nice.

(He starts to head her toward the cottage, but she pulls away.)

MAGGIE: No, I don't want to go inside.

JOE: Huh? Why not?

MAGGIE: I don't . . . I'll see it. I'll see it.

JOE: But . . .

MAGGIE: How do I look? It's a new dress.

JOE: You look real pretty.

MAGGIE: I got dressed for the plane. I don't know. I should have worn pants. You get so tired, sitting, all pushed together like that. My ears hurt so bad. Steve loved it. I couldn't make him sit still. He was all over the place taking pictures. The stewardess was crazy about him. She was *pretty*, too. They look real nice. They wear . . . they smile. I asked her what to do about my ears and she just smiled. I don't think she heard me. So I smiled, too, but it didn't do any good . . .

JOE: You must be tired, huh?

MAGGIE: Yeah. I don't know.

JOE: *(Hugs her)* Come on in. You can rest.

MAGGIE: *(Ignores his offer)* One minute you're there. The next minute you're here. I still feel like I'm there. *(She pulls away from him and starts rummaging through the bags.)* What else? Three thousand miles, it must be. They . . . Oh, yeah. I made a ham . . . *(She pulls the monster out of the bag.)*

JOE: What?

MAGGIE: A ham. We can have it for lunch.

JOE: Christ!

MAGGIE: What's the matter? It's no good?

JOE: You mean you carried a ham three thousand miles across the country?

MAGGIE: No. I put it under the seat.

JOE: Well, what the hell are we going to do with it?

MAGGIE: I don't know . . . I thought it'd last, so . . .

JOE: *We got* everything we need. I told you.

MAGGIE: I don't remember. You can't eat this, huh?

JOE: No, I can eat it. I can eat it. That's not what I'm talking about.

MAGGIE: Then what *are* you talking about?

JOE: I'm talking about they got ham in California. They got stores like every place in the world and you go in and you buy whatever you want . . .

MAGGIE: *(Making a vain effort to hide the ham)* I'll take it back with me . . .

JOE: It's all right! It's here now.

MAGGIE: *(Overlapping)* It'll keep. I'll put it away. You don't have to look at it.

JOE: *(Overlapping)* No. It's fine. It's all right. *What the hell are we talking about?!!*

MAGGIE: *(All upset, still holding on to the ham)* You didn't say in the letter. And we talked and I couldn't remember. I tried. What the hell. They said to come and bring Steve. That's all. At first I thought that was it. Then I got your letter and you sound fine and I talk to you . . . so, I made the ham . . . I . . .

(She cries. JOE goes to her. Holds her and the ham in his arms)

JOE: I missed you, Maggie. I missed you real bad.

MAGGIE: You got to tell me what's going on. Don't make me feel so stupid. Like I'm supposed to know everything. I don't know nothing. I just know what I see.

JOE: Maggie . . .

MAGGIE: But you look real good. You're all right now, huh?

JOE: Maggie, listen . . .

MAGGIE: No. It's all right. You don't have to tell me. I can see it. You're fine. Huh? It's just I got so scared. Thinking about it. Making things up in my head. But it's all right now. I can see it's all right. I knew it would be when I got here.

JOE: *(Giving in)* Yes, Maggie. Everything's all right.

MAGGIE: I knew it. I knew it.

(Our focus shifts now to the Interview Area. BRIAN is talking)

BRIAN: . . . people don't want to let go. Do they?

VOICE OF INTERVIEWER: How do you mean, Brian?

BRIAN: They think it's a mistake, they think it's supposed to last forever. I'll never understand that. My God, it's the one thing in this world you can be sure of! No matter who you are, no matter what you do, no matter anything–sooner or later–it's going to happen. You're going to die.

(BRIAN is a graceful man . . . simple, direct, straightforward. He possesses an agile mind and a childlike joy about life.)

. . . and that's a relief—if you think about it. I should say if you think clearly about it.

VOICE OF INTERVIEWER: I'm not sure I follow you.

BRIAN: Well, the trouble is that most of us spend our entire lives trying to *forget* that we're going to die. And some of us even succeed. It's like pulling the cart *without* the horse. Or is that a poor analogy?

VOICE OF INTERVIEWER: No, Brian. I think it's fine.

BRIAN: Well, you get the gist of it anyway. I'm afraid I've really lost my touch with words. They don't add up as neatly as they used to.

VOICE OF INTERVIEWER: But you're still writing.

BRIAN: Oh, yes. With great abandon. I may have lost touch with the words, but I still have faith in them. Eventually they have to mean *something* . . . give or take a few thousand monkeys, a few thousand typewriters. I'm not particular. Am I being helpful or just boring?

VOICE OF INTERVIEWER: Very helpful.

BRIAN: Well, I don't see how. Too much thinking and talking. My former wife once said to me, "We've done enough thinking. Couldn't we just dance for a few years?" *(He laughs.)*

VOICE OF INTERVIEWER: Did you?

BRIAN: No. I have lousy feet. Instead, I started going on about music and mathematics, the difference between Apollonian airs and Dionysian rites, explaining to her the history of dance and the struggle with form . . . and before I finished the first paragraph, she was gone . . .

(The lights fade on the porch area of the cottage where JOE *and* MAGGIE *are. Then they start to come up on the living room area of the cottage.* BRIAN *continues his interview)*

VOICE OF INTERVIEWER: Gone for good?

BRIAN: Like a bat out of hell.

VOICE OF INTERVIEWER: I see.

BRIAN: So do I . . . now. But then I didn't. I became totally irrational . . . idiotic, in the Greek sense of the word. I blamed her, I damned her, I hated her . . . I missed her. I got so worked up I began to realize what she was talking about. You see, I'd lost the energy of it, the magic of it. No wonder she left. After all, the universe isn't a syllogism, it's a miracle. Isn't it? And if you can believe in one small part of it, then you can believe in all of it. And if you can believe in all of it . . . well, that *is* a reason for dancing, isn't it?

VOICE OF INTERVIEWER: What happened to her?

BRIAN: Beverly? Oh, she's still dancing as far as I know.

VOICE OF INTERVIEWER: I see.

BRIAN: Well, every life makes sense on its own terms, I suppose. She must be very happy. I'm sure of that. Otherwise she would have come back. There I go, rambling on again. I'm sorry.

VOICE OF INTERVIEWER: You seem to have everything so well thought out.

(In the living room area of the cottage, MARK *enters. He is a young man, passionately intelligent, sexually attractive.)*

BRIAN: *(Still talking to the* INTERVIEWER*)* Well, I think it's important to be sensible. Even about the miraculous. Otherwise you lose track of what it's all about.

VOICE OF INTERVIEWER: How is Mark?

BRIAN: *(Smiles)* Speaking of the miraculous . . . ? Well, he's fine.

MARK: *(In the living room, looking around)* Brian?

BRIAN: *(To* INTERVIEWER*)* What's the official line on him now?

VOICE OF INTERVIEWER: How do you mean?

BRIAN: Well, I know these are supposed to be strictly family situations. I'm curious. I mean, what are we calling him this week? Nephew? Cousin? Butler?

VOICE OF INTERVIEWER: No. I have him down as a friend.

BRIAN: I See.

VOICE OF INTERVIEWER: In the Greek sense of the word.

BRIAN: *(Laughs)* Very good. Very good.

VOICE OF INTERVIEWER: He's welcome to come and talk to us if he likes.

(In the living room area, MARK *takes off his jacket, throws it on a chair, sits down and takes out a package . . .)*

BRIAN: Well, we've talked a lot about it already. Generally, we have the same opinion on the subject. Wisdom doesn't always come with age. Occasionally the young can be as rational as you or I.

*(*MARK *carefully takes six or seven bottles of medication from the package. He makes notes of each label, copying down the information in a small pad.)*

VOICE OF INTERVIEWER: Yes. I suppose they can.

BRIAN: *(Checking his watch)* My watch is stopped. How long have I been babbling?

VOICE OF INTERVIEWER: It doesn't matter. There's no hurry.

BRIAN: Not for you, maybe. Some of us are on a tighter schedule.

VOICE OF INTERVIEWER: I am sorry. I didn't mean . . .

BRIAN: *(Laughs)* It's all right. It's all right. You mustn't take all of this too seriously. I don't . . . Our dreams are beautiful, our fate is sad. But day by day, it's generally pretty funny.

We can talk again tomorrow, if you want. I don't mind. It's a bit of a shock, that's all. You always think . . . no matter what they tell you . . . you always think you have more time. And you don't.

But I appreciate what you're trying to do here, and I do enjoy being a guinea pig.

VOICE OF INTERVIEWER: Good. Very good.

BRIAN: Tomorrow, then. If I'm still breathing. Or even if I'm not, I don't think it'll stop me from talking.

VOICE OF INTERVIEWER: Yes. Tomorrow.

(The lights fade on the Interview Area and come up on the living room. MARK *puts the medicine in a bookcase that is already loaded with bottles of pills and boxes of medical supplies.*

BEVERLY: *comes bursting into the living room, blowing a party horn.)*

BEVERLY: Surprise! Oh, who are you? I'm sorry. I'm looking for Brian . . . uh . . . Two. They said cottage two. I must have . . .

MARK: No, you didn't . . .

BEVERLY: I didn't?

MARK: No. This is two. This is cottage two.

BEVERLY: Oh.

MARK: Yes.

BEVERLY: Thank God. *(Pause)* Is . . . uh . . .

MARK: *(A little uncomfortable)* No. Not at the moment. But he should be back any minute.

BEVERLY: Good.

(Another pause. They look at each other.)

I wanted to surprise him and he's not here. Well . . . surprise!

*(*BEVERLY *starts to walk around the cottage. She is an extremely attractive woman. Middle-aged. She's dressed curiously in what was once a very expensive, chic evening dress. But it is now soiled and torn. She also has over and around the dress about twenty odd pieces of jewelry attached wherever there is room for them. In her hand a noisemaker that squeaks uncheerfully, and over everything, a yellow slicker raincoat and rubber boots. Looking around)*

BEVERLY: Hmn. Very nice. Very nice.

MARK: Glad you like it.

BEVERLY: All the comforts of home. Amazing what you can do with a coffin if you put your mind to it.

MARK: What?!?

BEVERLY: Oh, sorry. Sorry. Introductions first. That way you'll know who you're throwing out. *(She extends her hand in a handshake.)* I'm Beverly. No doubt you've . . .

MARK: Yes.

BEVERLY: That's what I figured.

MARK: Brian's wife.

BEVERLY: Ex-wife.

MARK: Former.

BEVERLY: Yes. Former. Former wife. He prefers former, doesn't he?

MARK: *(Shakes her hand)* Yes. I figured it was you.

BEVERLY: You did?

MARK: Yes . . . it wasn't hard.

BEVERLY: No, I guess not. *(She smiles)* And you're . . . uh . . .

MARK: Yes.

BEVERLY: Yes. I figured.

MARK: Mark.

BEVERLY: Great. Well.

MARK: Well. *(Pause)*

BEVERLY: Well, now that we know who we are . . . how about a drink.

MARK: A what?

BEVERLY: A drink. A drink.

MARK: Oh, no.

BEVERLY: No?

MARK: No. We don't keep any liquor here. I could get you some coffee or some penicillin, if you'd like.

BEVERLY: No. No. *I* was inviting *you.*

(Out of her tote bag she pulls a half finished bottle of Scotch.)

I had an accident with the Scotch on the way out here. There's quite a dent in it. *(She laughs.* MARK *doesn't.)* Anyway, we both look like we could use a little. Hmn?

MARK: No. I don't drink.

BEVERLY: *(Rummaging in her bag)* Ah, a dope man.

MARK: Neither. I like to avoid as much poison as possible.

BEVERLY: I see.

MARK: Anyway, it's really not the time or place, is it?

BEVERLY: Oh, I don't know.

MARK: Well, you go ahead. If you feel you have to.

BEVERLY: No. No, really. I don't *need* it. I mean, I'm not . . . forget it.

(She looks remorsefully at the bottle, takes off the cap, takes a swig, replaces the cap and puts the bottle back in the tote bag.

MARK *stares at her, obviously displeased by the action. There is a pause.*

BEVERLY *smiles.* MARK *does not.)*

So. How is he?

MARK: Dying. How are you?

BEVERLY: *(Taken aback)* Oooops. Let's start again. Is he feeling any pain?

MARK: Are you?

BEVERLY: Strike two. Well, I think we've got it all straight now. He's dying. I'm drunk. And you're pissed off. Did I leave anything out?

MARK: No, I think that just about covers it.

BEVERLY: Tell me. How is he?

MARK: Hard to say. One day he's flat on his ass, the next day he's running around like a two year old. But he is terminal–officially. They moved him down to these cottages because there's nothing they can do for him in the hospital. But he can't go home, either.

There's some pain. But it's tolerable. At least he makes it seem tolerable. They keep shooting him full of cortisone.

BEVERLY: Ouch!

MARK: Yes. Ouch. You should be prepared, I guess.

BEVERLY: Prepared for what?

MARK: The cortisone.

BEVERLY: Why? They don't give it to the visitors, do they?

MARK: No. I mean it has side effects. It . . . well, you may not notice it, but the skin goes sort of white and puffy. It changed the shape of his face for a while, and he started to get really fat.

BEVERLY: His whole body?

MARK: Yes. His whole body.

BEVERLY: Charming.

MARK: Well, don't get too upset. A lot of it's been corrected, but he's still very pale. And he has fainting spells. They're harmless. Well, that's what they tell me. But it's embarrassing for him because he falls down a lot and his face gets a little purple for a minute.

BEVERLY: All the details. You're very graphic.

MARK: It happens a lot. The details aren't easy to forget.

BEVERLY: I guess not.

MARK: I just want you to know. If you're staying around. I mean, I think it would hurt him if people noticed.

BEVERLY: Well, if he turns purple and falls on the floor, it'd be sort of difficult not to notice, wouldn't it?

MARK: *(Taken aback)* What?

BEVERLY: I mean, what do people *usually* do when it happens?

MARK: I don't know. I mean, there hasn't been anyone here except me and . . .

BEVERLY: And you have everything pretty much under control.

MARK: I do my best.

BEVERLY: I'm sure you do.

MARK: Look. I don't mean to be rude or stupid about this . . .

BEVERLY: Why not? I like people to be rude and stupid. It's one of the ways you can be sure they're still alive.

Oh dear, I did it again, didn't I?

MARK: Yes. You have to understand–I mean, you will be careful, won't you?

BEVERLY: About what?

MARK: That's exactly what I mean. You're . . . I'm sorry, but you're very stoned, aren't you? And you're dressed in funny clothes, and you're saying a lot of funny things but I'm just not sure, frankly, what the fuck you're doing here.

BEVERLY: *(Still flip)* Neither am I. You sure you wouldn't like a drink?

MARK: Positive. Look, please, don't you think it'd be better if you came back some other time, like tomorrow or next year or something?

BEVERLY: I'd just have to get drunk all over again.

MARK: I mean, it's sort of a delicate situation, right now. He's had a very bad time of it and any kind of, well, disturbance . . .

BEVERLY: Such as me? Oh, you'll get used to it. You just have to think of me as your average tramp.

MARK: . . . any disturbance might be dangerous, especially psychologically and . . . Shit! I sound like an idiot, the way I'm talking. But you don't seem to be understanding a goddamn word I'm saying!

BEVERLY: No. I am. I am. You know, you don't *look* like a faggot.

MARK: Oh, for Christ's sake!

BEVERLY: No, I mean it . . . I mean, I didn't expect . . .

MARK: Well, you'll get used to it. You just have to think of me as your average cocksucker. All right?

BEVERLY: Good. Now we're getting someplace. Are you sure you wouldn't like a drink?

MARK: *No!* I would not like a drink. *You* have a drink. Have two. Take off your clothes. Make yourself at home. *(He grabs his jacket and beads for the door.)* When you're ready to throw up, the bathroom is in there. *(He exits.)*

BEVERLY: *(Left with the bottle)* Hey!

(The lights come up on the porch area where STEVE is just coming out of the cottage to join MAGGIE and JOE.)

STEVE: Hey! Is this place bugged or what?

JOE: Bugged?

MAGGIE: *(Reaching into a shopping bag)* I brought some Lysol. Here.

STEVE: No. Bugged. *Wired.* What do they do? Listen in with hidden cameras?

JOE: *(Laughing)* Yeah. Every move. Every word.

MAGGIE: Joe, cut it out.

(Meanwhile, as this scene continues, AGNES wheels FELICITY on stage and to the kitchen area. AGNES sings softly as she is pushing the wheelchair.)

AGNES: Holy God, we praise thy name.

STEVE: *(Continuing)* But they got wires near the bed.

JOE: That's for me. Don't worry about it.

MAGGIE: *(Changing the subject)* Here. *(To* STEVE*)* You take this stuff inside. And keep the noise down.

JOE: *(To* MAGGIE*)* Come on in, Maggie, I'll show you around.

MAGGIE: No. I want to stay outside. For a while, it's nice.

STEVE: *(Runs back into the cottage)* I'll get my guitar . . .

JOE: You like it, don't you?

MAGGIE: Sure. It's nice. *(Calling)* Stephen, you help me with this . . .

JOE: *(Overlapping)* I knew you would. I'll take you for a walk later. They got a swimming pool. And a tennis court. There's a little river, just a little one, runs back through the trees. Over there. I'll show you later. We got time. There's no hurry.

MAGGIE: Stephen!

JOE: Ah, leave him be. I'll get this. *(He starts to pick up the bags.)*

MAGGIE: No, you rest. Stephen!

JOE: I can get it. The more exercise I get, the better I feel.

MAGGIE: *(Stopping him)* There's no sense pushing it, huh? Steve can do it. *(*STEVE *comes out of the cottage with his guitar. He sits down and starts to play it.)*

MAGGIE: Put that thing down and give your father a hand.

JOE: *(To* STEVE*)* Wait till you see, dad. From the north side, near the gate when you come in, you can see the whole valley. All squared off and patched up with farms like a quilt. Hundreds of them. I'll show you.

STEVE: Farms? They got farms?

JOE: Yeah. Hundreds of them.

MAGGIE: Stephen, take this bag inside. Put this one in the kitchen. *(To* JOE*)* You got a kitchen?

JOE: Sure. A kitchen, a bathroom, two bedrooms, a living room . . .

STEVE: *(Overlapping)* We never did get our farm. We should do that. We should get that farm. *(He takes bag inside)*

JOE: Well, maybe we should have. A little place . . .

MAGGIE: *(To* STEVE*)* There's more here, when you're finished, so hurry up.

JOE: A little place like this . . .

MAGGIE: Don't start on the farm, for God's sake. It always ends up bad when you start on the farm.

STEVE: *(Returning)* We could sit out every night, singing and howling at the moon. *(He howls like a wolf.)*

MAGGIE: *(Getting more and more agitated)* Stephen, be quiet. Where do you think you are? This goes in the bedroom.

STEVE: Aren't you ever coming in?

MAGGIE: *(A little too firmly)* I'll go in when I'm good and ready.
(STEVE exits with suitcase)
JOE: *(Noticing MAGGIE's nervousness, trying to keep things happy.)* It might have worked, Maggie. See me all dressed up in coveralls. Early morning, up with the sun. What do you think?
MAGGIE: What do you know about running a farm?
JOE: Nothing. What do *you* know?
MAGGIE: Nothing. *(More irritated)* It's a lot of work. I don't want to hear about it.
JOE: A little hard work'll never kill you.
MAGGIE: Don't tell me about hard work.
JOE: It's good for you.
MAGGIE: Good for *you.* Not for me. Milk the cows, clean the chicken coop, who would have done that, huh?
STEVE: *(Returning)* We could have had a couple hundred acres . . .
JOE: No, someplace small, something we could keep our hands on. Al and Lena had that place, we used to go every Sunday.
MAGGIE: It was dirty.
STEVE: No, it wasn't.
MAGGIE: And I never had anything to say to them, anyway. Out there in the sticks. Who do you see out there? Chickens and pigs.
JOE: They had neighbors.
MAGGIE: Chickens and pigs.
JOE: You get used to all that . . .
MAGGIE: I don't want to hear about it. Here, Stephen. It's the last one. Put it anywhere.
STEVE: *(To MAGGIE)* You would too have liked it. Get a little chicken shit between your toes, kiss a few pigs . . . It'd change your whole disposition . . .
(He grabs the bag and MAGGIE and starts whirling her around)
MAGGIE: *(Almost laughing)* Cut it out! Stephen!
STEVE: *(Starts to tickle her and push her toward the cottage)* Come on inside, Chicken Lady. I'll show you the roost!
(MAGGIE is laughing hard now. STEVE clucks like a chicken, tickling her, and steering her toward the cottage. JOE laughs and joins them.)
JOE: Come on, Maggie. We got you.
(He grabs her hand and pulls her toward the cottage.)
MAGGIE: *(Laughing hysterically)* Joe . . . ! No . . . I don't . . . !
STEVE: Chickens and pigs! Chickens and pigs!
JOE: Come on inside, Maggie. Come on!
MAGGIE: No . . . I don't . . . want to go inside . . . No . . . ! Joe!

(Suddenly MAGGIE *turns and slaps* STEVE *hard across the face. She is terrified.)*

I'm not going in there! Now stop it!

(Nobody moves for a moment. STEVE *is stunned.* MAGGIE *turns away from them.* JOE *goes to* STEVE *and puts his arm around him.)*

STEVE: I'm going inside to practice . . .

JOE: Sure. *(He musses* STEVE's *hair and kisses him on the cheek.)*

STEVE: *(Picks up his guitar and goes to the cottage door. Then he turns, looks at* MAGGIE. *Then he says to* JOE . . . *)* There's a . . . there's a whole lot of shit I got to tell you. We can talk, huh? Not to worry you, but just so you know . . . There's a whole lot . . . well, we can talk, huh?

JOE: Sure, dad.

*(*STEVE *goes inside,* JOE *looks at* MAGGIE, *not knowing what came over her.)* Maggie?

MAGGIE: I didn't tell him.

JOE: What?

MAGGIE: *(Still turned away from him)* I didn't tell him. Stephen. I didn't . . .

JOE: Oh, no. No, Maggie. What's the matter with you?

MAGGIE: I couldn't.

JOE: He doesn't know?

*(*MAGGIE *shakes her head "No.")*

What does he think? He thinks I'm going home with you? Maggie? Why didn't you tell him?

MAGGIE: I couldn't.

JOE: Why not?

MAGGIE: Because . . . It isn't true. It isn't true. It isn't . . .

(She runs off away from the cottage. JOE *is stunned. He sits down on the porch* steps and puts his head in his hands.

The lights come up on the Interview Area. AGNES *is pushing* FELICITY *to the area.* FELICITY *is wide awake now. She is about sixty or seventy years old. She is singing vaguely to herself. The* INTERVIEWER *is with her, trying to get her attention.)*

INTERVIEWER: . . . but you don't have to talk to us if you don't want to. Felicity?

(She continues to sing to herself.)

If you'd rather not talk now, we can wait until tomorrow.

(She pays no attention to him.)

Shall we do that? Shall we wait until tomorrow?

(No response.)

Felicity?

(No response.)

Well, why don't we do that, then? Why don't we wait, and later if you feel . . .

FELICITY: Piss poor.

INTERVIEWER: What?

FELICITY: Your attitude. It's a piss poor way to treat people.

INTERVIEWER: But, Felicity . . .

(AGNES returns to the kitchen area of the cottage.)

FELICITY: But, but, but!

INTERVIEWER: Please . . .

FELICITY: Please what?! All right. All right. You want to talk? Let's talk. "I feel fine." Is that what you want to hear? Of course it is. I feel fine, there's no pain, I'm as blind as I was yesterday, my bowels are working–and that's all I got to say about it.

INTERVIEWER: We're only trying to help.

FELICITY: Well I don't need any more help from you. Do I?

INTERVIEWER: Well, we don't know.

FELICITY: Of course you know. I've just told you. I've just said it, haven't I?

INTERVIEWER: Yes.

FELICITY: Well, then . . . there you are. You should learn to listen.

INTERVIEWER: Yes.

FELICITY: What, have you got your friends out there again? All come to look at the dead people.

INTERVIEWER: Felicity . . .

FELICITY: He doesn't like me to say things like that. He's sensitive. Why don't you go hide yourself out there with the rest of them?

INTERVIEWER: Would you like me to . . . ?

FELICITY: No. *(Beat)* No. You stay where you are.

INTERVIEWER: All right.

FELICITY: How do I look today?

INTERVIEWER: You look fine.

FELICITY: You're a liar. I look like I feel. I smell, too. *(She turns away from him)*

INTERVIEWER: Are you tired, Felicity?

FELICITY: No.

INTERVIEWER: Do you want to talk some more today?

FELICITY: No.

INTERVIEWER: All right then. Do you want to go back to the cottage?

FELICITY: No.

INTERVIEWER: Will you tell us if you're in pain?

FELICITY: No.

INTERVIEWER: You could help us if you talked to us.

FELICITY: Help you? Help you? Which one of us is kicking the bucket? Me? Me or you?

INTERVIEWER: Well . . .

FELICITY: Come on. Spit it out. Don't be shy. You're not stupid on top of everything else, are you? One of us is dying and it isn't you, is it?

INTERVIEWER: No. You are the patient.

FELICITY: Patient?! Patient, hell! I'm the corpse. I have one lung, one plastic bag for a stomach, and two springs and a battery where my heart used to be. You cut me up and took everything that wasn't nailed down. Sons of bitches.

INTERVIEWER: But we're not your doctors, Mrs. Thomas. We have nothing to do with . . .

FELICITY: (Overlapping) We're not your doctors . . . Claire . . .

INTERVIEWER: What?

FELICITY: Claire . . .

INTERVIEWER: Mrs. Thomas? Are you all right?

FELICITY: I'm all right! I'm all right! I'll tell you when I'm not all right. It isn't five, is it? Is it five yet?

INTERVIEWER: Five?

FELICITY: Sons of bitches . . . my daughter, Claire.

INTERVIEWER: Yes.

FELICITY: She writes to me regularly. A letter almost every day. I have them at the cottage.

INTERVIEWER: That's very nice!

FELICITY: Yes!

INTERVIEWER: Where does she live?

FELICITY: Who?

INTERVIEWER: Your daughter, Claire.

FELICITY: Yes. I've kept them all–every letter she ever sent me.

INTERVIEWER: That's a good idea.

FELICITY: So I'll have them when I go home. She's a good girl, my Claire.

INTERVIEWER: Where is she now?

FELICITY: Now?

INTERVIEWER: Yes.

FELICITY: She's with me.

INTERVIEWER: Where?

FELICITY: Here. At the house.

INTERVIEWER: The house?

FELICITY: Yes. You don't run a place like this on dreams. It takes hard work. The property isn't much but the stock is good. We showed a clear profit in '63. Nobody was more surprised than I was–but we did it. How do I look today?

INTERVIEWER: You look fine. Do you want to talk about Claire?

FELICITY: I look terrible.

INTERVIEWER: The more we know, the easier it is for us to understand how you feel.

FELICITY: No. Claire isn't with me anymore. She'll be here soon. But she isn't here now. Agnes is with me now . . . *(She calls out)* Agnes! *(To the* INTERVIEWER*)* Agnes is my oldest.

INTERVIEWER: Yes, we . . .

FELICITY: *(Calling again)* Agnes!!

(The lights come up on the cottage behind FELICITY. AGNES *is discovered inside, writing at a table. When she hears her mother's voice, she gets up slowly, folds the paper she has been writing on, puts it into an envelope, seals the envelope and puts it into her pocket.*

AGNES *is a middle-aged woman–very neat, very tense, very tired. She has tried all her life to do the right thing, and the attempt has left her confused, awkward, and unsure of herself.*

When she hears her mother call, she goes to her.)

FELICITY: Agnes!

INTERVIEWER: Mrs. Thomas . . . ?

FELICITY: *(Her voice and manner growing harder again)* Claire has two children now, two beautiful, twin angels . . . *(Calling)* Agnes! *(To* INTER-VIEWER*)* Agnes has me.

AGNES: *(Approaching the Interview Area)* Yes, Mama. I'm coming.

FELICITY: She's a little slow. It's not her fault. She takes after her father. Not too pretty and not too bright. Is she here yet?

AGNES: *(Standing behind* FELICITY*'s wheelchair)* Yes, Mama. I'm here.

FELICITY: *(To* INTERVIEWER*)* There. You see what I mean? You be careful of Agnes. She's jealous.

AGNES: *(A little embarrassed)* Mama . . . please.

FELICITY: Get me out of here.

AGNES: *(To* INTERVIEWER*)* Is that all for today?

INTERVIEWER: Yes, thank you, Agnes, that's . . .

FELICITY: *(Overlapping)* That's all. That's all! Now take me back.

AGNES: Yes, Mama.

(She turns the wheelchair and starts to push it toward the cottage.)

FELICITY: Easy! Easy! You'll upset my internal wire works.

AGNES: I'm sorry. *(Turning back to the* INTERVIEWER*)* Same time tomorrow?

INTERVIEWER: Yes. And if you have time, Agnes, we'd like to talk to you.

AGNES: Me?

FELICITY: We'll see about tomorrow. You sons of bitches.

AGNES: *(To* INTERVIEWER*)* All right.

FELICITY: Push, Agnes. Push!

AGNES: Yes, Mama. Off we go.

(They go up to the kitchen area of the cottage.)

FELICITY: That's the spirit. Put some balls into it!

(Back in the cottage, BRIAN *enters the living room area where* BEVERLY *is waiting.)*

BEVERLY: Caro! Caro! You old tart! Vieni qua!

BRIAN: *(Delighted)* Sweet Jesus! Beverly!

BEVERLY: My God, he even remembers my name! What a mind! *(She hugs and kisses him.)*

BRIAN: What a picture!

BEVERLY: *(Taking off her coat to show her dress and jewels)* All my medals. All of them! I wore as many of them as I could fit.

BRIAN: Fantastic.

BEVERLY: Everything I could carry. I tried to get X-rays done but there wasn't time. Inside and out. I'll strip later and show you all of it.

BRIAN: *(Laughing)* Good. Good. What a surprise! *(Another embrace)* I'm so happy you've come. Where's Mark? Have you met him?

BEVERLY: Oh, yes. He's beautiful. A little cool, but I'm sure there's a heart in there somewhere.

BRIAN: Where is he?

BEVERLY: Well . . . he's gone.

BRIAN: What?

BEVERLY: It's my fault. I made a very sloppy entrance. I think he left in lieu of punching me in the mouth.

BRIAN: I don't believe it.

BEVERLY: It's true. But I do like him.

BRIAN: Good. So do I.

BEVERLY: *(Insinuating)* So I gather.

BRIAN: *(Cheerfully)* Uh-uh. Careful.

BEVERLY: Is he any good?

BRIAN: Beverly!

BEVERLY: Well, what's it like?

BRIAN: "It?"

BEVERLY: Yes. Him, you, it . . . you know I'm a glutton for pornography. Tell me, quick.

BRIAN: *(Laughs)* Oh, no.

BEVERLY: No?

BRIAN: No. And that's final. I refuse to discuss it.

BEVERLY: Brian, that's not fair. Here I am all damp in my panties and you're changing the subject. Now come on. Tell me all about it.

BRIAN: Absolutely not. I'm much too happy.

BEVERLY: Brian . . . I was married to you, I deserve an explanation. Isn't that what I'm supposed to say?

BRIAN: Yes, but you're too late. No excuses, no explanations. *(Singing)* He is my sunshine, my only sunshine . . . He's the–pardon the expression–cream in my coffee–the milk in my tea–He will always be my necessity . . .

BEVERLY: Ah, but is he enough?

BRIAN: More than enough.

BEVERLY: Shucks.

BRIAN: *(Laughs)* Sorry, but it's out of my hands. All of it. Some supreme logic has taken hold of my life. And in the absence of any refutable tomorrow, every insane thing I do today seems to make a great deal of sense.

BEVERLY: What the hell does that mean?

BRIAN: It means there are more important things in this world.

BEVERLY: More important than what?

BRIAN: More important than worrying about who is fucking whom.

BEVERLY: You *are* happy, aren't you?

BRIAN: Ecstatic. I'm even writing again.

BEVERLY: Oh, my God. You couldn't be *that* happy!

BRIAN: Why not?

BEVERLY: Brian, you're a terrible writer, and you know it.

BRIAN: So?

BEVERLY: Outside of that wonderful book of crossword puzzles, your greatest contribution to the literary world was your retirement.

BRIAN: *(Finishes the sentence with her)* . . . was my retirement. Yes. Well, the literary world, such as it is, will have to brave the storm. Because I'm back.

BEVERLY: But why?

BRIAN: Pure and unadulterated masochism. No. It's just that when they told me I was on the way out . . . so to speak . . . I realized that there was a lot to do that I hadn't done yet. So I figured I better get off my ass and start working.

BEVERLY: Doing what?

BRIAN: Everything! Everything! It's amazing what you can accomplish. Two rotten novels, twenty-seven boring short stories, several volumes of tortured verse–including twelve Italian sonnets and one epic investigation of the Firth of Forth Bridge . . .

BEVERLY: The what?

BRIAN: The bridge. The railroad bridge in Scotland. The one Hitchcock used in *The Thirty-nine Steps*. You remember. We saw the picture on our honeymoon.

BEVERLY: Oh, yes.

BRIAN: And I swore that one day I would do a poem about it. Well, I've done it.

BEVERLY: Thank God.

BRIAN: Yes. Four hundred stanzas–trochaic hexameters with rhymed couplets. *(He demonstrates the rhythm)* Da-da-da, Da-da-da, Da-da-da, Da-da-da, Da-da-da, Da-da-da, Da-da-da-Dee! It's perfectly ghastly. But it's done. I've also completed nearly one hundred and thirty-six epitaphs, the largest contribution to the Forest Lawn catalogue since Edna St. Vincent Millay, and four autobiographies.

BEVERLY: Four?!

BRIAN: Yes. Each one under a different name. There's a huge market for dying people right now. My agent assured me.

BEVERLY: I don't believe it.

BRIAN: It's true. And then we thought we'd give them each one of those insipid dirty titles–like *Sex . . . And the Dying Man!*

BEVERLY: Or *The Sensuous Corpse.*

BRIAN: Very good.

BEVERLY: *(Affectionately)* You idiot. What else?

BRIAN: Not too much. For a while they were giving me this drug and my vision was doubled. I couldn't really see to write. So I started to paint.

BEVERLY: Paint?

BRIAN: Pictures. I did fourteen of them. Really extraordinary stuff. I was amazed. I mean, you know I can't draw a straight line. But with my vision all cockeyed–I could do a bowl of fruit that sent people screaming from the room.

BEVERLY: I can believe it. So now you're painting.

BRIAN: No, no. They changed the medication again and now all the fruit just looks like fruit again. But I did learn to drive.

BEVERLY: A car?

BRIAN: Yes.

BEVERLY: Good grief.

BRIAN: Not very well, but with a certain style and sufficient accuracy to keep myself alive–although that is beside the point, isn't it? Let's see, what else? I've become a master at chess, bridge, poker and mahjongg, I finally bought a television set, I sold the house and everything that was in it, closed all bank accounts, got rid of all stocks, bonds, securities, everything.

BEVERLY: What did you do with the money?

BRIAN: I put it in a sock and buried it on Staten Island.

BEVERLY: You did, didn't you?

BRIAN: Almost. I gave back my American Express card, my BankAmericard–severed all my patriotic connections. I even closed my account at Bloomingdale's.

BEVERLY: This is serious.

BRIAN: You're damn right it is. I sleep only three hours a day, I never miss a dawn or a sunset, I say and do everything that comes into my head. I even sent letters to everyone I know and told them exactly what I think of them . . . just so none of the wrong people show up for the funeral. And finally . . . I went to Passaic, New Jersey.

BEVERLY: For God's sake, why?!

BRIAN: Because I had no desire to go there.

BEVERLY: Then why did you go?

BRIAN: Because I wanted to be absolutely sure I had no desire to go there.

BEVERLY: And now you know.

BRIAN: Yes. I spent two weeks at a Holiday Inn and had all my meals at Howard Johnson.

BEVERLY: Jesus! You've really gone the limit.

BRIAN: Believe me, Passaic is beyond the limit. Anyway, that's what I've been doing. Every day in everyway, I get smaller and smaller. There's practically nothing left of me.

BEVERLY: You're disappearing before my very eyes.

BRIAN: Good. You see, the only way to beat this thing is to leave absolutely nothing behind. I don't want to leave anything unsaid, undone . . . not a word, not even a lonely, obscure, silly, worthless thought. I want it all used up. All of it. That's not too much to ask, is it?

BEVERLY: No.

BRIAN: That's what I thought. Then I can happily leap into my coffin and call it a day. Lie down, close my eyes, shut my mouth and disappear into eternity.

BEVERLY: As easy as that?

BRIAN: Like falling off a log.

(BRIAN *laughs.* BEVERLY *laughs. And then the laughter slowly dies.*

BEVERLY: *goes to him, takes his hands, holds them for a moment. Long pause.)*

It shows. Doesn't it?

BEVERLY: You're shaking.

BRIAN: I can't help it. I'm scared to death.

BEVERLY: It's a lot to deal with.

BRIAN: No. Not really. It's a little thing. I mean, all this . . . this is easy. Pain, discomfort . . . that's all part of living. And I'm just as alive now as I ever was. And I *will* be alive right up to the last moment. *That's* the hard part, that last fraction of a second—when you know that the next fraction of a second—I can't seem to fit that moment into my life . . . You're absolutely alone facing an absolute unknown and there is absolutely nothing you can do about it . . . except give in.

(Pause)

BEVERLY: That's how I felt the first time I lost my virginity.

BRIAN: *(Smiles)* How was it the second time?

BEVERLY: Much easier.

BRIAN: There. You see? The real trouble with dying is you only get to do it once. (BRIAN *drifts into the thought.)*

BEVERLY: *(Pulling him back)* I brought you some champagne.

BRIAN: I'm sorry. I must be the most tedious person alive.

BEVERLY: As a matter of fact, you are. Thank God you won't be around much longer.

BRIAN: *(Looking at the champagne)* I hope you don't think I'm going to pass away drunk. I intend to be cold sober.

BEVERLY: No. No. I thought we could break it on your ass and shove you off with a great bon voyage, confetti and streamers all over the grave.

BRIAN: *(Laughing)* Perfect. Perfect. I've missed your foolishness.

BEVERLY: You hated my foolishness.

BRIAN: I never understood it.

BEVERLY: Neither did I. But it was the only way. The only way I knew.

BRIAN: Well, all those roads, they all go to Rome, as they say.

BEVERLY: Yes. But why is it I always seem to end up in Naples?

(BRIAN *and* BEVERLY *embrace.)*

(*The lights come up on the kitchen area of the cottage where* AGNES *is singing quietly.)*

AGNES: *(Singing)*

Holy God, we praise thy name

Lord of all, we bow before Thee

All on earth thy scepter claim

All in heaven above adore thee.

FELICITY: *(Who appeared to be asleep)* What the hell is that?

AGNES: It's a hymn, Mama.

FELICITY: Hymn! The time for hymns is when I'm in the coffin. Sing us a song!

AGNES: A song?

FELICITY: You know what a song *is,* don't you?

AGNES: Of course I know what a song is, but I don't think I know anything . . .

FELICITY: *(Singing)* "Roll me over, in the clover, Lay me down, roll me over, do it again . . ."

AGNES: Mama, people can hear you.

FELICITY: Do them good.

"This is a number one and the fun is just begun

Lay me down, roll me over, do it again . . ."

AGNES: All right, Mama. I'll get you some tea.

FELICITY: *(Ignoring her)*

"Roll me over, in the clover

Lay me down, roll me over, do it again . . ."

AGNES: Would you like that? Would you like some tea, Mama?

FELICITY: Put me by the table.

FELICITY: *(More singing)* "This is number two and his hand is on my shoe. Lay me down, roll me over, do it again . . ."	AGNES: You should try to rest, Mama. This medicine does no good if you exhaust yourself . . .

(AGNES wheels her to the table)

FELICITY: Other side! Other side

(AGNES moves her to the other side of the table)

FELICITY: "This is number three and his hand is on my knee. Lay me down, roll me over . . ."	AGNES: We've done enough singing now, Mama. I want you to stop. Please.

(FELICITY feels for the edge of the table.)

FELICITY: Closer! Closer!

AGNES: *(Pushing her closer to the table)* There. Is that all right?

FELICITY: *(Ignoring her)* "This is number four and . . ." I don't remember four. What's four?

AGNES: *(Setting up a game of checkers)* I don't know, Mama. I don't think I know this song.

FELICITY: "This is number five and his hand is on my thigh . . ." Do you
   know that one?

AGNES: No, Mama. I don't.

FELICITY: They'll pass you by, Agnes. They will.

AGNES: Who, Mama?

FELICITY: They'll leave you at the station with your suitcase in your hand
   and a big gardenia tacked onto your collar. Sons of bitches.

AGNES: I'm not anxious to be going anywhere.

FELICITY: "This is number six and his hands are on my tits . . ."

AGNES: Mama!

FELICITY: Does *that* make you anxious?

AGNES: No.

FELICITY: Well, it makes *me* anxious. And I haven't even *got* tits anymore.

AGNES: I'll get you some tea, Mama.

FELICITY: Tea . . . tea . . . tea . . . !

AGNES: Please, Mama. I'm very tired.

FELICITY: *(At the top of her lungs)* "This is number seven and we're on our
   way to heaven . . . !"

AGNES: *(Suddenly and violently screams at her)* Mama!!!! *Stop it!!*

(FELICITY *stops singing. She looks hurt, confused. She seems to drift off again
   as she did earlier, all her energy draining away.*

AGNES: *covers her mouth quickly, immediately ashamed and sorry for her
   outburst.*

There is a long silence. BRIAN *goes to the stage left porch.* JOE *crosses to the
   downstage porch and sits on the bench.*

FELICITY: *(Very gentle, very weak)* Put 'em away. Put 'em away. Shoot 'em
   and bury them. You can't get good milk from sick cows. Can you?

AGNES: No, Mama, You can't.

FELICITY: They're not doing anybody any good. Standing around, making
   noises like it mattered. Bursting their bellies and there's nothing good
   inside. Just a lot of bad milk. Put 'em away. You see to that machinery.

AGNES: Yes, Mama. I will.

FELICITY: It wants attention.

AGNES: We'll manage. We can sell off some of the land, if we have to.

FELICITY: But not the house.

AGNES: No, not the house. We'll keep the house.

FELICITY: What . . . what time did you say it was?

AGNES: Oh . . . about four. Four-fifteen.

FELICITY: Claire? Claire . . . ?

AGNES: No, Mama. It's Agnes.

FELICITY: It hurts . . . hurts now.

AGNES: I know, Mama . . .

FELICITY: Make it stop. Make it stop now . . .

AGNES: I'll give you some of the medicine.

FELICITY: Yes. With some tea. Could I have it with some tea?

AGNES: Yes, Mama. I think so.

FELICITY: Just one cup. Very weak.

AGNES: Yes, Mama. I'll make it for you. *(She goes to make the tea.)*

FELICITY: *(A sudden small panic)* Agnes . . . ! ?

AGNES: Here, Mama, here. I'm just going to make the tea.

FELICITY: Yes. All right. *(She panics again)* Agnes!

AGNES: *(Takes a wet cloth and wrings it out)* Yes, Mama. I'm here. *(She goes to* FELICITY *and wipes her brow with the cloth)* It's all right. I'll get you your tea and then I'll read you your letter.

*(*STEVE *starts to play "Goodnight Irene" on his guitar.* MARK *crosses to the down right Interview area.)*

FELICITY: Where are they now?

AGNES: Let me check the calendar.

MARK: I don't want to talk about it. It doesn't do any good to talk about it. I mean, it's just words. Isn't it? Little mirrors. You keep hanging them up like they mean something. You put labels on them. This one is true. This one is false. This one is broken . . . You can see right through it. Well, it all depends on how you look at it. Doesn't it?

FELICITY: When did they say they were coming?

AGNES: Let's see. Today is the fifth. The fifth of May.

MAGGIE: I called home. I told them we got here all right. I told them . . . I don't know . . . I wanted to talk to Pop. But he was asleep. He takes naps now. He gets up every morning at seven and he goes to church. All his life–since the day he was married–you couldn't get him near a church. Now he's seventy-five and he's there every morning. I asked him why, he said it was between him and God. What does that mean?

FELICITY: When did they say they were coming?

AGNES: Yes. Mexico. They should be passing right through the center of Mexico today.

FELICITY: They're moving awfully slow, don't you think?

AGNES: Well, it's difficult for them, I imagine. Trying to get so much organized, a family, a whole family and everything else . . . You can't just drop everything and leave. Especially if you live in a foreign country, as they do . . .

BRIAN: I asked one of the doctors. I said, why do I shake like this? He said

he didn't know . . . I said, well . . . is it a symptom or is it because of the
drugs? He said, no. And I said, well, why then? I don't seem to have any
control of it. I'm feeling perfectly all right and then I shake.

And he said, try to think if it's ever happened before . . . that kind of
thing. And I couldn't. For a long time. And then I remembered being
very young . . . I was—oh—five years old. My father was taking me to
Coney Island. And we got separated on the train. And I kept trying to
ask for directions but I couldn't talk because I was shaking so badly.
It was because I was frightened. That . . . uh . . . That's why I shake now.
Isn't it?

FELICITY: *(In great pain)* Agnes . . . !!! Agnes.

AGNES: Yes, Mama, here. It's all right.

FELICITY: Agnes! Sons of bitches . . .

JOE: I get dreams now. Every night. I get dreams so big. I never used to dream.
But now, every night so big. Every person I ever knew in my life coming
through my room, talking and talking and sometimes singing and dancing.
Jumping all around my bed. And I get up to go with them, but I can't. The
sheets are too heavy and I can't move to save my life. And they keep talking
and calling my name, whispering so loud it hurts my ears . . ."Joe" and "Joe"
and laughing and singing and I know every one of them and they pull at my
arms and my legs and I still can't move. And I'm laughing and singing, too,
inside, where you can't hear it . . . And it hurts so bad, but I can't feel it. And
I yell back at them, every person I ever knew, and they don't hear me, either,
and then the room gets brighter and brighter. So bright I can't see anything
anymore. Nobody. Not even me. It's all gone. All white. All gone.

FELICITY: Agnes . . . !!

AGNES: Yes, Mama.

FELICITY: When did they say they were coming?

AGNES: I don't know, Mama. Soon. Soon.

FELICITY: As long as we know . . . As long as we know they're coming.

AGNES: Well, of course they're coming. You wait and see . . . One afternoon,
we'll be sitting here, having tea, and that door will fly open like the gates
of heaven and there they'll be . . .

*(She takes a capsule from a small bottle and adds the medication to the cup
of tea.)*

. . . two twin angels and our bright-eyed little girl. You wait and see, Mama.
You wait . . .

(She takes the cup to FELICITY *and then notices that she is asleep.)* Mama?
Oh, Mama.

BRIAN: *(Going to* BEVERLY*)* Dance with me, Bev.

BEVERLY: My pleasure, sir.

MAGGIE: Joe?

JOE: We got to tell him, Maggie. We got to tell him.

AGNES: Rest, Mama . . . rest . . .

MARK: It'll all be over in a minute. It just seems to take forever.

(The lights fade out.)

ACT II

Evening.

Music is coming from the living room area . . . a recording of "Don't Sit Under The Apple Tree." BEVERLY is dancing around alone, BRIAN is sitting on the sofa watching her. MARK is in the kitchen area getting a glass of milk.

As the lights come up, however, we focus on the porch area where MAGGIE is seated, staring off at the sunset. JOE comes down to her, carrying a cup of coffee.

JOE: It's getting dark, Maggie.

MAGGIE: *(Very distant)* It's pretty.

JOE: Yeah. *(Pause)* You can't sit out here all night. Huh? *(MAGGIE doesn't answer.)* I brought you some coffee. *(MAGGIE takes it.)*

MAGGIE: I'm all right. I'm all right. I just need some time, that's all.

JOE: I'll get you a sweater

(JOE goes back into the cottage, to the UC room and sits. Our focus shifts now into the living room area. It looks like a small party. BEVERLY is carrying on and BRIAN is enjoying every minute of it. MARK is not.)

BRIAN: Another drink for Beverly and then she can show us her scars.

BEVERLY: Medals, medals! Not scars.

BRIAN: Well, we won't argue the perspective.

MARK: *(Giving her a drink)* I don't understand.

BEVERLY: Dancing contests. That's a euphemism for balling. First prize, second prize, third prize . . . sometimes just a citation for style. I like to keep Brian informed.

MARK: You lost me.

BEVERLY: Look. *(She takes off an earring.)* Peter somebody. Diamonds. Really. very pure, very idealistic, an architect. Form follows function . . . never understood it. *(She tosses the earring into her tote bag.)*

BRIAN: *(Toasting with his milk)* To Peter!

BEVERLY: *(Drinks)* One among many. *(She takes off a bracelet.)* This one's copper. A doctor in Colorado Springs. Said it would cure my arthritis and he'd take care of the rest. He didn't. *(She drops the bracelet on the floor.)*

BRIAN: *(Toasting again)* Colorado Springs!

BEVERLY: *(Drinks)* Anyway, I didn't have arthritis. *(She points to a brooch.)* This one, God knows. A family heirloom and would I join the collection. No, thank you. *(Takes off a chain necklace with a tooth on it and swings it in a circle.)* Claus. Norwegian shark tooth or something. A thousand and one positions, and each one lasted several hours. I couldn't. *(She drops it.)*

BRIAN: I should hope not.

BEVERLY: But I tried. *(Takes another, very similar to the previous one, but smaller.)* Claus' brother. If at first you don't succeed . . . *(Points at a bracelet)* A Russian in Paris. *(Another bracelet)* A Frenchman in Moscow. *(Taking off an ankle bracelet)* Ah . . . a Tunisian in Newfoundland. Really. We met at an airport and made it between flights under his grass skirt. *(Drops it on the couch and then takes off two tiaras)* Two lovely ladies in Biarritz. No comment, thank you. *(Drops it on the sofa)* Oh . . . yes. The Jean Jacques collection. *(Taking off several other pieces)* Jean Jacques. Jean Jacques. Jean Jacques. Jean Jacques. Jean Jacques. You might say I took him for everything he was worth. You'd be wrong. There was a whole lot more I couldn't get my hands on. *(Toasting)* A big one for Jean Jacques.

BRIAN: *(Toasting)* Jean Jacques!

BEVERLY: *(A little dizzy)* I'm getting sloppy. I tried. Dear Brian, how, I tried. *(To MARK)* You're the scholar. What's the exact declension of incompatibility? I tried, they tried, we tried . . .

MARK: That's not a declension. That's a conjugation.

BEVERLY: No, it wasn't. Not once. Not a single conjugator in the bunch. Not one real dancer. Not one real jump to the music, flat out, no count, foot stomping crazy-man . . . just a lot of tired "declining" people who really didn't want to do anything but sit the next one out. What else? Oh. Last and least, my favorite dress. A gap here, a stain there, a spilled drink, a catch, a tear . . . spots you can hardly see, that won't come out . . . people hardly knew.

MARK: It looks walked over.

BEVERLY: Over and over again. stitch it up, tie it up, wrap it up . . . it keeps coming back for more. Greedy little bitch. Here's a good one. A very well dressed man on a train. Put his hand here, on my leg, kept saying over and over again, "Trust me, trust me," and all the time he was beating off under his coat.

MARK: That's pathetic.

BEVERLY: Oh, I don't know. I think he liked me. Don't you think so? I mean the car was full of attractive younger women and the bastard chose me.

MARK: You must have been his type.

BRIAN: Mark!

MARK: I'm sorry. It just came out.

BEVERLY: That's all right.

MARK: It's not all right, it stinks.

BEVERLY: Okay. It stinks. Forget it. Here's to all of them. The young, the old, the black, the white, the yellow, the lame, the hale, the feebleminded, the poor, the rich, the small and the well endowed . . . all of them. Here's hoping there's better where *they* came from.

MARK: *(Getting his jacket and going toward, the door)* I'm going out for a walk.

BEVERLY: Oh, no. How are we ever going to get to know each other if you keep leaving the room?

BRIAN: Don't go, Mark.

MARK: I need some air. *(He starts to go.)*

BEVERLY: No. Stay. Come on. Please. *(She gets the champagne bottle.)*

MARK: Please what? You don't need me here, you've got a captive audience.

BEVERLY: Come on, We'll open the champagne and I'll shut up for a while.

MARK: Thanks, but I already told you . . .

BEVERLY: *(Forcing off the cork)* It's good stuff. I only *look* cheap. Really. Are you sure you wouldn't like . . .

(The cork flies off and BEVERLY *accidentally spills the contents of the bottle on* MARK*)*

. . . a drink?

MARK: *(Sopping wet)* No. Thank you.

BEVERLY: *(Really embarrassed, somewhere between giggling and crying)* Oh, God, I'm sorry. Talk about tedious people. I think I feel an exit coming up.

BRIAN: *(Goes to her, comforting)* You look very beautiful, Beverly. I should have noticed when I walked in.

BEVERLY: I'm tired and drunk.

BRIAN: And beautiful.

BEVERLY: *(Clings to him for an instant)* I'll miss you, you fucker.

BRIAN: I'll miss you, too.

BEVERLY: *(To* MARK*)* Look what I've done. *(She starts to take the jacket from him.)*

MARK: *(Not letting go)* It's all right.

BEVERLY: No. It's not. I've ruined it.

MARK: All right, you've ruined it

BEVERLY: I'll send you another one.

MARK: No, I'll have it cleaned.

BEVERLY: It won't come out.

MARK: Please!

BRIAN: *(Grabbing the jacket and throwing it down)* My God, it's only a jacket. Two sleeves, a collar, a piece of cloth. It was probably made by a machine in East Podunk. Why are we wasting this time?

MARK: Brian, take it easy . . .

BRIAN: No! Not easy. Not easy at all! At this very moment, twelve million stars are pumping light in and out of a three hundred and sixty degree notion of a limited universe. Not easy! At this very moment, a dozen Long Island oysters are stranded in some laboratory in Chicago, opening and closing to the rhythm of the tide–over a thousand miles away. Not easy! At this very moment, the sun is probably hurtling out of control, defying ninety percent of all organized religion–plummeting toward a massive world collision that was predicted simultaneously by three equally archaic cultures who had barely invented the wheel. At this very moment, some simple peasant in Mexico is planting seeds in his veins with the blind hope that flowers will bloom on his body before the frost kills him! And here we stand, the combined energy of our three magnificent minds focused irrevocably on this fucking jacket.

(He picks up the jacket and hands it to MARK.)

My God. There are more important things I promise you.

(MARK does not respond. BRIAN goes to BEVERLY and takes her in his arms.)

Come on, my beauty, I'll show you a dancer.

(They begin to do the Lindy. BRIAN turns on the tape recorder and "Don't Sit Under the Apple Tree" starts to play.)

BEVERLY: *(Laughing)* Brian! Stop!

(Suddenly BRIAN falters. Breathless, he starts to fall, catches himself, and then falls.

BEVERLY: *(goes to him.)*

Brian?! Are you all . . . ?

BRIAN: No! No. It's all right. I'm all right. He walks, he talks, he falls down, he gets up. Life goes on.

MARK: Let me give you a hand.

BRIAN: Leave me alone.

(Carefully he exits to the bedroom. BEVERLY looks anxiously at MARK.)

BEVERLY: Do you think you should . . . ?

MARK: No. No.

(MARK doesn't move. Finally, BEVERLY follows BRIAN to the bedroom. BEVERLY exits.

MARK: *picks up the bottle, turns off the recorder, sits down and starts drinking from the bottle.*

At the same time, AGNES *comes down to the stool at DR kitchen area, which becomes her Interview Area)*

AGNES: *(Speaking to the* INTERVIEWER*)* I shouldn't stay too long.

INTERVIEWER: *(At DL stool, but still miked)* Yes. We won't keep you.

AGNES: You said you wanted to see me. Are there people there?

INTERVIEWER: Yes.

AGNES: I don't know what I can tell you.

INTERVIEWER: Well . . .

AGNES: The doctors saw her yesterday. They said they were going to change the medication, and after that, they weren't sure . . . Oh, but they must have told you all this.

INTERVIEWER: Yes.

AGNES: Oh. What . . . what was it you wanted to know, then.

INTERVIEWER: Well, we wanted to know about you.

AGNES: *(Almost smiles)* Me? Oh, that's . . . *(Then worried)* Why? I've done everything that . . . just like the nurse tells me. I've been very careful to . . .

INTERVIEWER: No. No. It isn't that. You're doing very well with her. Much better than anyone could ask. We know that.

AGNES: Then . . . what?

INTERVIEWER: Well, we were just wondering how you were?

AGNES: *(Relieved)* Oh. I'm fine. Is that what you mean? I'm fine.

INTERVIEWER: Yes.

AGNES: I'm fine.

INTERVIEWER: Good.

AGNES: Yes. I'm a little tired. And sometimes a headache . . . I used to get headaches.

INTERVIEWER: Oh?

AGNES: Yes. Terrible headaches. Mama always said they were psychosomatic. She said if I concentrated hard enough, they would go away.

INTERVIEWER: And did they?

AGNES: As a matter of fact, they did, Not right away. But after a while . . .

INTERVIEWER: Do you still get them?

AGNES: What . . . ?

INTERVIEWER: The headaches. Do you still get them?

AGNES: I don't know. I used to get them so often. Now sometimes I don't know I have them–until they go away. You get used to them and you don't feel any different until they're gone. And I . . . what was it you wanted to ask me?

INTERVIEWER: Tell us about Claire.

AGNES: What?

INTERVIEWER: Claire. Felicity has been telling us that . . .

AGNES: Claire.

INTERVIEWER: Your sister.

AGNES: Oh, Claire . . .

INTERVIEWER: Yes.

AGNES: Claire is my sister.

INTERVIEWER: Yes.

AGNES: *(With great reluctance)* We were very close. Our whole family. Especially after my father died. We were just children then. Mama worked very hard to keep us together. We had a dairy farm. It was a beautiful place. Big, old house . . . 1873. And so much land. It seemed even bigger then . . . I was so little. We were very happy.

And then Claire . . . there was a boy . . . well, she left us . . . just like that. She was a lot like Mama. They would fight and yell and throw things at each other . . . they got along very well.

Claire was so beautiful. I would hide in my room. I got so frightened when they fought, but . . . I don't know . . . suddenly the fight would be over and Mama would throw open her arms and curse the day she bore children and Claire would laugh and then Mama would laugh and hug her close . . . and then all of us, we would laugh . . . I can still hear us . . .

But she left. And we never heard from her. Almost a year. The longest year I can remember. Mama waited and waited, but she never wrote or came back to visit . . . nothing. And then one morning, finally, we received a letter from a man in Louisiana. There was an accident . . . something. And Claire was dead. They said at first they thought she was going to be all right, but she was hemorrhaging and . . . This is very hard to remember.

INTERVIEWER: But these letters from Claire.

AGNES: Yes. You see, it was after Claire died that Mama started to get sick. All of a sudden, she was "old." And she isn't, you know. But she just seemed to give up. I couldn't bring her out of it. Claire could have. But I couldn't. We lost the farm, the house, everything. One thing led to another.

The letters . . . uh . . . It was after one of the last of the operations. Mama came home from the hospital and she seemed very happy. She was stronger than ever. She laughed and joked and made fun of me, just like she used to . . . and then she told me she had written a letter while she was in the hospital . . . to Claire . . . and she said she forgave her for not writing and keeping in touch and she asked her to come home to visit and to bring her children . . . Claire had been dead for a long time then.

I didn't know what to do. I tried to tell her . . . I tried . . . but she wouldn't listen . . .

And, of course, no letter came. No reply. And Mama asked every day for the mail. Every day I had to tell her no, there wasn't any. Every day. I kept hoping she would forget, but she didn't. And when there wasn't any letter for a long time, she started to get worse. She wouldn't talk and when she did she accused me of being jealous and hiding the letters and sometimes . . . I didn't know what to do . . . So . . . *(Pause)*

INTERVIEWER: How long have you been writing these letters?

AGNES: Almost two years . . . You're not angry with me, are you?

INTERVIEWER: No.

AGNES: It means so much to her. It's important to her. It's something to hope for. You have to have something. People *need* something to keep them going.

INTERVIEWER: Do they?

AGNES: Yes. Sometimes I think, if you can wait long enough, something will happen. Oh, not that Mama will get better, but something . . .

So I write the letters. I don't mind. It's not difficult. I read little things in books and newspapers and I make up what's happening. Sometimes I just write whatever comes into my head. You see, Mama doesn't really listen to them anymore. She used to. It used to be the only time I could talk to her. But now it doesn't matter what they say. It's just so she knows that Claire is coming.

INTERVIEWER: What happens when Claire doesn't show up?

AGNES: Oh, but I don't think that will happen. I mean, Mama . . . well, she won't . . . I mean, even if . . .

INTERVIEWER: You mean she'll probably die before she even finds out.

AGNES: *(Nods her head)* Yes.

INTERVIEWER: What will *you* do then, Agnes?

AGNES: *(Surprised by the question, she looks at the INTERVIEWER for a long time. Then . . .)* It makes her happy.

INTERVIEWER: Does it?

AGNES: *(More confused)* I don't know.

INTERVIEWER: What about you, Agnes?

AGNES: Me?

INTERVIEWER: Does it make you happy?

AGNES: Me?

INTERVIEWER: Yes.

AGNES: *(She touches her head lightly.)* Please, I . . . I should be getting back.

INTERVIEWER: Agnes?

AGNES: Sometimes she does things now, I don't know why . . . I . . . *(Trying to accuse the* INTERVIEWER*)* The pain is much worse. This medicine you've given her . . . it doesn't help.

INTERVIEWER: Yes, we know. It may be necessary to move her up to the hospital again.

AGNES: But you said before . . .

INTERVIEWER: I know.

AGNES: And now?

INTERVIEWER: It's hard to say.

AGNES: No.

INTERVIEWER: I'm sorry.

AGNES: No, you are not sorry. You don't know. You put her in some room. You do one more operation. You wrap her up in your machines. You scribble on her chart. And then you go away. You don't know anything about sorry.

INTERVIEWER: We hoped it wouldn't go on this long, but there's nothing we can do about it.

AGNES: But I don't *want* it to go on. You promised . . . it can't! Even when she's asleep now, she has dreams. I can tell. I hear them. You keep saying, a few days, a few days. But it's weeks and months . . . all winter and now the spring . . .

INTERVIEWER: She has a strong will.

AGNES: *(Almost laughs)* I know that.

INTERVIEWER: Sometimes that's enough to keep a very sick person alive for a long time.

AGNES: But why? Why? When it hurts so bad? Why does she want to keep going like this?

INTERVIEWER: She's waiting for Claire.

AGNES: *(Stunned)* What . . . ? What did you say?

INTERVIEWER: It's what we call "making a bargain." She's made up her mind that she's not going to die until Claire arrives.

AGNES: *(Denying it)* Oh, no . . . no . . .

INTERVIEWER: . . . it might easily be the reason. Now that you've explained about the letters.

AGNES: . . . no . . . no . . .

INTERVIEWER: Agnes . . . ?

AGNES: . . . no . . . It isn't true . . . It isn't . . .

INTERVIEWER: Perhaps it isn't . . .

(In the cottage, FELICITY *is slowly waking up. She mumbles.)*

FELICITY: . . . Claire . . .

AGNES: It isn't wrong to hope.

INTERVIEWER: Agnes . . . ?

AGNES: . . . waiting for . . .

FELICITY: . . . Claire . . .

AGNES: . . . no . . . she can't . . . she can't do that . . . she can't.

INTERVIEWER: Agnes . . .

AGNES: *(Rising)* No. Please. I have to go . . . I have to go back . . .

INTERVIEWER: Listen to me . . .

AGNES: No! . . . I don't want to.

INTERVIEWER: Will you come back tomorrow?

AGNES: Tomorrow?

FELICITY: . . . put 'em away . . .

AGNES: Yes .

FELICITY: Put 'em away.

INTERVIEWER: All right, then.

(AGNES turns quickly and goes back into the cottage.

The lights fade on the Interview Area.

At the same time, JOE comes out of the cottage and goes to MAGGIE and puts a sweater on her shoulders.

In the kitchen area, AGNES goes to FELICITY and tries to comfort her disturbed sleep.)

FELICITY: . . . Claire? . . . Claire? . . . Claire?

AGNES: . . . yes, Mama . . . I'm here . . . I'm here . . .

(The focus shifts down to the porch area.)

MAGGIE: I found a picture of us in New York. Kids. We were kids. Laughing. Standing on my head in Central Park. You were in uniform. What did we have? A few days in January was all. A little box camera, and that was broken, it didn't work all the time, you had to be so careful with it.

JOE: You were nervous all the time, you never stopped laughing.

MAGGIE: I was pretty in the picture. I had a head like a rock–headstands, handstands, cart wheels–Remember? I must have been crazy. I could run. I could sing . . . I was in the play one year. *The Red Mill.*

JOE: You got thrown out.

MAGGIE: I did not.

JOE: You got thrown out.

MAGGIE: No.

JOE: On your ass.

MAGGIE: All right, all right. It wasn't my fault. What was his name?

JOE: I don't know, Vice-principal, somebody.

MAGGIE: Son of a bitch kept putting his hands all over me. *(She almost laughs.)*

JOE: You were pretty.

MAGGIE: I loved it.

JOE: You punched him in the mouth.

MAGGIE: I was scared. What else could I do?

JOE: You got thrown out.

MAGGIE: I got thrown out.

(The words spill as they remember bits and pieces of their life together, searching for some solid ground.)

MAGGIE: I was still a virgin.

JOE: I never touched you until we were married.

MAGGIE: I wanted you to. I did.

JOE: Your mother would have killed me.

MAGGIE: We went to New York . . .

JOE: Sometimes Connecticut. With Steve . . .

MAGGIE: He doesn't remember . . .

JOE: In the fall, in the Plymouth . . .

MAGGIE: I tell him, but he doesn't remember . . .

JOE: Sundays and Saturdays, when I could get off . . .

MAGGIE: He should have had brothers and sisters . . .

JOE: We couldn't.

MAGGIE: I know.

JOE: They asked me all those questions. I was embarrassed, but I told them. They said, no, no more kids.

MAGGIE: It hurt so bad, I cried . . .

(In the kitchen, AGNES begins to talk to FELICITY, who is still asleep.)

AGNES: Mama . . . Mama . . . ?

(FELICITY continues to sleep.)

If I told you the truth, Mama, would you listen? If I told you the truth, would you think I was lying?

MAGGIE: *(Continues with JOE)* . . . I cried.

JOE: I built the house.

MAGGIE: Way out in the country, we thought . . . way out . . .

JOE: Something to *have,* we said. Where does it go?

AGNES: *(Continuing to the sleeping FELICITY)* I don't remember the good times anymore, Mama. I keep thinking we have something to go back to. But I don't remember what it is. All I can remember is this . . .

MAGGIE: What a house . . .

AGNES: This . . .

MAGGIE: Three bedrooms . . .

JOE: One and a half baths . . .

AGNES: . . . pushing and pulling and hurting . . . this is all I can remember . . .

JOE: I did it all myself.

MAGGIE: The first two years, nothing worked.

JOE: What do you mean, nothing worked? I built it good, damn good.

MAGGIE: The wiring, the roof was bad, the plumbing, we never had water
 ... (JOE *laughs*)

AGNES: It all went wrong. What happened, Mama? There must have been a
 time when I loved you. Oh, Mama, if 1 told you the truth, if I told you the
 truth now, would it matter?

MAGGIE: Then they put in the sidewalks, the sewers ...

JOE: They never worked, either ...

(They laugh.

In the living room area, MARK *is drinking heavily.* BEVERLY *enters from the
 bedroom where she has just left* BRIAN.*)*

BEVERLY: He's resting.

MARK: He'll be all right.

BEVERLY: How about you?

MARK: Better every minute. *(He downs another drink.)*

BEVERLY: You could fool me. (MARK *gives her a look.)* Okay, Okay. I'm
 going.

(She starts to collect her things.

In the porch area)

MAGGIE: More houses, more streets ... You couldn't breathe.

JOE: Overnight ... it happened overnight ...

MAGGIE: We had to build fences. All of a sudden, fences ...

(In the living room area)

BEVERLY: You're sure he's all right?

MARK: Of course he's all right. It's just this dying business, Beverly. It gets a
 little messy every now and then.

BEVERLY: I noticed.

MARK: Did you? Brian takes such pride in putting things in order, keeping
 things in their proper perspective, it's hard to tell. I mean, give him ten
 minutes and a few thousand words, and he'll make you think dying is the
 best thing that ever happened to him. Would you like a drink?

BEVERLY: No, thank you.

MARK: It's all words for Brian. And it's a little hard to keep up. One letter
 follows the next, one paragraph, one chapter, one book after another,
 close parenthesis, end of quote. Never mind what it's all about.

BEVERLY: That's not fair.

MARK: Isn't it? The way you two have been carrying on, I was beginning to
 think I was at a wedding. I mean, I enjoy a good joke as much as the next
 fellow, but dead people are pretty low on my list of funny topics.

BEVERLY: Let's not get angry, we'll spoil your metaphor.

MARK: Fuck my metaphor! It's true! *(Pause. Then quietly.)* My God, listen to me. You think you know something. You think you *have* something . . .

(In the porch area)

JOE: More houses, more streets.

MARK: And it all goes crazy.

JOE: So many goddamn things. Where do they go? The freezer, the washer and the dryer, a dishwasher for Christ's sake, the lawn mower, the barbe-cue, three bicycles, four, six lawn chairs and a chaise lounge—aluminum, last forever—the white table with the umbrella, the hammock, the bar, I put that wood paneling in the basement, we finished the attic—well, half of it, I got the insulation in—the patio, with screens . . . Jesus, it was a lot to let go of.

MAGGIE: I don't want to talk about it.

JOE: Before you know it, everything you *had* is gone. Not that it was ever yours but you feel it anyway when it's gone.

MAGGIE: I'm telling you, I don't want to talk about it.

JOE: *(He turns from her)* All right! All right! We won't talk about it.

MAGGIE: You get tired. You get old. My hands got too big. I got too fat. I don't know how it happens, I can't remember.

(In the living room)

MARK: . . . when I met Brian, I was hustling outside a bar in San Francisco. Right after the great "summer of love." You remember the summer of love . . . one of those many American revolutions that get about as far as *Time* magazine and then fart to a quick finish. Well, just after the summer of love, winter came. Which was the last thing anybody expected. And sud-denly it got very cold. People were starving to death in the streets.

BEVERLY: Sounds lovely.

MARK: Very colorful—you would have liked it. Anyway, like everybody else, I was very hungry, very desperate . . . the whole scene. So there I was one night, like many other nights, selling it down on Market Street, I wasn't very good at it, but it was paying the rent, and Brian walks up to me . . . I didn't know him of course . . . he walks up and asks me the *time*. Right?

Well, I did my little number about time for what and how much was it worth to him . . . I figured anybody who'd come on to me with an old line like that was good for a fast twenty.

And all of a sudden, he starts explaining exactly what time *was* worth to him . . . Philosophy! On Market Street.

And before I know it, he's into concepts of history, cyclical and lineal configurations, Hebraic and Greco-Roman attitudes, repetitive notions . . . time *warps*, even! Jesus, I thought, I've got a real freak on my hands!

BEVERLY: You did.

MARK: And he's talking and talking and talking and I'm thinking I've got to score soon because it's getting late and I need the bread and I'm hungry . . . but I can't get *rid* of him. I walk away, and he walks away *with* me. I go inside the bar and *he* goes inside the bar. A real "fuck bar." I figured this has got to shake him. Right? Nothing. He didn't even *notice*. People are humping on the tables practically and he's quoting Aristotle to me and Whitehead and elaborating on St. Thomas Aquinas' definition of sin . . . completely oblivious to everything around him! I thought I was losing my mind. Finally, I said, "Look, man, I haven't eaten in a long time, and I'm getting a headache. Why don't we talk some business before I starve to death?"

BEVERLY: What did he do?

MARK: He bought me dinner! I couldn't believe it. I mean, what the hell did he *want* from me? And he never stopped talking. Never.

BEVERLY: Perfect. And then he left.

MARK: Right.

BEVERLY: He didn't want *anything* from you.

MARK: But before he went, I lifted his wallet.

BEVERLY: I always warned him not to talk to strangers.

MARK: It doesn't matter, because the next day I returned it. I don't know why. I just did. And that's how I got to know him. I got interested in what he was doing . . . which as it turns out was nothing. But he was doing it so well. He gave me a room. I could use it whenever I wanted.

I started reading again . . . I thought to myself, my God, I could really *do* something. Salvation! We talked and talked endlessly . . . word equals idea equals action equals change equals time equals freedom equals . . . well, who knows? But the point is

. . . What am I talking about?

BEVERLY: Dead people.

MARK: Exactly! I mean, exactly!

BEVERLY: Exactly what?

MARK: I mean *it's not enough!* Ten thousand pages of paragraphed garbage . . . it's just words. We are dying here, lady. That's what it's about. We are dropping like flies. Look around you, one word after another, one life after another . . . Zap. Gone. Dead.

Don't sit there with your ass falling off and try to deny it. Because you can't.

Brian looks at me and I can see it in his eyes. One stone slab smack in the face, the rug is coming out from under, the light is going *out*. You can do the pills and the syringes and the "let's play games" with cotton swabs and x-rays, but it's not going to change it. You can wipe up the mucous and the blood and the piss and the excrement, you can burn the sheets and boil his clothes, but it's still there. You can smell it on him. You can smell it on me. It soaks into your hands when you touch him. It gets into your blood. It's stuck inside him, filling up inside his head, inside his skin, inside his mouth. You can taste it on him, you can swallow it and feel it inside your belly like a sewer.

You wake up at night and you shake and you spit. You try to vomit it out of you. But you can't. It doesn't go away. It stays inside you. Inside every word, every touch, every move, every day, every night, it lies down with you and gets in between you. It's sick and putrid and soft and rotten and it is killing me.

BEVERLY: It's killing him, too.

MARK: That's right, lady. And some of us have to watch it. Some of us have to live with it and clean up after it. I mean, you can waltz in and out of here like a fucking Christmas tree if you want to, but some of us are staying. Some of us are here for the duration.

And it is not easy.

BEVERLY: And some of us wouldn't mind changing places with you at all.

MARK: And some of us just don't care anymore.

BEVERLY: What?

MARK: Some of us just don't care.

BEVERLY: You're cute, Mark. But next to me, you are the most selfish son of a bitch I've ever met.

MARK: Oh, wonderful! That's what I needed. Yes, sir. That's just what I needed.

BEVERLY: You're welcome!

MARK: Look, don't you think it's time you picked up all your little screwing trophies and went home?

BEVERLY: Past time . . . way past time. The sign goes up and I can see "useless" printed all over it. Let me tell you something, as one whore to another–what you do with your ass is your business. You can drag it through every gutter from here to Morocco. You can trade it, sell it, or give it away. You can run it up a flagpole, paint it blue or cut it off if you feel like it.

I don't care. I'll even show you the best way to do it. That's the kind of person I am. But Brian is different. Because Brian is stupid. Because Brian is blind. Because Brian doesn't know where you come from or who you come from or why or how or even what you are coming to. Because Brian happens to need you.

And if that is not enough for you, then you get yourself out of his life–
fast. You take your delicate sensibilities and your fears and your disgust
and you pack it up and get out.

MARK: That simple, huh?

BEVERLY: Yes. That simple. A postcard at Christmas, a telegram for his
birthday, and maybe a phone call every few years . . . if he lives. But only
when it gets really bad.

When the money and the time and the people are all running out
faster than you care to count, and the reasons don't sound as good as
they used to and you don't remember anymore why . . . why you walked
out on the one person who said yes, you do what you have to because I
love you. And you can't remember anymore what it was you thought you
had to do or who the hell you thought you were that was so goddamn
important you couldn't hang around long enough to say goodbye or to
find out what it was you were saying goodbye to . . . Then you phone,
because you need to know that somewhere, for no good reason, there is
one poor stupid deluded human being who smells and rots and dies and
still believes in you. One human being who cares. My God, why isn't that
ever enough?

MARK: You want an answer to that?

BEVERLY: No. I want you to get yourself together or get yourself away from
him.

MARK: Just leave.

BEVERLY: Yes.

MARK: I can't.

BEVERLY: Why not?

MARK: He's dying.

BEVERLY: He doesn't need *you* for that. He can do it all by himself. You're
young, intelligent, not bad looking . . . probably good trade on a slow
market. Why hang around?

MARK: I can't leave him.

BEVERLY: Why not?

MARK: I owe him.

BEVERLY: What? Pity?

MARK: No.

BEVERLY: Then what? You don't make sense, Mark. I mean, what's in it for
you?

MARK: Nothing's in it for me.

BEVERLY: So what's keeping you here? You said it yourself. He's just a tired,
sick old man . . .

MARK: What?

BEVERLY: ... A tired old trick with some phony ideas that don't hold piss,
  let alone water ...

MARK: Get out of here.

BEVERLY: A broken-down sewer, that's all he is.

MARK: I didn't say that ...

BEVERLY: Yes, you did. Garbage. You can't even bear to look at him. You
  don't need that. You don't need to dirty your hands with that kind of
  rotten, putrid filth. Unless of course you need the money. What does he
  do—pay you by the month? Or does it depend on how much you put out?

(MARK *suddenly hits her in the face.* BEVERLY *quickly slaps him back–*
  hard–several times.

MARK *is stunned.*

So is BEVERLY.

A sudden silence.

Embarrassment.

Pain.

Finally, MARK *breaks down.)*

MARK: I don't want him to die. I don't ... Please ...

(BEVERLY *goes to him tentatively and puts her arms around him.)* I don't
  want him to die.

(JOE *is at up left.* MAGGIE *is at up right)*

JOE: Maggie ... ?

MAGGIE: *(Crossing to up left)* I'm here, Joe, It's all right.

JOE: Maggie ... ?

(In the kitchen area)

FELICITY: Claire ... ?

AGNES: Yes, Mama ...

(The lines overlap, coming from all three areas.)

MAGGIE: I'm here, Joe ...

BEVERLY: It's all right ...

FELICITY: Claire ... ?

AGNES: Yes, Mama ... I'm here ...

MAGGIE: It's all right now ...

BEVERLY: It's all right.

AGNES: It's all right ...

MAGGIE: Sshhh ...

BEVERLY: It's all right. It's all right.

MAGGIE: Sshhh ...

(Pause)

BEVERLY: *(Gently)* Hopes, baby. That's what you got. A bad case of the hopes. They sneaked up on you when you weren't looking. You think maybe it's not gonna happen. You think maybe you'll find some way out. Some word that's still alive, some word that will make it all different . . . Maybe, maybe, maybe . . .

FELICITY: *(Waking up)* Claire . . . ?

MAGGIE: It's all right . . .

AGNES: Yes, Mama . . .

MAGGIE: Sshhh . . .

BEVERLY: Please, baby. Just one favor you owe him. Don't hurt him Don't hurt him with your hope. *(MARK pulls away from BEVERLY.)* He needs somebody. *(MARK doesn't answer.)* Yeah. That was my answer, too. *(She gathers her things.)* 'Bye, baby.

MARK: Wait . . .

BEVERLY: No, no. Another two minutes and I'll be dancing you all over the floor.

MARK: I might not mind.

BEVERLY: Might not mind? You'd love it.

MARK: All right. I'd love it.

BEVERLY: Tell Brian goodbye for me.

MARK: Don't you want to see him?

BEVERLY: No. I've got a plane to catch. I want to get to Hawaii before the hangover hits me. *(She stops and turns to MARK.)* It's funny, he always makes the same mistake. He always cares about the wrong people.

(In the kitchen area)

FELICITY: Claire . . .

AGNES: What happened, Mama?

BEVERLY: Bye!

FELICITY: Claire . . .

AGNES: You sit down one day, and you get caught . . . you get caught somewhere in a chair . . . in some foreign room. Caught in slow motion . . .

(BEVERLY exits DL.)

   . . . stretched across the floor, listening to the windows and the doors. It's hard to remember sometimes what you're listening *for*. A whistle, maybe . . . or a shout . . . somebody calling your name. Or maybe just a few words. A few kind words. A ticket to Louisiana . . . a letter . . . something . . .

(In the porch area)

JOE: A farm would have been nice.

MAGGIE: We couldn't afford it.

JOE: Some place all our own.

AGNES: Something.

MAGGIE: Just to watch the sunset?

JOE: Every day a different job. Every day a different reason. Something grows, something . . . all in a day.

AGNES: Something . . .

MAGGIE: It would have been nice.

JOE: Something to have.

AGNES: Something . . .

JOE: Jesus Christ, we built the house, and before we finish, fifteen years, and it's gone.

MAGGIE: We didn't need it. It was more work to keep up than it was worth.

JOE: Maybe . . . maybe it was. But it was *something,* wasn't it? Something to have. You put in one more fucking tree, you fix up another room, I kept seeing grandchildren.

What the hell else was it for? Not right away, but someday, you figure, kids running around, falling down under it, when it's grown big enough to climb and you can chase them down, spend some time running around the goddamn house . . .

MAGGIE: *(Still detached)* The apartment is nice. It was closer to work.

JOE: *(Starting to get really angry)* Work? Shit. Fifty weeks a year in a flat-wire shop. Twenty-four years.

MAGGIE: We had the saloon in between. And the oil truck . . .

JOE: A bartender and a truck driver in between.

MAGGIE: We *owned* the bar. That was ours.

JOE: Gone.

MAGGIE: And the truck, we owned . . .

JOE: All gone. Christ, even the factory is gone.

MAGGIE: They couldn't get along without you.

JOE: Twenty-four years. Two weeks a year at the beach. One week off for Christmas . . . *(Pause)* Talk to me, Maggie. Talk to me.

MAGGIE: What? What can I say?

JOE: I don't know. Somebody walks up one day, one day, somebody walks up and tells you it's finished. And me . . . all I can say is "what?" . . . *what's* finished? What did I have that's finished? What?

MAGGIE: We give up too easy. We don't fight hard enough. We give up . . . too easy . . .

JOE: We got to tell him, Maggie. We got to face it and tell him. Some son of a bitch walks up one day and tells you it's finished. What? What did we have that's finished?

MAGGIE: *(Breaking down)* Us. Us. For Christ's sake, don't make me say things I don't understand. I don't want to hear them. I shake all over when I think about them. How long? Two weeks? Three? A month? And then what? What have I got *then?* An apartment full of some furniture I can't even keep clean for company, a closet full of some old pictures, some curtains I made out of my wedding dress that don't even fit the windows . . . What? What do I do? Sit down with the TV set every night, spill my coffee when I fall asleep on the sofa and burn holes in the carpet, dropping cigarettes?

JOE: Maggie . . .

MAGGIE: No. I want you to come home. What is this place, anyway? They make everything so nice. Why? So you forget? I can't. I want you to come home. I want you to stay out four nights a week bowling, and then come home so I can yell and not talk to you, you son of a bitch. I want to fight so you'll take me to a movie and by the time I get you to take me I'm so upset I can't enjoy the picture. I want to make too much noise in the bathroom because you go to bed too early and I don't care if you *are* asleep because I want somebody, somebody to hug me once before I go to bed. I want to get up too early, too goddamn early, and I'll let you know about it, too, because I have to make you breakfast, because you never, never once eat it, because you make me get up too early just to keep you company and talk to you, and it's cold, and my back aches, and I got nothing to say to you and we never talk and it's six-thirty in the morning, every morning, even Sunday morning and it's all right . . . it's all right . . . it's all right because I *want* to be there because you need me to be there because I want you to be there because I want you to come home.

JOE: Maggie . . .

MAGGIE: Come home, that's all. Come home.

JOE: I can't, Maggie. You know I can't.

MAGGIE: No, I don't know. I don't.

JOE: I can't.

MAGGIE: You can. Don't believe what they tell you. What do they know? We've been through worse than this. You look fine. I can see it.

JOE: No, Maggie.

MAGGIE: You get stronger every day.

JOE: It gets worse.

MAGGIE: No. I can see it.

JOE: Every day, it gets worse.

MAGGIE: We'll go home, tomorrow. I got another ticket. We can get a plane tomorrow.

JOE: Don't do this, Maggie.

MAGGIE: I put a new chair in the apartment. You'll like. It's red. You always said we should have a big red chair. I got it for you. It's a surprise.

JOE: No! It won't work.

MAGGIE: We'll get dressed up. I'll get my hair done. We'll go out someplace. What do we need? A little time, that's all.

JOE: It's not going to change anything.

MAGGIE: No. It's too fast. Too fast. What'll I do? I can't remember tomorrow. It's no good. We'll look around. Maybe we *can* find a little place.
Something we like.

JOE: No. This is all. This is all we got.

MAGGIE: No. Something farther out. Not big. Just a little place we like. *All
right, a farm, if you want. I don't care. Tomorrow!*

JOE: *(Angry and frustrated)* Tomorrow is nothing, Maggie! Nothing! It's not
going to change. You don't snap your fingers and it disappears. You don't
buy a ticket and it goes away. It's here. Now.

MAGGIE: No.

JOE: Look at me, Maggie.

MAGGIE: No.

JOE: *Look* at me. You want magic to happen? Is that what you want? Go
ahead. Make it happen. I'm waiting. Make it happen!

MAGGIE: I can't.

JOE: Make it happen!

MAGGIE: I can't. I can't.

(STEVE comes out of the cottage. MAGGIE and JOE look at him.
MAGGIE crosses away from STEVE. He speaks quietly, sensing that he's inter-
rupted something.)

STEVE: Hey, I'm ready to play for you now. If you want to hear?

JOE: Sure, dad. I'll be right in.

STEVE: It's not great, but it's not bad, either.

JOE: Good.

STEVE: *(To MAGGIE, tentatively)* Mom, I'm sorry.

MAGGIE: What?

STEVE: I'm sorry for fucking around like that. I didn't mean to upset you.

MAGGIE: That's okay.

STEVE: Yeah?

MAGGIE: *(Smiles and goes to him)* Yeah, yeah, yeah. *(She throws her arms*
around him and holds him tightly)

JOE: You get tuned up, and I'll be right in.

STEVE: Better hurry up before I lose my nerve.

(He exists. After a moment he tunes up and we hear "Good Night, Irene" being
played on the guitar.)

JOE: I'm going inside now, Maggie. I'm going to tell him.

MAGGIE: Tell me. Say it out loud.

JOE: I'm going to die, Maggie.

MAGGIE: *(After a moment)* Why?

JOE: I don't know. I don't know. I don't know. Like everything else, I don't know. Come inside.

MAGGIE: What'll we do in there?

JOE: Try. That's all. Just try. Live with it. Look at it. Don't make me do it alone.

MAGGIE: I can't promise . . .

JOE: Don't promise. Just come inside.

(MAGGIE *doesn't move for a long time.* STEVE *continues to play the guitar softly. Finally* MAGGIE *turns and walks slowly toward the cottage.* JOE *joins her and together they walk inside.*

As they pass through the living room, MARK *checks his watch, rises from the couch and goes to the bookcase. He begins to prepare some medicine for* BRIAN, *but instead he picks up the medicine and throws it violently.*

After a beat, BRIAN *enters.)*

BRIAN: *(Looking at the mess)* What happened?

MARK: Nothing. Nothing. I had an accident.

BRIAN: Oh. Me too.

MARK: What?

BRIAN: I need some help.

MARK: What happened?

BRIAN: I . . . uh . . . I fell asleep and I wet the bed.

MARK: Come and sit down.

BRIAN: I'm embarrassed.

MARK: I'm drunk.

BRIAN: Pleased to meet you.

MARK: Sit down. Before you fall down.

BRIAN: *(Starts to sit, but then stops.)* I am truly disgusting.

MARK: No, you're not. Just wet.

(BRIAN *reaches out his hand to* MARK, *they embrace. Then* MARK *helps him off to the bedroom.*

And our focus shifts to the kitchen.)

FELICITY: *(Calling out in her sleep)* Agnes.

AGNES: *(Putting one capsule of the medicine into a cup)* Mama, if I told you the truth now, would it matter?

FELICITY: *(Waking up)* Agnes!

AGNES: *(When medicine is finished)* Yes, Mama?

FELICITY: What . . . what time is it . . . ?

AGNES: I don't know, Mama.

FELICITY: . . . sons of bitches . . . Did we get any mail today, Agnes?

AGNES: *(Every word of this lie is now more and more unbearable.)* Yes, Mama
    . . . we did . . .

FELICITY: From Claire?

AGNES: Yes, we did. Another letter from Claire. Another . . .

FELICITY: *(As if she never said it before)* I get so lonesome for Claire . . .

AGNES: *(Cutting her off)* I know, Mama . . .

FELICITY: Will you read it to me, Agnes?

AGNES: Yes, Mama.

FELICITY: *(Like a phonograph, skipping back)* I get so lonesome for Claire . . .

AGNES: *(Unable to bear any more)* Mama, please . . .

FELICITY: I get so lonesome for Claire . . .

AGNES: Please.

FELICITY: I get so lonesome . . .

AGNES: Mama. *(And then silence)*

FELICITY: Agnes?

AGNES: Yes.

FELICITY: Could I have some tea?

AGNES: *(Pours the tea and carefully puts the cup in* FELICITY's *hands)* Yes.

FELICITY: *(Holding the cup, but not drinking from it yet)* Could you read
    me the letter, now?

AGNES: Yes.

FELICITY: The letter from Claire.

AGNES: Yes. Yes. Yes.

*(She takes the letter from her pocket—the one she was writing earlier. She
    opens the envelope and begins reading . . .)*
    Dear Mama, I am writing today from Mexico. We are finally out of the
    swamp and onto high dry ground. What a relief after so much rain and
    dampness . . . Because of some unexplainable mechanical difficulties,
    we found ourselves stranded today in a beautiful little mountain village
    called San Miguel . . . It's a lovely little town clinging for dear life to the
    side of a great ghostly mountain in the middle of nowhere . . . a very
    curious place to be. Nothing has changed in hundreds of years and noth-
    ing *will* change, I guess, for hundreds more . . .

FELICITY: *(Mumbling)* . . . my bright-eyed . . . girl . . .

AGNES: . . . There are so many things to see during the day, but then the
    nights grow bitter cold . . .

(AGNES watches her, making up the words to the letter.)
    . . . and I can hear the wind blowing . . . outside the door, whistling and
    . . . and whispering . . . and when I look out the window, nothing is

there . . . nothing . . . Mama . . . I think . . . I think it's because I miss you because it hurts not being close to you . . . and . . . and touching you . . . *(AGNES breaks down and can't go any further.)*

FELICITY: Agnes?

AGNES: Yes, Mama. Yes.

FELICITY: What time is it now?

AGNES: Oh, four . . . five . . . I don't know.

FELICITY: *(Still holding her cup)* Could I have some tea, Agnes? *(AGNES just looks at her.)* Could you read me the letter now?

AGNES: Mama . . .

FELICITY: Could you read me the letter now?

AGNES: Mama . . .

FELICITY: The letter from Claire?

(Pause)

AGNES: Yes. Yes. *(She starts to read the letter again)* Dear Mama, I am writing today from Mexico. We are finally out of the swamp and onto high dry ground. What a relief after so much rain and dampness . . . Because of some unexplainable mechanical difficulties . . .

(She continues reading under the following:

In the shadows, JOE and BRIAN slowly become visible. They are standing in isolated areas, facing the audience as if they were speaking to the INTER-VIEWER.

The coda music begins)

BRIAN: People don't want to let go. Do they. They think it's a mistake. They think it's supposed to last forever . . .

JOE: There's a few things–I could talk to you about them . . .

BRIAN: I suppose it's because . . .

JOE: . . . you don't expect it to happen.

BRIAN: You don't expect it to happen to you.

JOE: But it happens anyway, doesn't it? It doesn't matter what you do, you can't stop it.

BRIAN: You try.

MARK: *(In the living room)* You keep thinking, there's got to be some way out of this.

BRIAN: You want to strike a bargain . . . make a deal.

MARK: You don't want to give in.

JOE: You want to say no.

MAGGIE: . . . no . . .

MARK: . . . no . . .

BRIAN: Your whole life goes by–it feels like it was only a minute.

BEVERLY: You try to remember what it was you believed in.

MARK: What was so important?

MAGGIE: What was it?

BEVERLY: You want it to make a difference.

MAGGIE: You want to blame somebody.

BRIAN: You want to be angry.

JOE: You want to shout, "Not me!"

BRIAN: Not me!

MAGGIE: Not me!

FELICITY: What time is it, Agnes?

AGNES: I don't know, Mama.

BRIAN: And then you think, someone should have said it sooner.

MARK: Someone should have said it a long time ago.

BEVERLY: When you were young.

BRIAN: Someone should have said, this living . . .

MARK: . . . this life . . .

BEVERLY: . . . this lifetime . . .

BRIAN: It doesn't last forever.

MAGGIE: A few days, a few minutes . . . that's all.

BRIAN: It has an end.

JOE: Yes.

MARK: This face.

BEVERLY: These hands.

MARK: This word.

JOE: It doesn't last forever.

BRIAN: This air.

MARK: This light.

BRIAN: This earth.

BEVERLY: These things you love.

MAGGIE: These children.

BEVERLY: This smile.

MAGGIE: This pain.

BRIAN: It doesn't last forever.

JOE: It was never supposed to last forever.

MARK: This day.

MAGGIE: This morning.

BEVERLY: This afternoon.

MARK: This evening.

FELICITY: What time is it, Agnes?

AGNES: I don't know, Mama. It's time to stop. Please, Mama. It's time to
stop.

BRIAN: These eyes . . .

MARK: These things you see.

MAGGIE: It's pretty.

JOE: Yes.

MARK: Yes.

BRIAN: These things you hear.

MARK: This noise.

BEVERLY: This music.

STEVE: I can play for you now. It's not good, but it's not bad either.

MAGGIE: Yes.

BEVERLY: Yes.

BRIAN: They tell you you're dying, and you say all right. But if I *am* dying . . .
    I must still be alive.

FELICITY: What time is it?

MARK: These things you have.

MAGGIE: Yes.

JOE: This smell, this touch.

MARK: Yes.

BEVERLY: This taste.

BRIAN: Yes.

MAGGIE: This breath.

STEVE: Yes.

MARK: Yes.

BRIAN: Yes.

MAGGIE: Yes.

BEVERLY: Yes.

JOE: Yes.

BRIAN: This moment.

(Long pause.
Lights fade.)

Before It Hits Home

ॐ

Cheryl L. West

INTRODUCTION

Before It Hits Home, written by Cheryl L. West, is a culturally sensitive work. It is the first major drama to address the subject of AIDS from the black perspective, charting the emotional geography of an African American family forced to face the issue when the oldest son, a jazz musician, becomes ill. Writing the play proved a challenge for the dramatist, who withstood criticism from within her own community for creating images that could be interpreted by white America as typical of the entire black community. While statistics indicate that HIV/AIDS has disproportionately affected African Americans across the United States, there has been a "collusion of denial" regarding AIDS among a population that is stigmatized by an increasing number of cases and fearful regarding the consequent threat to a favorable image of self, family, and community. An illusion has been nourished by African Americans that AIDS, bisexuality, and homosexuality are not to be found in their midst; the denial is coupled with the fear that acknowledging the prevalence of the disease could provide justification for further excluding a people who have had to confront racial bias. While recent surveys indicate that African Americans view HIV/AIDS as the nation's most urgent health problem, stigma remains one of the primary obstacles preventing people from getting tested and seeking medical treatment. West's goal in writing her play was to generate a dialogue aimed at exposing stereotypes and correcting misconceptions of gay life, familial relationships in the presence of AIDS, and courses of action to take if the catastrophe "hits home." The protagonist in West's play, Wendal Bailey, is a jazz musician who faces social ostracism on multiple counts: he is Black; he is gay; he pursues a bisexual life, cause for conflict throughout the drama; and he has AIDS. He is morally bankrupt in taking a married man with a family as a lover, with both men living on the "down low," a term in the black community to signify the lifestyle of men who lead heterosexual

251

lives while maintaining secret sexual relationships with other men. Wendal has impregnated his girlfriend without telling her that he is infected, and he has withheld knowledge of his illness from his family, further distancing him from those who care most for him.

Structurally, West dispenses with linear narration and presents the action in short scenes that blend into one another as indicated by the lighting. A particularly effective device is introduced in the first act where the scenes between Wendal and each of his lovers overlap as both Douglass and Simone compete for his exclusive attention. His vacillation between the two is rendered visual as is his desperation in trying to inform them of the truth while knowing that the revelation will sever him from each forever. Initially, Wendal is in denial. He distrusts the medical profession, and in the scene where a white female Jewish doctor confirms the diagnosis he fears, the racial tension is palpable. Wendal's reaction reflects the mistrust and wariness felt by many African Americans toward the medical establishment for tolerating racial disparities in the provision of health care. The feeling persists that whites are privileged over blacks in receiving health-related services. During his conversation with the doctor, Wendal voices the view of many when he blurts out, "You know this whole AIDS thing is some kind of conspiracy" (19). The widely held view is that the government created AIDS to control the African American population and is withholding any information about the nature of the disease, including a cure. Irrational though the feeling may seem, it has its roots in the memory of an infamous case of racial discrimination that was an element of government-sponsored research. Wendal recalls it for us: "remember ol' Tuskegee?" (20). The reference is to the Tuskegee experiment during which poor African American men in Alabama were denied treatment for syphilis while being told that they were being treated for "bad blood." Wendal feels that his diagnosis of "bad blood" links him to the men in Alabama in opposition to the medical establishment. Yet his hostility toward his doctor vanishes at her unexpected gift of a desired music cassette and her comforting touch. Later Wendal admits, "It's nice to be touched with a hand instead of rubber gloves" (33).

In contrast to the doctor, Wendal's mother becomes irrational upon learning the truth of her son's illness, suddenly viewing her entire home as contaminated. She fears to touch the very walls. While the play addresses the issue of AIDS in a general way, it is mainly exploratory of family and the conflicts and ruptured relationships generated by catastrophic illness (Russo 38). In presenting Wendal's mother, Reba, as a woman incapable of dealing with AIDS in her family, the dramatist is exposing as stereotype the notion of the black woman as martyr, able to bear any tribulation. It is fact, however, that primary among cultural values of African Americans is family as the essential institution related to care and survival. African Americans rely on loved ones as their main means of providing care when physically or terminally ill.[1] Acting as expected, Reba assumes at first the role of matriarch, affirming her identity, "I ain't never been nothing but somebody's mother" (51). Her first impulse on seeing her son in physical decline is to assume the responsibility of nursing him back to health. Upon learning of the nature of his illness and how he contracted it, she acts atypically. Her homophobic response in rejecting her son extends to her abandoning her home altogether. Her exit recalls that of an earlier heroine, Nora in Ibsen's *A Doll House,* and generates the same controversy among spectators regarding the role of women in domestic life. The major distinction between Reba's action and that of Nora's is that in leaving her home Reba is betraying her culturally inscribed obligations as caregiver. She does violence to the concept of family in denying the primacy of blood ties. She rejects the key values of her community.

Exhibiting a female sensibility, West draws female characters whose behavior follows conventional gender lines. Two women characters, Reba and Angel, are drawn exclusively in terms of their maternal identities. Simone, Wendal's fiancée, is represented as a temptress who lures her reluctant prey with sexual favors when he attempts to break off their relationship; her goal is marriage and, presumably, motherhood. The first image of Angel is that of a "very pregnant" woman whose impatience with the delay in her treatment at the clinic and her accompanying hostility suggest that she feels disadvantaged as a black woman receiving care in a predominantly white facility. Aware of her haggard appearance, she applies cosmetics to her face in an attempt to mislead the doctor, since "they don't seem to find as much wrong with you when you look pretty" (12). Her feminine wiles are exercised in her flirtation with Wendal, or "cutie pie," as she calls him at first glance. Angel's appearance explodes the myth that the disease affects only gay men. She calls attention to the fastest growing group of those with HIV, women of color.

While creating credible female characters, West draws convincing male figures as well. Homophobia in Wendal's family is not confined to his mother. His father, brother, and young son each turn from him on learning of his illness. The strongest of the male figures, Wendal's father, Bailey, is also the most complex. On learning the truth, he renounces his son and, in a violent scene, throws Wendal to the ground shouting, "Take your sissy fairy ass and get the hell out of my house" (63). When he sees that Wendal lacks the strength to lift himself up, his anger turns to grief; he drops to his knees and cradles his son in his arms.

In a surprising reversal, he assumes the role of caregiver relinquished by his wife; where his initial response had been to cast Wendal out, the last scene of the drama finds him pleading with God to give him "just one more day" with his dying son.

Bailey's transformation is owed to a deep-rooted sense of family that surfaces even as he would put aside his son. His love for Wendal overpowers his bias toward homosexuals. Revealing himself to be stronger than his wife, Bailey remains true to the value of the primacy of blood ties. Reba's vehement and irrational rejection of the altered circumstances of her household points to emotional instability that soon manifests itself in compulsive and neurotic behavior. *Before It Hits Home* explores the nature of family life, examines everyday relationships. While the victim remains the center of dramatic interest, other characters are tested as they react to the threat to health and image posed by the maverick. Both the limitations as well as the power of familial love are revealed. All the while treating a specific challenge to specific individuals, Cheryl L. West presents a view of family that transcends race and culture.

NOTES

1. The results of a study examining the caregiving process and context of African American families are noted by William L. Turner, et al. in "The Last Mile of the Way: Understanding Caregiving in African American Families at the End-of-Life," *Journal of Marital and Family Therapy* 30.4 (Oct. 2004): 427–38.

WORKS CITED

Russo, Ann. "Exploring AIDS in the Black Community." *Sojourner: The Women's Forum* 15.1 (1989): 37–38.

Turner, William L., et al. "The Last Mile of the Way: Understanding Caregiving in African American Families at the End-of-Life." *Journal of Marital and Family Therapy* 30.4 (Oct. 2004): 427–38.

West, Cheryl L. *Before It Hits Home*. New York: Dramatists Play Service, 1993.

———. *New Traditions Compendium Forums and Commentaries: 1992–96*. 1994. http://www. ntcp.org/compendium/artists/CHERYL.html. Accessed May 31, 2005.

BEFORE IT HITS HOME

By Cheryl L. West

This play is dedicated to those who have to hide
and to those who refuse to

CHARACTERS

WENDAL, Black male in his early 30s
REBA, Black woman in her 50s, Wendal's mother
BAILEY, Black man in his late 50s, Wendal's father
MAYBELLE, Black woman in her 50s, Reba's best friend
SIMONE, Black woman in her early 20s, Wendal's lover
ANGEL PETERSON, Black woman in her early 20s, Woman in clinic
DOUGLASS, Black man in his early 40s, Wendal's lover
JUNIOR, Black male in his late 20s, Wendal's younger brother
DWAYNE, Black boy, 12, Wendal's son
DOCTOR, White woman in her 40s or 50s
NURSE, A middle-age Hispanic or Asian woman

** The following part is played by the above:
ANGEL PETERSON (should be played by whoever plays Simone)
TWO ATTENDANTS (Attendants can be used as part of the crew, but their primary actions are to assist Wendal on stage.)

AUTHOR'S NOTE

There is a tendency to be seduced by the Bailey family, thus having the focus of the play be on them. This is not my intention. Wendal's two worlds—before he gets home and after he gets home—are equally important and at times, equally fractured. Douglass and Simone are not "social" characters and should not be portrayed as such. The action shifts frequently and the pacing between scenes should be quick, and in some scenes (as noted), action juxtaposed. To expedite this, whenever possible, actors should remain on stage while other scenes are taking place and remain true to the overlapping dialogue in the play.

PROLOGUE

WENDAL *is in a bar playing his saxophone.* WENDAL *is in to it, feeling the power, his power. Each note punctuates how "bad" he is. He's one fine confident specimen.*
Sound cue of audience clapping.
WENDAL: Thank you. Thank you. I dedicate that song for a special lady, Mrs. Reba Bailey, and since today is her birthday and I can't be with her . . . that

one's for you Mama. You know we talk about first love, but we got it wrong. I'm here to tell you, your first love connection is Mama, that first love journey is with her. And usually it's the one kinda love that out lasts the test of time. Home boy over there says I heard that. *(Chuckles.)* I know that's right. Don't get me wrong, I love my woman, I ain't no Oedipus or some sick shit like that, but I ain't shamed to tell you, I got one of them Sadie Mamas. Can't touch her. Yeah, you know what I'm talkin' 'bout. So happy birthday Mama . . . *(Coughs.)* This next tune, a ballad. We're gonna play it deep, deep as your Mama's soul . . . *(He plays saxophone again.)*

SIMONE: *(Crosses.)* Baby I told you that cough is getting worse. Flu doesn't hang on this long. Do I need to call the doctor for you? Is that what you're waiting on? Ok, Simone's going to call the doctor for her big baby. Make him an appointment . . . but mister baby better take his sick behind down there. No more excuses Wendal. Ok? *(Suggestively.)* Hey baby it's been a while. . . . Do I have to start hanging my panties out to dry on your horn? *(SIMONE exits.)*

WENDAL: For those of you who don't know, I'm Wendal Bailey and we're Sojourn. We're glad you came out tonight. Fellas and me gon' take a short break. So, have another drink, don't forget to tip the ladies and we'll be right back at you. *(Just then DOUGLASS strikes a match, lights a cigarette. WENDAL crosses to DOUGLASS and takes a drag off of DOUGLASS's cigarette, silence for a moment. The silence is not awkward; instead these are two people used to communicating in whatever form, even abbreviated, if and when their environment dictates to do such.)*

DOUGLASS: You have any time later?

WENDAL: I don't know. I promised Simone I'd be home early. Breaks over. You gon' wait around?

DOUGLASS: Probably. I liked that last song. What's the name of it?

WENDAL: Hell if I know. The shit defies a title. If you knew my old girl, you'd know what I mean. *(WENDAL starts to play, his sound is eerie in its need, its desperation.)*

ACT ONE

Clinic reception area. Sound of WENDAL *singing before lights. Waiting is a very pregnant* ANGEL PETERSON. *A half-finished lunch is at her side. She is tired looking, haggard.* NURSE *is sitting at the desk.*

ANGEL: *(Slamming the magazine.)* How long she gon' be? I can't be sitting up here all day.

NURSE: Like I told you before Ms. Peterson, the doctor will be with you as soon as possible.

ANGEL: That's what you said two hours ago. *(Grumbling to herself.)* All
   day sittin' up in somebody's f 'ing clinic, with nothing to look at but you
   white folks.
NURSE: Ms. Peterson, first of all I'm not white.
ANGEL: Same difference. *(WENDAL enters loudly singing so cool—so full of
   himself.)*
WENDAL: *(To NURSE.)* Excuse me, I have an appointment with a Dr. Wein-
   berg. Bailey . . .
NURSE: Yes . . . you can fill out this medical history form *(Hands him a
   clipboard.)* and the doctor will be with you in a few minutes.
ANGEL: She lying.
WENDAL: *(To ANGEL.)* What's up? How you doing?
ANGEL: Hangin'. *(WENDAL sits, works on the clipboard, starts humming and
   singing again. After a moment, to WENDAL.)* Hey. *(Louder.)* Hey. Yeah,
   I'm talking to you cutie pie. This first time here?
WENDAL: Un-hum.
ANGEL: Could tell. You too damn happy to be in the family. *(Pause.)* Tau-
   rus!
WENDAL: What?
ANGEL: Naw don't tell me. Sag, Cancer, Gemini . . . Gemini! You's a Gemini
   if I ever saw one. My old man was a Gemini. All you fine mutherfuckers
   are Geminis. Can tell by the way you walk. You think yo shit don't stink.
WENDAL: Scorpio. And I been told my shit smells better than most
   colognes, 'specially them expensive kind.
ANGEL: *(Laughs.)* Umph! I heard that. *(WENDAL laughs too.)* Man, what's
   your name?
WENDAL: Wendal. Wendal Bailey.
ANGEL: My name Angel. Angel Peterson.
WENDAL: *(Eyeing her stomach.)* So when's the big day?
ANGEL: Soon. Just holdin' on till it gits here, then I'm gittin' on board, catch-
   ing the first thing smokin' 'tween this hell and heaven's door. *(Angel has
   a coughing fit, WENDAL hands her a handkerchief. She wipes her mouth,
   then takes out a compact and lipstick, applies make-up, a little too much,
   which gives her a garish appearance. She continues while looking in the
   compact mirror.)* I don't know what I'd do without this shit. *(Re: Make-up.)*
   How I look?
WENDAL: Fine.
ANGEL: You ain't a good liar Wendal Bailey. See the secret is they don't
   seem to find as much wrong with you when you look pretty. *(Holds out
   the compact to him.)* You wanna try some?
WENDAL: I'll pass.

ANGEL: So Mr. Shit-smell-better-than-cologne, what you here to see the AIDS doctor for?

WENDAL: Who said who I was here to see? What I'm here for ain't really none of your business. . . .

ANGEL: Oh-oh. Got me a live one here. I love you first time boys. Some indignant mutherfuckers. Well you better come offa that pride Mr. Bailey, 'cause you gon' git your feelings hurt . . . *(Yelling to* NURSE.*)* Tell this sick mutherfucker he's got AIDS and put him out of his misery . . . so he can stop walking around foolin' himself . . .

NURSE: Ms. Peterson . . . we do not discuss a patient's medical history with another patient.

WENDAL: You got a nasty mouth on you, you know that?

ANGEL: Un-hun . . . it finally caught up with the rest of me.

WENDAL: Well I don't appreciate it.

ANGEL: Me neither. *(A beat.)* Solid. I was just trying to help you out brother. Welcome you into the family.

WENDAL: What are you talking about? What family?

ANGEL: You'll see . . .

NURSE: Ms. Peterson, you can come in now . . .

ANGEL: I'll see you around . . .

WENDAL: I doubt it. . . .

ANGEL: Oh yeah, we'll see each other again . . . just like the train . . . there's always a new one coming in and another one going out . . . *(She exits singing the same song* WENDAL *was singing when he entered.* NURSE *looks at* WENDAL. WENDAL *starts to laugh. It is an uneasy laugh.)*

WENDAL: She's a trip. *(Laughs again.)* I don't think the chick's playing with a full deck. Kept calling me part of some family. *(Laughs again as his laugh fades into* REBA*'s and* MAYBELLE*'s laughter. Fade in to* BAILEY *household.* MAYBELLE *is in the mirror trying to see her backside.* REBA *is standing behind her.)*

MAYBELLE: I don't see what you talkin' about Reba . . .

REBA: That's because you don't wanna see . . .

MAYBELLE: That ain't nothing . . . nothing but a curve.

REBA: Well that curve is ten pounds with dimples. You oughtta get here early so you can get on the floor with me and do some exercise.

MAYBELLE: That floor is hard.

REBA: And so is your head.

MAYBELLE: *(Pouting.)* I don't 'preciate you talking 'bout me like this. You done gone an' hurt my feelings. I oughtta keep what I brought over for myself.

REBA: What you done made now, Maybelle?

MAYBELLE: Nuttin'. It don't concern you. It's got my name on it now.

REBA: Come on. *(Tickles her.)* You ain't mad at your Reba now, are you?

MAYBELLE: *(Giving in, laughing out loud.)* Stop, stop Reba, you know I'm ticklish. Stop Reba.

REBA: *(Stops tickling her.)* I ain't got time to be carrying on like this. I got work to do. You pick some beans for me?

MAYBELLE: Yeah, but don't you want your surprise now?

REBA: *(Absentmindedly.)* What surprise?

MAYBELLE: Where's your mind Reba?

REBA: I don't know.

MAYBELLE: I told you I had got you something . . . wait till you see what . . .

REBA: *(Not really listening to her.)* Don't say nothing to Bailey but I had me one of those dreams again. My child was playing Maybelle, playing his horn, I declare he was, playing it like his life depended on it.

MAYBELLE: He's fine Reba. You would've heard if something was wrong. But wait . . . wait till you see what I got. It'll cheer you right up. *(Takes out a big box, hands it to* REBA.*)* Voila.

REBA: You didn't. I thought you brought something to eat. *(Stomps her feet.)* I know you didn't.

MAYBELLE: Well you know more than I know. Go 'head, open it up.

REBA: *(Excited like a child, goes through a ritual of balling her fists and stomping her feet, wanting to take the box, but holding back.)* I . . . I can't. I can't. I just can't. I know you didn't get it. You didn't, did you? Well, did you? I just can't. I know what it is . . . I told you I didn't need it. You did it, didn't you? You got it? I can't stand it. Naw, don't tell me . . .

MAYBELLE: Half the joy of giving you a present Reba is watching you go through this stupid ass ritual. You ain't changed since you were five years old.

REBA: Oh shut up.

MAYBELLE: Go 'head, take the box.

REBA: Well, give it here. *(Takes the box.)* Maybelle, you shouldn't spend your money on me like this.

MAYBELLE: And miss this? *(*REBA *opens the box, it's a beautiful dress.)*

REBA: Oh Maybelle.

MAYBELLE: Yeah, it's the same one. Told you to buy it but you was too cheap. I had the girl put it on lay-a-way. Go on, slip it on. *(*REBA *takes off her housecoat and slips on the dress.)*

REBA: It's beautiful.

MAYBELLE: Lord, it was meant for you. That dressmaker knew what she was doing! Go look in the mirror. *(*REBA *looks in the mirror.)*

REBA: I'm ready. *(Sings.)* "Put on your red dress baby 'cause we going out tonight. . . . Put on your high heeled sneakers . . ." *(*MAYBELLE *joins in, they sing and do an old-time dance with silly sequential steps. After a moment and unbeknownst to the two,* BAILEY *and* DWAYNE *enter.* BAILEY *is carrying two suits in a cleaning bag, which he makes a big deal about hiding from* MAYBELLE. *They watch* MAYBELLE *and* REBA *a moment, enjoying the show.)*

MAYBELLE: Whew, I done worked up a sweat. That's my exercise for the day.

REBA: *(Kisses her.)* What would I do without you?

MAYBELLE: Well, I never plan for you to find out. *(*REBA *takes off the dress and slips back into her housecoat.)*

BAILEY: *(Gruffly, for he is always jealous witness when it comes to the intimacy between the two women.)* For once I'd like to walk through this door and not find you sittin' up in my house.

MAYBELLE: You know I brighten up your day Luke Bailey . . . *(*MAYBELLE *takes out fingernail polish and an emery board, starts doing her nails.)*

REBA: *(Folding up the dress and putting it in the box.)* Bailey, call the Center. They called 'bout an hour ago.

DWAYNE: *(Overlapping, kissing her.)* Hi Aunt May.

MAYBELLE: Hi baby.

DWAYNE: Aunt May, you need me to cut the grass again this weekend?

MAYBELLE: Well, I don't know.

DWAYNE: How about trimming the hedges?

MAYBELLE: Boy, you sure is enterprising. *(*BAILEY *is almost comical as he attempts to hide the suits from* MAYBELLE *while getting* REBA *to notice them.)*

BAILEY: *(To* REBA.*)* Which one?

DWAYNE: I'm going to see my Dad if he doesn't come home soon.

BAILEY: If your father wanted you to come, he'd send for you.

REBA: Bailey!

BAILEY: Well he would. Now Reba which . . .

DWAYNE: Can I be excused?

REBA: *(Busying herself straightening up the house.)* Where you going?

DWAYNE: Watch TV.

BAILEY: *(Overlapping, whispering.)* Reba, which suit?

REBA: You do your homework?

DWAYNE: It's Saturday.

REBA: What, you don't learn nothing except Monday through Friday?

BAILEY: Boy, get it over with.

DWAYNE: But, Daddy, I can do it tomorrow.

BAILEY: Well, I was thinking that tomorrow a certain young man might want to go with his Daddy fishing.

DWAYNE: *(Excited.)* Really?

BAILEY: Yeah really, really. Reba which one? You know I got this thing coming up, you know, which suit?

REBA: I don't know Bailey. You decide. *(To DWAYNE.)* And Mister, you ain't going nowhere if I don't see you crack a book before the day is out. I mean that Dwayne. Maybelle, did you know that Bailey got nominated . . .

BAILEY: Reba.

REBA: . . . as volunteer of the year . . .

BAILEY: Reba don't . . .

REBA: . . . down at the Boy's Club.

BAILEY: Reba! Shit! *(Throws the suits on his chair, pouts.)* You getting to be just like her, can't keep nothing to yourself.

REBA: Well it ain't no secret Bailey. He's got to give a speech.

MAYBELLE: *(Crossing to BAILEY.)* Well, that's good Bailey. That's why you been trying to hide them two suits looking silly? Ain't that one your funeral suit?

BAILEY: Leave me alone.

MAYBELLE: Wish that husband of mine would volunteer at something.

REBA: He just enjoying his retirement.

MAYBELLE: Wish he'd do it some other kinda way. All he wants to do is eat and sleep and pat on me, makes me sick. Let me get on out of here. Been up in here all day.

BAILEY: Today ain't no different than any other. Don't know why you pretending you in a hurry now. Don't know how you keep a husband . . . 'cause if you was my wife. . . .

MAYBELLE: I wouldn't wish that on nobody. No offense Reba.

BAILEY: Un-humm. Keep on talkin'.

MAYBELLE: Bailey, I bet you didn't hear 'bout Thelma Butts? Heard tell her husband put her out on the corner . . .

BAILEY: *(Clearly interested.)* On the corner? Say what?

MAYBELLE: That's right. And she ain't passing out leaflets either. Passing out something else though. . . . And cheap!

REBA: *(Overlapping sharply.)* Maybelle, don't start that mess. I don't allow that kinda talk in my house, you know that. Need to stay out of other people's business, 'specially somebody nasty and trifling like that.

MAYBELLE: *(Taken aback, sputtering.)* I was . . . I . . .

REBA: I mean it.

BAILEY: *(Conspiratorially to Maybelle.)* Tell me later.

REBA: I heard that Bailey.

BAILEY: Anybody else call?

REBA: No, but I thought we'd hear from . . . *(Catches herself.)*

BAILEY: From who?

REBA: Nothing.

BAILEY: *(Annoyed.)* You on that again?

REBA: On what Bailey?

BAILEY: We ain't callin' him. Hear me? I mean that. If he got a dime to his name, Wendal can pick up the damn phone and call us . . .

REBA: Dwayne, what I tell you 'bout listening around grown folks talking? That's why you too grown now.

DWAYNE: I wasn't listening.

BAILEY: Boy, what your Grandma tell you? You better get them feet to marching. *(DWAYNE exits.)*

REBA: Wish you wouldn't talk about his father like that in front of him.

BAILEY: Why not? Call a spade a spade, son or no son. His father is worthless. Playing in two-bit clubs, talking that funny talk.

REBA: He's a musician and if he's happy . . .

BAILEY: Happy! How you know he's happy? He don't bother to call here and tell you he's happy. *(To MAYBELLE.)* He rather play somewhere in a juke joint than make an honest living, he could've helped me down at the store . . .

REBA: *(Angry.)* That store ain't everything Bailey.

BAILEY: It puts food on this table and in that boy's mouth upstairs. Ain't no damn music feedin' him . . . ain't seen a horn blow no food this way . . .

REBA: Hush Bailey, he'll hear you.

BAILEY: I don't give a damn. I don't want him growing up pretending that Wendal is something he's not . . . making excuses for him all the time. You do that enough for everybody.

MAYBELLE: Well sir . . . like I said I guess I better be getting on out of here . . .

BAILEY: Hey, hey Maybelle, Reba tell you Junior coming home?

REBA: I forgot.

MAYBELLE: Really? Can't wait to see my boy.

BAILEY: Yeah, I'm gonna have him come down to the store and help me get those new shelves up. Think we gon' expand to that back room, start selling small appliances . . .

REBA: He's only going to be here a few days Bailey. He's on leave, not work release.

BAILEY: Little hard work never hurt nobody and Junior, that boy, ain't never been scared of hard work. Not like Mr. Music man.

REBA: Crossing the line Bailey. I'm not in the mood today to be tangling with you about them boys.

BAILEY: Thirty years and you still don't see that boy for what he is. *(Exits in a huff.)*

REBA: I get so sick of him comparing Wendal to Junior.

MAYBELLE: Well Reba, honey, you know a man don't like softness in his sons.

REBA: Well, a man gets what he makes. (*Lights down on* BAILEY *household and up on* WENDAL *sitting on examination table.*)

WENDAL: Lord Jesus. God . . . I ain't got no words. Just need a little favor. I know I'm in no position to bargain, but just let this one be different. I need it to be negative. So why don't you help me out here. . . . Oh shit. (*The* DOCTOR *enters and starts listening to his lungs. Nervous and with forced humor.*) It's just a little cough. You know, between you and me Doc, I don't believe that test was right, somebody in that lab must have screwed up. Should've had it redone, but me and the band was on the move. You know how that is. We don't stay in one place too long.

DOCTOR: How long have you been seropositive?

WENDAL: You mean when did I test?

DOCTOR: Yes.

WENDAL: About seven months ago. It wasn't here. I think it was in Florida. Don't know why I'm even here. You see I can't have AIDS. Look, I got a woman . . . we thinking about getting married . . .

DOCTOR: Any history of IV drug use?

WENDAL: What?

DOCTOR: I'm trying to ascertain Mr. Bailey if you have engaged in any risk behavior.

WENDAL: Smoke a little weed every now and then. . . .

DOCTOR: So if I understand you correctly, you believe you contracted the virus through sexual intercourse?

WENDAL: No, you don't understand me correctly . . .

DOCTOR: I know this is uncomfortable Mr. Bailey. . . .

WENDAL: (*Putting on his shirt.*) All you doctors are alike. You my fourth one and every one of you trying to make me believe I'm dying.

DOCTOR: I didn't say anything about dying. . . . If you would just sit . . .

WENDAL: You know this whole AIDS thing is some kind of conspiracy. Some more of ya'lls genocide. . . . Try and lay everything on us, cancer, drugs, whatever y'all think up. Well I'm here to tell you, y'alls AIDS better take a number, get in line. And you might as well wipe that silly grin off your face 'cause this is one nigger that ain't gon' lay down and die. Call it what you want, but I ain't sick. (*Yelling.*) You hear me? I'm fine . . . (*Collapses with a coughing spell.*) I'm fine . . .

DOCTOR: (*After a moment.*) Mr. Bailey, I think you and I both know that you are not fine . . . now if we . . .

WENDAL: Ya'll some cold mutherfuckers.

DOCTOR: Who do you think you're talking to?

WENDAL: All you had to do was tell us, didn't cost you nothing . . . not a damn thing . . .

DOCTOR: I'm not responsible for . . .

WENDAL: Then who is? Now let me see if I got this right. You telling me I got bad blood . . . well now . . . remember ol' Tuskegee? I recall you told 'em they had bad blood too . . . and then watched 'em rot to death. Ya'll got a history of this bad blood shit, don't you?

DOCTOR: Hey, hey time out. I tell you what, it's the end of the day . . . the end of a very long day . . . I've seen more patients today than most doctors see in a week so why don't you do us both a favor and cut the shit. You've seen four doctors, if you want I'll refer you to a fifth. I've been working in this epidemic for a long time and it's not because I have an affinity for your suffering or for that matter, my own. You understand? The bottom line: you screwed somebody, you didn't protect yourself, and that's your responsibility, not mine. Your partners will have to be notified. You can do it or you can have the State do it. Which will it be?

WENDAL: Just tell me how long I've been infected.

DOCTOR: I can't. Were any of your partners gay or bisexual men?

WENDAL: Naw. I don't mess with no men. *(Getting up, putting on his shirt.)* Time's up Doc, I gotta go.

DOCTOR: Wait. What about your girlfriend? I know it's difficult, but you have a responsibility to inform your partners. *(Loud.)* Mr. Bailey, you have a responsibility to inform your partners . . . *(Repeats until WEN-DAL phones home; he is using a public phone. It's a difficult conversation for him. Lights up on the BAILEY household. He is practicing his speech. Phone rings, BAILEY crosses to answer, carrying speech cards.)*

BAILEY: I'll get it. Hello. *(WENDAL hesitates, is tempted to hang up.)* Hello?

WENDAL: Hello.

BAILEY: Speak up. I can hardly hear you. *(The following exchange is much talking at once and escalated voices as each tries to be heard.)*

WENDAL: Hello. Hello Dad.

BAILEY: Wendal?

REBA: *(Crowding near the phone.)* Is that Wendal?

DWAYNE: *(Overlapping on the upstairs extension.)* Daddy?

BAILEY: *(Yelling in the phone.)* Boy, what are you doing up?

REBA: He's a grown man Bailey.

BAILEY: I'm talking about Dwayne. Dwayne's on that phone upstairs.

REBA: He's supposed to be sleep.

WENDAL: Dad, you still there?

BAILEY: Yes. *(Phone.)* Wendal where are you?

DWAYNE: Hi Daddy. How you doing? . . .

WENDAL: Hey man, I thought you'd be sleep.

BAILEY: He should be. Get off that phone Dwayne.

REBA: Let the boy talk to his father.

DWAYNE: I almost got enough money to come . . . I wanna come see you.

REBA: Is he ok? Is he coming?

WENDAL: I may be coming there. Dad, you still there?

BAILEY: *(To* REBA, *irritated.)* Yes. Yes.

REBA: *(Whispers to* BAILEY.*)* Be nice. Try to get along.

BAILEY: *(In phone.)* Wendal? *(Irritated, quickly before interrupted again.)* I'm here, got this dinner to go to, got to give a speech . . . getting honored . . . volunteer of the year . . . all the boys voted for me . . . role model . . .

REBA: Bailey, you ain't got to shout, he ain't hard of hearing. Let me talk.

BAILEY: And Dwayne and I going fishing.

DWAYNE: I'm getting straight As, except for a few Cs and couple of Bs.

BAILEY: I can't hear myself think. DWAYNE GET OFF THAT PHONE NOW.

WENDAL: *(Overlapping.)* I want you to know that I love you Dwayne.

BAILEY: Didn't I tell you to hang up? It's past his bedtime. HANG THAT PHONE UP DWAYNE. *(*DWAYNE *hangs up.)*

WENDAL: *(Overlapping.)* Did you hear me Dwayne?

REBA: Let me talk Bailey.

BAILEY: Just a minute. Well, you sound good. Your brother coming home.

WENDAL: I was thinking about coming home . . . I'd like to see you . . . Dad I. . . .

BAILEY: *(Overlapping.)* Coming home a sergeant. Service made a man of him. I always did say that boy was gonna 'mount to something.

WENDAL: Yeah, you always did. Dad . . .

BAILEY: Yeah, I'm real proud of him. You don't sound right. You in some kind of trouble?

WENDAL: Why do you always ask me that? Why do I always have to be in some kind of trouble to call home.

BAILEY: So you not in trouble. You working?

WENDAL: Yeah. We're trying to get a record deal. Looks like it might come through. Supposed to have a meeting with this producer . . .

BAILEY: *(Obviously disgusted.)* Your mother is here. She's right here. Let me let you talk to her.

WENDAL: Dad wait.

BAILEY: *(Overlapping.)* Wait. Wait just a moment. Here she is. *(Hands the phone to* REBA, *clearly exasperated, exits.)*

REBA: Before you say a word, Mama's gon' tell you what's waiting on you. Fried corn, candied yams. Your mouth watering? Chicken and dressing, greens that'll make you shout, beef so tender the butcher wanna buy it back. Then we gon' finish it all off with some 7-Up pound cake and Neapolitan ice cream, trim it with Maybelle's sweet potato pie.

WENDAL: Have mercy!

REBA: You just say when. I'm a get that guest room dolled up for Simone. Dwayne done moved most of your stuff from the attic in his room so you can probably bunk in with him. . . . Lord, the house is gon' be full again. . . . I can't wait. Simone cooking any better?

WENDAL: *(WENDAL starts coughing uncontrollably.)* I gotta go. Talk to you later Mama. *(He hangs up, she exits. Lights to DOUGLASS and SIMONE area. DOUGLASS is sitting at a desk. SIMONE enters singing. She has just bathed and is wearing WENDAL's robe. She surveys the house with pleasure, maybe puffing up the pillows, straightening things for the umpteenth time. WENDAL watches both of them for a minute, clearly debating whom he should approach first. The following scene should be paced so that the dialogue and action overlap. WENDAL's world is literally split between the two relationships.)*

DOUGLASS: How did you get in?

WENDAL: The door was open. I saw her leave.

DOUGLASS: I thought we agreed . . .

SIMONE: *(Finally)* What do you think? Pretty proud of myself. What do you think about the color? I got this serious vision about wallpapering the whole place.

DOUGLASS: Wendal, did you hear me? We've been through this before. I thought we agreed . . .

WENDAL: This couldn't wait. *(Kissing him, holds on.)*

DOUGLASS: Well, I'm glad to see you too.

SIMONE: How 'bout a kiss? Lay one on me. *(She kisses WENDAL.)*

SIMONE and DOUGLASS: You ok?

WENDAL: Yeah. You smell good.

DOUGLASS: Yeah, I thought I'd try a new scent.

SIMONE: Just got out the shower. Boy, where did you get that cologne? I like it.

DOUGLASS: I went by the club last night. Where were you?

WENDAL: Somebody was supposed to sit in for me. I went away for a few days. Needed to think.

SIMONE: How come you didn't call?

WENDAL: We got through late every night. I thought you'd be studying.

SIMONE: How considerate. *(Hands* WENDAL *the lotion.* WENDAL *kneels and starts applying the lotion and massaging her feet.)* I thought we could fix up a spare room for Dwayne when he comes to visit. . . . Hello in there, a spare room for Dwayne, your son. . . .

DOUGLASS: What's her name go with you?

WENDAL: You know her name.

SIMONE: I may have some good news. A teacher is leaving. They're going to recommend me to replace her. My own classroom! Isn't that great?

WENDAL: How long is she gon' be gone?

DOUGLASS: I don't know.

SIMONE: It's a big class, but I'll have an aide.

WENDAL: Where's the kids?

DOUGLASS: She let them go to some concert that I suspect will give them permanent hearing damage.

SIMONE: Of course I might not get it. But think positive, that's what you're always telling me . . . *(She moans with pleasure.)* That feels good. Nobody has hands like you.

DOUGLASS: I just found out today that Alison needs braces: At her age! I told Beth maybe we should try a pair of pliers . . .

WENDAL: Pliers! That's cold blooded Douglass. *(*DOUGLASS *laughs;* SIMONE *laughs at the same time.)* What? What is it?

DOUGLASS: You're right.

WENDAL: I have something to tell you.

SIMONE: *(Overlapping.)* Oh, just that the kids were teasing me about you today. You were a big hit with them. You should see them strutting around, they all think they're sax players now . . . and of course the girls all want to grow up and marry you. *(*SIMONE *laughs again, is bubbling over with excitement.)*

DOUGLASS: Beth is taking the kids to see her mother. I'll be a free man for a week, one whole glorious week with no demands.

WENDAL: I have something to tell you. There's something else. Come on Simone, what's up?

DOUGLASS: I have to see a few clients in the morning. Why people wait to the last minute to file. . . . You could tell Simone you had a gig. . . . Thought maybe we could go somewhere . . .

WENDAL: Will you shut up for a minute?

DOUGLASS: What did I say?

SIMONE: Touchy. Touchy.

WENDAL: Nothing . . . I just . . .

DOUGLASS: Let me fix you a drink.

WENDAL: How about a beer?

DOUGLASS and SIMONE: *(Both exit to get a beer.)* Ok.

WENDAL: But I can get it.

SIMONE: That's ok.

DOUGLASS: *(Off.)* You want something to eat? You've lost weight.

SIMONE: *(Off.)* Dwayne called but it was a strange message. He said your father said to call your mother but not to tell your mother . . . something like that. You see the doctor before you left on Friday? Did they find out what's wrong with you?

DOUGLASS: I cooked. The roast would melt in your mouth.

SIMONE: I tried a new recipe, but I took pity on you and threw it out.

DOUGLASS: You sure I can't tempt you?

WENDAL: *(Irritated.)* No.

DOUGLASS: *(Entering hands him a beer.)* It was just a simple question?

SIMONE: *(Entering.)* No?

WENDAL: They want to run some more tests.

SIMONE: Sorry, we're out of beer.

WENDAL: That's ok.

SIMONE: More tests?

WENDAL: What's with the silent treatment? You know how I feel about her. And you're the one that said it was just a good time. . . . And for seven years, we've been having a real swell time, haven't we? . . . You ever get the seven year itch Douglass?

SIMONE: You telling me everything?

WENDAL: *(Sharply.)* You think I'm lying?

SIMONE: Is that a challenge or an answer?

WENDAL: No.

DOUGLASS: You could have spared me this dark mood you're in. . . . Why don't you take it on home to Simone.

SIMONE: *(Snuggling.)* I'm glad you're home. I missed you.

WENDAL: I needed to talk to you.

DOUGLASS: My back's been bothering me again. Will you do my shoulders? (WENDAL *massages his shoulders.*)

WENDAL: How's that?

DOUGLASS: Good. You really ought to go in business. (DOUGLASS *moans with pleasure.*)

WENDAL: You wanna hear a joke?

SIMONE: My sister may stay with us for a few days. That husband of hers is acting up again.

DOUGLASS: Not particularly.

WENDAL: What's the difference between a black man and a fag.

DOUGLASS: I can hardly wait for this punch line.

SIMONE: I don't know why she doesn't leave him. I keep telling her she can do better.

WENDAL: One doesn't have to tell his mother. *(Laughs, seeing* DOUGLASS *didn't get it.)* You don't get it?

SIMONE: I have another surprise for you. *(Dramatically opens her robe revealing a sexy nightgowm.)* Voila! *(In a Dracula voice, she parades around him.)* I want to make love to you my sweet.

WENDAL: Be still my heart.

DOUGLASS: Wendal?

SIMONE: *(In the same Dracula voice.)* Your heart can be still, but I was hoping something else would get to moving. *(Continues to parade around and tease him.)*

WENDAL: What am I going to do with you?

DOUGLASS: Now can we talk about something else? I can make reservations . . .

SIMONE: I can think of something my sweet.

WENDAL: See, my mother is not the only one I have to tell. I'm trying to tell you. . . .

DOUGLASS: Tell me what Wendal?

SIMONE: Tell me.

WENDAL: What?

SIMONE: Go 'head tell me. When were you planning to ask me? The answer is yes, yes, yes, yes.

WENDAL: I don't think we should see each other anymore. At least . . . not like . . . you know what I mean . . .

DOUGLASS: No, I don't know what you mean.

SIMONE: I found it. You know. . . .

WENDAL: Don't be dense.

DOUGLASS: Well, talk English.

SIMONE: I wasn't snooping, not exactly. I was just straightening out your night stand and I just happened across. . . .

DOUGLASS: *(Pause.)* I knew this day was coming. Trust you to be creative in breaking the news. Fag jokes, no less. So, you decided to marry her, huh?

SIMONE: It's a tad expensive, but I'm sure it's really beautiful. *(Hugs him.)* I love you so much. All weekend I've been on cloud nine. When were you going to ask me?

WENDAL: Marry? I got AIDS Douglass.

SIMONE: When?

WENDAL: Well, this certainly wasn't what I had in mind.

DOUGLASS: Where did I put that brochure?

WENDAL: I can't believe you went rummaging through my things.

DOUGLASS: I figured we could go to that same place . . . maybe even get the same room. . . . Now, where did I put it?

WENDAL: What?

SIMONE: I wasn't rummaging . . . I was looking for a number . . . this ring, it's on lay-a-way for me, isn't it?

WENDAL: Who else?

DOUGLASS: (Looking, somewhat frantically for the brochure.) Remember how we jumped on that bed so it would look like you slept in it. . . .

WENDAL: We broke it. But Douglass what's that got to do . . .

SIMONE: I know it was supposed to be a surprise. If you want, I'll be surprised again . . . over and over again. . . .

DOUGLASS: I felt like a kid again. The maid, what was her name again?

WENDAL: Why do you always have to push?

SIMONE: (Annoyed.) 'Cause somebody needs to jump-start your ass.

DOUGLASS: What was her name?

WENDAL: I don't know Douglass . . . I'm really not in a mood for a trip down memory lane. . . . Didn't you hear what I said? I tested positive . . .

SIMONE: You're right, maybe I am pushing. I just don't understand this. What's happening to us Wendal?

DOUGLASS: She was a doll. I think she knew. I'm sure she knew. Two black men traveling alone together . . .

SIMONE: I live with you. I sleep with you. I used to make love with you, at least until you started shutting me out.

DOUGLASS: "You boys sure know how to mess up a room. Look like you been riding the devil in here."

SIMONE: I moved in here because that's what you said you wanted . . .

WENDAL: Douglass . . .

DOUGLASS: Jasmine. That was her name. Jasmine.

WENDAL: It was what you wanted.

SIMONE: I thought it was what we both wanted. I've tried not to push, tried like hell but you always knew I wanted more . . . I never made that a secret . . . I have no desire to be somebody's trial wife or trial roommate or trial nothing . . . understand? It's either shit or get off the pot baby.

DOUGLASS: (Finding the brochure, crosses to WENDAL with it.) Here it is. I found it.

WENDAL: I can't. I'm sorry . . .

SIMONE: I'm sure there's some humor in this somewhere.

WENDAL: This virus is kicking my ass Douglass . . . I guess it's a test of my faith . . . I know death is a part of life . . .

SIMONE: Can't you at least be a little more original? You're sorry. That's all you can say is you're sorry.

DOUGLASS: When'd you find out?

WENDAL: A couple days ago.

SIMONE: I don't believe you. Why did you buy the ring in the first place?

DOUGLASS: And you're just now telling me?

WENDAL: You have to believe me. I wanted things to work. I love you. I wanted you to be my wife. With you I thought I had a future.

DOUGLASS: I don't believe you.

SIMONE: Past tense?

WENDAL: No. But you're the one who set the rules, way in the beginning. No strings, no commitment.

SIMONE: I want a commitment.

WENDAL: Me too. But everything has changed.

DOUGLASS: This can't be happening.

WENDAL: I knew I had to tell you and I'm still trying to find the right words to tell Simone . . .

DOUGLASS: Well, you didn't seem to have any problem finding the right words to tell me . . .

SIMONE: Prove it.

WENDAL: She has no idea.

SIMONE: I said prove it. Make love to me.

WENDAL: I'm scared, real scared Douglass.

SIMONE: I need you.

WENDAL: I need you too. (SIMONE *starts to undress him.* DOUGLASS *slowly tears the brochure into little pieces.*)

DOUGLASS: You know I'm not sick. I've been gaining weight. Just this morning Beth told me I was getting fat.

WENDAL: I can't do that to you.

DOUGLASS: You think I gave you this shit, don't you?

WENDAL: I just want to settle down.

DOUGLASS: You think it was me?

SIMONE: You are my best friend.

WENDAL: You know you're my best friend.

DOUGLASS: Don't use that word. I am your lover!

WENDAL: I need a friend.

DOUGLASS: And I didn't give it to you.

WENDAL: Right now Douglass that's the least of my worries. It really
doesn't matter . . .

SIMONE: I'm not letting go.

DOUGLASS: It most certainly does matter.

SIMONE: I can't let go. Hold me Wendal.

WENDAL: Simone, baby don't. I can't. (WENDAL *and* SIMONE *kiss deeply.*)

DOUGLASS: I trusted you.

WENDAL: God, give me strength. I'm . . . so scared. . . .

DOUGLASS: I trusted you.

WENDAL: That goes both ways.

DOUGLASS: I'm the one with the family . . .

SIMONE: I want to be your family. (*He struggles, they struggle, but ultimately need
and passion win out.* WENDAL *and* SIMONE *lie back on the bed or floor.*)

DOUGLASS: We were careful . . . (*Softer to himself*) we were, weren't we
Wendal? (*Lights shift to* SIMONE *and* WENDAL *in bed. At lights,* SIMONE
is sitting in bed, clutching the sheet for protection, for comfort. WENDAL
*is smoking a cigarette. Neither looks at the other. Silence for a moment,
clearly they're both in pain, however* SIMONE's *pain is more obvious in its
physical expression.*)

SIMONE: I wanted you so bad . . . I've been waiting weeks . . . for this?
You've never . . .

WENDAL: (*Reaching to touch her.*) Simone, I . . .

SIMONE: (*Recoils at his touch.*) There's this little boy in my class—Raymond.
I don't know if you remember him. He stutters, so he's real shy. The
kids make fun of him, even the teacher loses patience, but every time I
see him I just want to take him in my arms and hold him, protect him
because I know no one sticks around too long with somebody who can't
communicate. Not enough love in the world that can withstand that kind
of stinginess, that kind of terror. You hear what I'm saying Wendal? The
teacher says I'm not helping him by not making him speak, but the real
message always seems to come through when the words are moved out
of the way . . . don't you think? Like now, how I heard you, for the first
time loud and clear . . . it's been good Wendal, but I can do better. You
know what I'm saying? . . . I can do better with someone, someone who
cares, at least even tries to stutter. (Waits, no response.) Hope you can get
your money back on the ring. (*She exits while we watch* WENDAL *come
to grips with what has just happened.*)

WENDAL: (*To himself.*) What have I done? Simone, forgive me. (*Lights shift
to* WENDAL *in hospital. Hospital intercom sound.* WENDAL *is hooked up
to IV and oxygen. As much as his strength allows, he's having a full fledged*

tantrum, knocking things off his bed table, pushing intercom buttons.) I'm sick of this. Wendal you getting out of here today. Where's the fucking nurse? *(Into the bedside intercom.)* Will one of you devil's angels get in here and get this shit out of my arm? I want out of this fucking hell hole.

NURSE'S VOICE: Mr. Bailey, now we've been through this before. Relax. You're not well enough to be discharged . . . just relax, the doctor is on her way . . .

WENDAL: *(Pulls the cannula out.)* I don't want to see the fucking doctor, I want my fucking clothes. (DOCTOR *enters.)*

DOCTOR: *(Firmly.)* WENDAL STOP. RIGHT NOW.

NURSE'S VOICE: Mr. Bailey, do you want a shot? *(*WENDAL *collapses in the bed.)* Mr. Bailey. . . . Do you need something to relax you?

DOCTOR: *(Into intercom.)* It's ok nurse. It's Dr. Weinberg. *(To* WENDAL *as she readjusts the cannula.)* I see we're in a good mood today. *(No response.)* Such a charming patient . . . It does my heart good to see you every day.

WENDAL: I wish I could say the same. (DOCTOR *laughs.)* It doesn't take much to get you people to laugh, does it?

DOCTOR: Wendal, I do believe you're getting better . . .

WENDAL: I bet you say that to all the guys . . .

DOCTOR: Try and have a little more patience . . . *(Takes out a jazz music cassette out of her pocket.)* I'll just leave this right here.

WENDAL: *(Brightening considerably.)* You got it?

DOCTOR: Yes.

WENDAL: You didn't have to do that Doc.

DOCTOR: I know. But music has a way of soothing the soul, making one more patient, a little less likely to throw things around a room, don't you think? . . .

WENDAL: Just tired Doc, that's all. Soon's I think things are getting better, ya'll find something else . . . tired of these tubes and I'm real tired of them nurses talking to me like I'm two. I hate feeling so . . . *(Pause.)* I don't know . . .

DOCTOR: (Touches him.) You'll be out of here soon, after we isolate what's causing this recent bout of diarrhea. Until then, give the room and the nurses a break. Ok? *(*WENDAL *nods yes.)* Have you told anyone you're in here? What about your family? (DOUGLASS *appears laden with gifts.)*

WENDAL: I told him.

DOUGLASS: *(Whispering.)* I brought you a few things. Some flowers. I thought you might want some candy . . . a bible . . . I won't stay long. I have to pick up Alison from school.

DOCTOR: Sir, this is a hospital, not a mausoleum. You can speak up.

WENDAL: *(To* DOUGLASS.*)* Fuck you.

DOCTOR: Right now, Wendal, I don't think you're able. *(Laughs loudly, no response from* WENDAL *or* DOUGLASS.*)* Well, it was just a little doctor humor. *(Extends her hand to* DOUGLASS.*)* Hi, I'm Dr. Weinberg.

DOUGLASS: *(Hesitates, not sure if he should reveal his name.)* Dennis . . . Dennis Smith.

DOCTOR: Smith did you say? We see a lot of Smith's in here. I was beginning to wonder if our buddy here had any friends. Well, good to meet you Dennis. *(To* WENDAL.*)* Check on you later Wendal. *(Exits.)*

WENDAL: Dennis? Dennis Smith? You couldn't be a little more creative, like Dennis "Coward."

DOUGLASS: I would've come sooner. I just came by to tell you I was negative.

WENDAL: Haven't seen you in weeks . . . and the only reason you here now is to deliver me a bible and a bulletin about you being negative. Well, who cares?

DOUGLASS: Maybe I shouldn't have come.

WENDAL: Bingo. So, you're negative. Maybe your antibodies are a little on the slow side.

DOUGLASS: Just came by to see how you were doing.

WENDAL: Now you've seen.

DOUGLASS: Where's Simone?

WENDAL: It's over.

DOUGLASS: Is she. . . . Is she ok?

WENDAL: Haven't heard from her.

DOUGLASS: I mean . . . you know . . . does she know?

WENDAL: We all know what we want to know.

DOUGLASS: But . . .

WENDAL: *(Defensive.)* But nothing. Now if you came in here to inquire about Simone I suggest you . . . *(*WENDAL *gags, spits up in pan.)*

DOUGLASS: *(Wiping his brow.)* I'm sorry. I didn't mean to get you so upset.

WENDAL: You tell Beth? *(No response, pause.)* I didn't think so. So what's all that?

DOUGLASS: I stopped by the bookstore, picked up some books for you. I know how much you like to read and I thought . . .

WENDAL: *(Reading one of the titles.)* "When Bad Things Happen To Good People . . ."

DOUGLASS: See, I think Wendal the secret is thinking positively. . . . You really got to change your attitude . . . meet this head on . . . that's how my father beat cancer . . . he never gave up.

WENDAL: *(Irritated)* And where is he now? Six feet under, still thinking positive. Don't bring that shit in here. I don't get it. Everybody talking 'bout positive attitude, like people ain't still dying. What the fuck is wrong with you people? Guess if you die it's 'cause you didn't have enough positive attitude. Well I'll grin all day long but the bottom line is I'm still gon' die. And if I wanna be pissy about it along the way, that's my right. So why don't you take that jolly attitude shit down to the morgue, maybe they can use your ass down there.

DOUGLASS: I'd say something if I could think of something redeeming . . .

WENDAL: (Suddenly starts thrashing with his feet and moaning.) Shit . . . . . . dammit . . .

DOUGLASS: What's wrong?

WENDAL: My feet. Shit. Goddamn! (DOUGLASS removes the covers, for a moment is taken aback by the sight, but then starts to massage WENDAL's feet.) They hurt so bad sometimes, other times I can't feel them at all. Look like little ape feet, don't they? Done turned blue black. Think I'm dying from the bottom up. That feels good. It's nice to be touched with a hand instead of rubber gloves. (A beat.) I need a favor. Can you buy me a train ticket?

DOUGLASS: A what?

WENDAL: I'm going home, to my parent's home. If I'm going to beat this thing . . .

DOUGLASS: That's it. Now you're talking. . . . You got to fight Wendal . . .

WENDAL: I believe I could get stronger at home . . . Mama would feed the fight back in me and my father, well . . . he don't take no for an answer . . . (BAILEY appears either through the audience or on the other side of the stage. He is dressed in one of the suits we saw earlier. He has some yellow pad papers in his hands. He delivers the following to the audience. For the following exchange, WENDAL and BAILEY's speeches overlap on line end words. Light focuses tighter on just WENDAL.)

BAILEY: Fathers, men, you have to take up time with these here boys. If they don't turn out right you don't have nobody to blame but yourselves.

WENDAL: I want to take the train.

BAILEY: I took my son on a train ride once . . .

WENDAL: When I was a kid, I loved the train. My father took me once to Mississippi on it . . .

BAILEY: I was born in Mississippi. All my people's from there . . .

WENDAL: We were going to see his folks . . .

BAILEY: That was when my mother and father was still living . . .

WENDAL: Just the two of us. Junior stayed home with Mama . . .

BAILEY: It was just me and him . . .

WENDAL: I can't tell you how much I loved having him all to myself.

BAILEY: It was our time. Wendal needed to come to some understanding . . .

WENDAL: Everybody knew him. I was so proud of him . . .

BAILEY: To know my roots, if you will. You see he was spoiled, not by me . . .

WENDAL: Let me eat, drink as much pop as I wanted . . .

BAILEY: His Mama. . . . The two of them was some kind of special together . . .

WENDAL: He was so excited, showed me every sight along the way, wouldn't even let me sleep . . .

BAILEY: You kids have it easy. I wanted Wendal to see what hard work was about . . .

WENDAL: Soon's I'd drift off, he'd wake me up and say, look Wendal. Look at that Wendal . . .

BAILEY: You see I love my son, both my sons . . .

WENDAL: Sometimes it wouldn't be nothing but a field . . .

BAILEY: They and their Mama is what I works hard for. . . . See, I didn't really want him working at the store. Wendal was special, different from Junior. That boy, from day one, was destined for bigger things . . . you could see it in his eyes . . . by the time Wendal was in grade school, shoot, he was reading better than me . . . I just knew he'd be an astronaut or some kind of scientist . . .

WENDAL: I don't think he ever thought I'd amount to anything. Now I gotta tell him this . . .

BAILEY: Fathers have to set an example for their children, specially them boys. . . . My father was everything to me . . .

WENDAL: Wish I'd told him how much I enjoyed myself. . . . Soon's we got there, I started crying, told him I wanted to go home and never go back . . .

BAILEY: He had so much fun when it was time to leave, he told me naw, he was staying. Ain't that something? *(Folds up the paper.)* It was our time. *(Walking off.)* I'll have to ask Wendal one day if he remembers when we took the train that time . . . *(Blackout on BAILEY. Broad lights on hospital scene.)*

DOUGLASS: You're tired. I'll get you that train ticket.

WENDAL: Thank you. *(Closes his eyes.)* They're waiting on me.

DOUGLASS: Who?

WENDAL: My family. *(Lights to Bailey household. BAILEY and JUNIOR enter laughing loudly.)*

DWAYNE: *(Hugging him; immediately works at monopolizing JUNIOR's attention.)* Uncle Luke.

JUNIOR: Boy, you ain't nothing but a bean sprouting. Look at this head. Ouch!

REBA: *(Overlapping.)* Junior.

BAILEY: Don't he look good, Reba? A sergeant.

REBA: Yes indeed.

JUNIOR: Where's Wendal, Mama?

REBA: He's not here . . . not yet.

BAILEY: *(Irritated)* Reba

REBA: Don't Reba me, Luke Bailey.

DWAYNE: He's coming. He promised this time.

BAILEY: *(To JUNIOR.)* That brother of yours did it again. Called weeks ago making his empty promises, he's coming home and gets your mother all upset . . .

JUNIOR: Whoa, I didn't mean to start another world war.

REBA: You oughtta stop acting like you don't get disappointed too. Every time that phone ring, you jumping.

JUNIOR: So, is he coming?

REBA: He said he was. It'll be so good to have both of you home.

JUNIOR: Well, I got presents for everybody.

BAILEY: Oh, you didn't have to do that.

JUNIOR: *(Overlapping.)* I didn't have time to wrap anything. This is for you Mama. *(Gives her a small box.)*

REBA: Oh Junior, you shouldn't have. I . . . I. . . . You didn't have to buy me . . .

JUNIOR: Mama, before you start, I know I didn't have to, but how 'bout saving us a little time and taking the present anyway. *(Retrieves a wind-breaker for DWAYNE.)* See if it fits little man. Mama, you can open the box now.

REBA: Ok, ok. *(Takes out a bracelet.)* Oh Junior. It's beautiful.

JUNIOR: Put it on.

REBA: I'll try it on but I have to put this up for safe keeping.

JUNIOR: Mama, I didn't buy it for you to keep it in a box under the bed.

REBA: Well, maybe I'll wear it to church . . .

JUNIOR: Why don't you, wear it tonight so I can see it on you.

BAILEY: You know your Mama ain't gon' change. Under our bed still look like a department store, don't throw nothing away. Thirty years I been buying for this woman and she still act like she ain't never had nothing.

REBA: Ya'll can laugh if you want, but I appreciate everything I get in this life. Ain't nothing promised. . . . When you been poor . . .

JUNIOR: Before you start preaching Mama, what you cook?

REBA: *(Laughs in spite of herself.)* Ok boy.

DWAYNE: Thanks man. *(Tries it on.)* It fits.

REBA: That's nice. The color really suits him. This boy gets more handsome by the day. Don't he put you in mind of Wendal when he was this age?

BAILEY: I don't see it myself. Um . . . Junior, son, it doesn't seem like you brought enough clothes. Is that all you brought what's in that bag? You know, this time of year the weather can be tricky.

JUNIOR: I'm set. Got plenty of clothes Dad.

BAILEY: Oh I see. Just didn't look like much in that bag.

JUNIOR: Yeah, I got something in there for Wendal and Auntie May too. *(Deliberately teasing* BAILEY, *stretches out, loosens his clothes.)* Dad, you got any beer? *(*REBA *and* DWAYNE *look over at* BAILEY *who is making a big deal about hiding his disappointment.)*

BAILEY: What ya'll looking at me like that for?

JUNIOR: *(Laughs.)* Old man, you know I got you something.

BAILEY: Well, it wasn't like I was looking for something. . . . You know I don't put much store in getting presents. It ain't even Christmas.

JUNIOR: Here. *(Hands him a box.)* Try this on for size.

BAILEY: What is it?

JUNIOR: Open it up and see.

BAILEY: *(Opens the box.)* A watch.

JUNIOR: A watch that ain't cheap. It's got an alarm and the date. . . .

BAILEY: Is this diamond real?

JUNIOR: They told me it was.

BAILEY: Look Reba.

DWAYNE: Boy, that's sharp.

REBA: It sure is. Junior, you shouldn't spend all your money on us like this.

JUNIOR: Always make some more money Mama. They ain't nothing much.

BAILEY: Good-bye Timex! Ain't gon' be able to hit me in the butt with a red apple.

JUNIOR: I'm glad you like it Dad.

REBA: What you get your brother?

JUNIOR: A chain and I got this box of candy for Auntie May.

BAILEY: That's one thing Maybelle don't need is candy. Anybody wanna know what time it is?

DWAYNE: Three o'clock.

BAILEY: Who asked the question Dwayne?

JUNIOR: *(Noticing the plaque for* BAILEY.) What's this?

BAILEY: Oh just something else I got from them boys.

REBA: Your father won. . . .

BAILEY: It was no big thing, you know something like being, oh I don't know . . . father of the year . . . no big thing.

JUNIOR: That's great Dad.

REBA: He had to give a speech.

JUNIOR: You did? I bet you got a standing ovation.

BAILEY: Naw, but they clapped real hard. Reba tell him.

REBA: Tell him what Bailey?

DWAYNE: And they was hooting. *(Starts making a hooting sound.)*

BAILEY: You know, about my speech.

REBA: Bailey, you can tell him. *(Moving to the phone.)* Let me call Maybelle. She'll be sick if she ain't included. *(Starts to dial.)*

JUNIOR: *(Overlapping.)* Maybe I'll go down there while I'm here . . . shoot some hoops. Me and Wendal used to practically live down there.

BAILEY: *(Overlapping, looking for a beer in the refrigerator.)* It ain't changed much. Different boys, same stink, but I'll take you down there. You'd be a good example to them boys. You know, while you're here I want you to help me finish some cabinets . . . *(Fade to hospital waiting area. WENDAL is sitting, looks around hopefully, yet impatiently, clearly he's been waiting for a while. Next to him is his suitcase and his sax case. There's something pitiful about the change in him, the weakness, the unsteady deliberation.)*

DOUGLASS: *(Enters.)* What are you doing in here? I went to your room first. Am I late?

WENDAL: Yes.

DOUGLASS: You said noon. It's only a few minutes after.

NURSE: *(Enters.)* Here's your medicine Mr. Bailey.

DOUGLASS: Why don't you just send him home with the whole pharmacy?

NURSE: I'll be back in a few minutes with your wheelchair.

WENDAL: Not necessary.

NURSE: Hospital rules. *(She exits.)*

DOUGLASS: I don't know why you insist on boarding a train today. You sure this trip is ok with your doctor?

WENDAL: Yes Douglass.

DOUGLASS: I wish you wouldn't go until you're feeling stronger.

WENDAL: I'm going Douglass.

DOUGLASS: I can get you a hotel room for a few days . . .

WENDAL: Douglass I'm going. I can't wait. Few home cooked meals, my family, be good as new.

DOUGLASS: Maybe you're expecting too much Wendal.

WENDAL: I have to.

DOUGLASS: Just don't want to see you hurt . . . *(WENDAL laughs.)* What's so funny?

WENDAL: AIDS done already hurt my feelings Douglass. I don't know how much more hurt I can get. *(Pause.)* Appreciate you taking care of things . . . figure you ain't such a bad guy, outside of my family, you the longest relationship I've had . . . that oughtta count for something . . . *(Hugs him.)*

DOUGLASS: Hey, I hope you aren't getting sentimental on me. I'm trying my damnest to be butch here. *(They both laugh a moment while they grapple with the loss.)* And look at you, you got your shirt buttoned all wrong. *(Re-buttons his shirt.)*

WENDAL: Thought it looked funny. You know, you'd make somebody a good husband.

DOUGLASS: Real cute. *(Finishing the buttoning.)* There. *(Pause.)* I may never see you again.

WENDAL: Don't.

DOUGLASS: Don't what?

WENDAL: Come on let's get out of here. I don't need a wheelchair. *(WENDAL picks up the suitcase.)*

DOUGLASS: Don't try to lift that. I can get it.

WENDAL: I can get it.

DOUGLASS: I said I would get it.

WENDAL: I'm not helpless Douglass.

DOUGLASS: *(They struggle.)* Would you let me carry the damn suitcase?!!!

WENDAL: Yeah, I'll let you carry it and I love you too. *(A moment as they both struggle with the loss, regrouping, teasing.)* Just psyching you out. Carry the damn thing so I can strut out of here looking like my old fine cute self. Who knows, somebody may look my way, give me a little play . . .

DOUGLASS: *(Laughing with him.)* Nigger please, not hardly . . .

NURSE: *(Rolling the wheelchair.)* Time to go home Mr. Bailey.

DOUGLASS: *(Helping WENDAL in the chair.)* That's right Mr. Bailey, time for you to go home. *(They exit.)*

END OF ACT ONE

ACT TWO

Lights up on Bailey household.

WENDAL, JUNIOR *and* DWAYNE *are in the kitchen preparing dinner.* REBA, MAYBELLE *and* BAILEY *are in the living room;* REBA *is dressed in her gifts, the red dress, the bracelet.*

REBA: I feel so useless. You all don't need any help in there?

DWAYNE, WENDAL and JUNIOR: *(Off, in unison.)* No.

WENDAL: *(Off.)* That's the third time Mama.

MAYBELLE: It sure is good to have them home. And they got the place looking so good.

REBA: They got most of the upstairs painted and they supposed to paint in here before Junior leave out.

BAILEY: *(Mumbling.)* I still got them cabinets down at the store I want done.

MAYBELLE: *(Overlapping.)* Wendal helping out too?

REBA: Oh yeah.

MAYBELLE: He don't look too well to me.

REBA: Trying to fatten him up a little.

BAILEY: He look OK. Don't you all start borrowing trouble with all that fussing over him. *(DWAYNE enters, starts setting the table.)*

MAYBELLE: *(To DWAYNE.)* How's it going in there? *(To REBA and BAILEY.)* Whatever they cooking, I hope we gon' be able to eat it. *(To DWAYNE.)* Honey, do it look edible?

DWAYNE: I don't know. It look OK.

BAILEY: Junior's a pretty good cook. It's Wendal ain't never learned his way 'round a kitchen.

REBA: Father like son.

MAYBELLE: *(Laughs.)* You got that right. She got you there Bailey.

BAILEY: I can cook. Reba know I can cook, she just don't let me.

REBA: Bailey please. *(DWAYNE moves MAYBELLE's purse on the floor, MAYBELLE screeches.)*

MAYBELLE: Un-Un. Un-Un child. Don't put my purse on that floor. That's bad luck. Put a woman's purse on the floor and she'll never have any money.

DWAYNE: Sorry.

MAYBELLE: Just hand it here. *(DWAYNE hands her her purse.)*

BAILEY: I don't know why you clutching that purse so, you know you ain't got nothing but a dollar in it. All your money if you got any is up between them bosoms.

REBA: Bailey!

BAILEY: Why you Baileying me. I ain't never seen Maybelle pull money from no purse. Maybelle need money she going between them pillows up there.

MAYBELLE: I got my money where I know it's safe. You just jealous. Some fool steal your wallet, you's a man without a dime. Somebody steal my purse, *(Cups her breasts.)* I'm still loaded.

REBA: *(Laughs out loud.)* Now that's the truth.

MAYBELLE: And you oughtta be complimenting your wife on how nice she looks instead of worrying 'bout where I put my money. She look real sexy in that dress, don't she?

BAILEY: Little flashy, I think, for Reba.

WENDAL: *(Enters, has overheard the last comment.)* I think she looks beautiful, real special tonight.

REBA: Well thank you son.

BAILEY: *(Defensive.)* I didn't say she didn't look beautiful. *(To REBA.)* That bracelet Junior bought you, now it look nice with that dress. *(To WENDAL.)* Did you see the bracelet your brother bought your Mama?

WENDAL: No. *(Admires the bracelet.)* That's nice.

BAILEY: And he got me this watch. Did I show it you? It's got a real diamond.

WENDAL: Yeah. You showed it to me when I first got home.

BAILEY: And he got Dwayne a little jacket. Did you show your father your jacket Dwayne?

REBA: He can show him later Bailey.

BAILEY: Oh. OK. That's fine with me. Junior just bought us home such nice things . . . I just thought Wendal might like to see 'em.

DWAYNE: Daddy's buying me some skates.

BAILEY: I don't know nothing 'bout that.

WENDAL: *(His arm around* DWAYNE.*)* That's because I'm buying 'em.

BAILEY: Oh.

JUNIOR: *(Enters with a big fork and spatula, deadpan serious.)* We got a fire extinguisher?

REBA: What?

MAYBELLE: Lord. Lord. I knew I should have eaten before I left home.

JUNIOR: Wendal kinda set fire to the chicken.

WENDAL: *(Laughing.)* Quit lying on me man. (BAILEY *realizes* JUNIOR*'s kidding, starts to laugh.)*

JUNIOR: *(Laughing out hilariously.)* And the potatoes . . .

BAILEY: I ain't surprised.

WENDAL: Man stop . . .

JUNIOR: And the pot holder . . . the kitchen curtains . . .

WENDAL: He's lying Mama. He's lying . . .

REBA: *(Getting up, on her way to the kitchen.)* What have you all done to my kitchen?

JUNIOR: *(Stopping her.)* I'm kidding. I'm kidding. Everything's cool.

REBA: Get out of my way Junior. I don't know what made me take leave of my senses, letting ya'll cook.

JUNIOR: Come on Mama. I'm kidding. The kitchen still in one piece. This your party, you shouldn't have to cook. All you supposed to do is sit right down here and enjoy this masterpiece or burnt pieces your two sons and grandson have concocted. Wendal's specialty this evening is A'LA crisp.

WENDAL: OK man.

MAYBELLE: That's OK. Wendal's a star. He ain't meant to do common labor, ain't that right baby? *(Kisses him.)*

WENDAL: Yeah. That's right. Thank you Aunt May.

BAILEY and JUNIOR: Shit.

MAYBELLE: So, what's the entertainment this evening? I know you and Junior gon' sing.

JUNIOR: Well . . .

REBA: Maybe you can play something on your horn for us.

BAILEY: That horn'll wake up the whole neighborhood this time of night . . .

MAYBELLE: Ya'll come on and sing a song, sing the song that used to make me wanna holler. Ya'll gon' do that for your Auntie May?

WENDAL: Well, I don't know. My throat's been bothering me.

BAILEY: I thought that's how you made your living boy. How you gon' work playing music when you complaining about your throat bothering you?

REBA: Ya'll sing a little bit. It would do me good to hear ya'll sing together.

MAYBELLE: It'll do me good too.

JUNIOR: Ok. How 'bout it man?

WENDAL: Ok.

JUNIOR: What's the song Auntie May?

WENDAL: Start us off.

MAYBELLE: Ok, I'll help you out. (MAYBELLE *starts humming a blues song such as "Kiddeo."** WENDAL joins in and takes the lead. JUNIOR accompanies, then everybody joins in. BAILEY gets up and starts dancing a wild exaggerated dance, maybe the funky chicken.)*

REBA: Go on Bailey. Go on now . . .

BAILEY: Come on Maybelle. Come on here.

MAYBELLE: *(Getting up and dancing with him.)* What are you doing Luke Bailey? You better sit down before I embarrass you. You know you can't keep up with a young woman like me. Come on and dance with me Junior.

BAILEY: *(Dancing with* DWAYNE.) Come on boy. (WENDAL *dances with his mother; clearly everybody is enjoying themselves;* MAYBELLE *becomes winded from* JUNIOR *spinning her around, sits down exhausted.)*

MAYBELLE: Oh Lordy . . . ooh . . .

BAILEY: What's wrong Maybelle, you can't keep up with the old man? I thought you was gon' embarrass somebody this evening.

MAYBELLE: I know when to stop making a fool of myself, something you oughtta learn Luke Bailey. You know you ain't gon' be able to move in the morning.

JUNIOR: I ain't sang that in years.

MAYBELLE: It still sound good.

JUNIOR: *(To* WENDAL.) Man, I see you ain't lost your touch. Still know how to croon.

BAILEY: Yeah, sound pretty good if I say so myself.

WENDAL: *(Surprised, pleasantly.)* Thanks Dad.

BAILEY: Yeah, sound damn good. Never said you didn't have a voice. You

* See Special Note on copyright page.

know we having this program down at the Center on the twenty-first. Maybe you can sing at it. People down there always asking me 'bout you, wanting to know when you gon' make a record, you know how people are, wanna make you out more than you is. You don't have to answer me now, just think about it. . . . They may have me do another speech . . . I told you 'bout my speech . . .

JUNIOR: Man you been telling us 'bout that speech . . .

MAYBELLE: Yes Jesus!

WENDAL: *(Seeing that* BAILEY *looks a little hurt.)* I'd like to hear you speak Dad. Never heard you before an audience. It can be tricky.

BAILEY: You got that right.

WENDAL: Let me know what you want me to sing.

JUNIOR: Well, what about me? Maybe I can do a little background. *(Starts doing some riffs; clearly carrying a tune is not* JUNIOR's *strong point.)* Do wah do wha . . .

BAILEY: *(Cutting him off.)* I want you to do a solo, it ain't gon' be but a few minutes . . .

REBA: *(Noticing how much* WENDAL *is sweating.)* Wendal, you ok?

BAILEY: He's fine. Now Wendal . . .

WENDAL: *(Overlapping.)* Fine Mama, just need a little water. Better change my shirt too. Be right back. *(He exits.)*

MAYBELLE: Oh Lord, look now how this knee done swole . . .

BAILEY: That knee ain't swole, that's just fat Maybelle! *(Falls out laughing.)*

JUNIOR: *(Trying to conceal his laughter.)* Nothing like a woman with a little flesh on her bones, though, ain't that right Auntie May?

MAYBELLE: That's right and I wanna thank you Junior. Your father eyesight just failing him. And you know what they say . . . every time a fat woman shakes, a skinny woman looses her home.

REBA: Please, don't you two get started.

MAYBELLE: I ain't getting nothing started. I feel too good this evening. My boys are home.

BAILEY: They's mens Maybelle, face it. You getting old.

MAYBELLE: They'll always be my boys. I don't make no difference between them and my own four.

WENDAL: *(Enters, he has changed his shirt.)* How they doing?

MAYBELLE: Got 'em all married off. They they wives' problems now. Speaking of wives, you and that child looking to get hooked up? What's her name again?

WENDAL: Simone.

MAYBELLE: Yeah. Pretty black thang.

WENDAL: *(A little uncomfortable.)* Well right now she's back there and I'm here. I just wanted to come home for a while. Didn't realize how much I missed everybody.

REBA: Well we missed you too. Didn't we Bailey?

BAILEY: Yeah, I'm glad he's here. Now that you sleeping through the night again maybe I can finally get some decent shut-eye.

MAYBELLE: Yeah Wendal having you home does this house good. This place needed livening up. All Auntie May need now is a little sustenance. Junior, ain't there no cheese slices or bread sticks? Ain't seen no dinner party without no hor-de-derves.

WENDAL: Won't be long. *(Exits to the kitchen.)*

BAILEY: *(Overlapping.)* Maybelle, you can't even pronounce the word.

MAYBELLE: Aw shut up Bailey.

JUNIOR: *(Overlapping.)* You have to talk to Wendal. This his thang, I'm just following orders.

WENDAL: *(Enters with fancy folded napkins which he places on the table.)* Everything's almost ready. We'll seat you now. *(With much formality, WENDAL seats his mother at the table, JUNIOR seats MAYBELLE while DWAYNE attempts to seat BAILEY.)*

BAILEY: *(To DWAYNE.)* I can manage my chair on my own, thank you.

WENDAL: *(Switches the forks around.)* Table looks nice Dwayne.

MAYBELLE: Where you learn how to do all this?

WENDAL: I've done my share of waiting tables. First course: shrimp cocktail. *(Snaps his finger in the air for JUNIOR and DWAYNE to follow him.)* Gentlemen, if you please . . .

JUNIOR: *(Grumbling good naturedly as he exits.)* Now Mr. Head Waiter, I didn't know you snapping your fingers at me was part of the deal. I don't see why we can't eat buffet style, should've set up a soup kitchen . . . *(DWAYNE and JUNIOR exit behind WENDAL.)*

MAYBELLE: *(Shaking her head.)* Umph, that's not a good sign. Whenever the service is too fancy, the food ain't worth shit. I bet we gon' get one shrimp.

BAILEY: You lucky to have that. Now you eat everything else and you gon' eat what these boys done cooked with a smile on your face. Ain't that right?

MAYBELLE: Yes sir massa.

BAILEY: Think it's kinda nice they giving their Mama a break.

REBA: That's more life I've seen in Wendal since he been here. And I love to hear my boy sing.

BAILEY: Yeah. Kinda put me in mind of the old days. Every Saturday, remember how he used to put on them little shows for us . . . ?

REBA: Yeah.

MAYBELLE: And that sorry James Brown act ya'll used to do. I used to have to drag my boys over here so ya'll would have a little audience.

REBA: Honey, yeah, Bailey and that cape.

MAYBELLE: Wendal falling down to the ground squealing like a pig and there come Bailey trying to get on the good foot with that toilet paper roll. . . . 'Member that Bailey? How you'd drape Wendal? When you was younger you used to have a lot more spirit.

BAILEY: I still do. *(Getting excited.)* Maybe after dinner I'll see if Wendal still remember our little routine we used to' do . . .

MAYBELLE: Oh Lord we gon' be subjected to that again. *(REBA suddenly reaches over and kisses BAILEY.)*

BAILEY: What's that for?

REBA: Nothing. I'm just so damn happy.

MAYBELLE: Reba, honey, did you say damn?

REBA: Yes. Damn. Damn. Damn. Damn happy!

JUNIOR: *(Enters carrying a covered platter, sets it down in the middle of the table.)* Un Un Un. Don't touch. Wendal says no unveiling till he's present. Forgot how bossy he is. Been leading me around all day, shopping and practicing . . . made me read every label, on every can, on every aisle . . . took us three hours . . . three hours in somebody's grocery store . . . I'm 'bout to fall out and he's whistling Dixie . . .

WENDAL: *(Off.)* Junior. Hey bro' . . .

JUNIOR: See? I got to get on back to the Army so I can get me some rest. *(He exits.)*

MAYBELLE: That boy know he love his brother. *(Reaches for the cover of the platter.)* Shoot. I need to prepare my stomach.

BAILEY: *(Smacks her hands.)* Wendal wants us to wait so we gon' wait. *(WENDAL brings in another dish.)* Everything smells good son.

WENDAL: Hope it tastes good. I don't know if Junior read the recipes right. *(He exits.)*

MAYBELLE: Umph! Did you hear that. They got to read while they cook. Lord, maybe I got a candy bar in my purse.

BAILEY: *(Laughing.)* I ain't got a candy bar but I got some peanuts in the basement. *(They all crack up laughing.)*

WENDAL: *(Enters.)* What's so funny?

MAYBELLE and REBA: Nothing.

BAILEY: *(Overlapping.)* Nothing son. Nothing. Just enjoying ourselves in here. (DWAYNE *comes out carrying a pot with sauce dripping, he's soiled the front of his shirt.* WENDAL *is behind him carrying a casserole dish.)*

REBA: Dwayne you done spilled something on your shirt.

DWAYNE: Oh.

MAYBELLE: You have to be careful. Watch what you doing.

BAILEY: Leave the boy alone, it'll wash out.

WENDAL: I'll get him something.

REBA: Maybe you should've cooked in some old clothes.

JUNIOR: *(Enters with another dish)* Last one. Ready to dig in?

WENDAL: *(Enters with an apron, a frilly type.)* No, remember, we're serving 'em.

MAYBELLE: We getting served? Well can I make me a special order?

REBA: Maybelle.

WENDAL: Here Dwayne. Put on Mama's apron while you serve. *(Ties apron around* DWAYNE.*)* There.

BAILEY: Now he looks like a little sissy faggot. (JUNIOR *laughs loud, every- body snickers except* WENDAL *whose whole demeanor has changed.)*

REBA: I think he looks kinda cute.

WENDAL: I don't see anything funny.

DWAYNE: *(With much disdain.)* I don't look like no fag. *(Takes the apron off.)*

WENDAL: *(Trying to control his rage.)* What you say? (DWAYNE *looks scared, knows his father is angry, is confused and embarrassed. Grabbing him.)* Answer me. I said what did you say?

DWAYNE: *(Slightly indignant.)* I said I didn't look like no fag.

WENDAL: I don't ever want to hear you say something like that again. You understand me?

BAILEY: I don't know why you jumping all over the boy. They call they- selves that

WENDAL: So! We call ourselves nigger, but that don't mean we are one. You don't allow him to use that word in this house. Do you? Go on Dwayne say nigger to your grandfather. Say nigger like you said fag. . . . Go on, say it . . .

BAILEY: Dwayne you bet not say one word . . .

WENDAL: Why the silence now? Dwayne, I told you . . .

REBA: I'd like to talk about something else, like this dinner.

JUNIOR: Yeah man, I don't know why you all upset, ain't nobody called you a fag. It was just a joke.

MAYBELLE: I sure am ready to eat this food.

WENDAL: *(Overlapping.)* You'll never change. I guess it's just a joke you raising him like you tried to do me . . . with the same small minded . . .

BAILEY: At least I'm raising him.

WENDAL: Is that what you call it?

REBA: Wendal!

JUNIOR: Whoa! You need to back up man. *(JUNIOR sits at the table.)* Come on. Everybody let's eat.

BAILEY: *(Angry.)* I don't know why in the Sam hell you come home. You ain't satisfied unless you upsetting everybody. Gotta defy me no matter what. Thank God I got me one son that's got some sense, but you, you wanna ram that crazy shit down my damn throat every time I turn around, well who needs it? This is my house . . . you hear me? Mine. And the door swings both ways. If you don't like it Mister, then let the door hit you where the good Lord split you. You can take your narrow ass back where. . . .

REBA: Bailey! That's enough.

DWAYNE: I'm sorry Dad. I didn't mean to make you mad.

WENDAL: I'm not mad at you Dwayne.

DWAYNE: You not getting ready to leave again, are you?

REBA: No. Your Dad is gon' be right here. Now everybody let's eat. We letting the food get cold. *(Puts on the apron, starts serving, in silence everybody passes food.)* Dwayne sit down. *(DWAYNE hesitates, looks at his father expectantly.)* I said sit down Dwayne. *(DWAYNE takes his seat at the table.)* What part of the chicken you want Bailey?

BAILEY: *(Still angry.)* I don't care.

JUNIOR: Old man, you better care. Me and Wendal went through a lot of trouble. Ain't that right Bro? Wendal had me inspecting every chicken in the store.

MAYBELLE: Wendal, baby you and Junior done cooked a feast here. Yes Lord! I may have to hurt myself.

REBA: *(Looks up at WENDAL who's still standing away from the table.)* Wendal?

WENDAL: *(Looks at all of them for a moment, hesitates.)* Sorry Mama. I think I lost my appetite. *(WENDAL exits. Lights. Later on that night. WENDAL comes downstairs. He's sick. With much effort, he moves to the kitchen and gets ice water from the refrigerator. Takes his medicine, moves back to the living room. REBA enters wearing a robe. WENDAL quickly hides the medicine.)*

REBA: I didn't know anyone was down here. You feeling any better?

WENDAL: A little.

REBA: How 'bout some ginger ale? I don't know why, I just woke up and had a taste for some pop. You want some?

WENDAL: No.

REBA: Sorry everything didn't work out like you planned this evening. *(Pause.)* Everything was going fine. Why'd you have to fight with him?

WENDAL: *(Moving to the couch.)* Why don't you ask him that question?

REBA: *(Walking around the room.)* I'm glad you and Junior gon' paint in here. I'm a help. Since you all been here I feel kinda useful again. Lately, I seem to have a lot of time on my hands. Sometimes I catch myself sitting all day right there on that couch and Lord this house can get so quiet. With Dwayne not needing me as much . . . don't get me wrong, I'm not complaining. He's got a mind of his own, just like you did. Scares your father. Sometimes a father can't see his son for his own failings. You ever think about that?

WENDAL: Oh Mama. Why do you always defend him?

REBA: *(As if she didn't hear him.)* Oh me and Maybelle go but sometimes I think about what if . . . what if something happened to your father . . . he never wanted me to work. I ain't never been nothing but somebody's mother. And today I wondered if I had even been good at that. *(WEN-DAL looks at her directly and she at him.)* I defend him for the same reason I defend you . . . because you both a part of me. Now why don't you tell Mama what's bothering you. I let it go for a week but something's eating you alive, I saw it when you first walked through that door.

WENDAL: Nothing.

REBA: *(Firmly.)* I asked you a question. Don't let me have to ask you twice.

WENDAL: I haven't been well Mama. Been a little under the weather.

REBA: *(Relieved.)* Well, we'll just have to get you better. It's probably one of them flu bugs going around . . .

WENDAL: It's not that simple.

REBA: I'll make an appointment the first thing in the morning with Dr. Miller and . . .

WENDAL: Has he ever treated an AIDS patient?

REBA: *(Not registering.)* Oh, he's treated all kinds of things. *(What he said sinking in.)* A what?

WENDAL: I have AIDS Mama.

REBA: Well we'll just get you there and have him check you out.

WENDAL: Mama, do you ever hear what people really say? Did you hear me say I have AIDS?

REBA: No Wendal. AIDS, I don't know nothing about it. You ain't got that.

WENDAL: I do.

REBA: What I just say? I don't know nothing about no . . .

WENDAL: I'm sorry.

REBA: Oh my God, tell me you kidding Wendal.

WENDAL: I wish.

REBA: Bailey . . .

WENDAL: I haven't figured out how to tell him.

REBA: How? How did you get something like this?

WENDAL: I don't know.

REBA: *(Her anger and fear out of control, loud.)* What do you mean you don't know? You come home and you're dying of some disease and you don't know how the hell you got it.

WENDAL: I'm not dying. I have . . .

REBA: Did you have some kind of surgery and they gave you bad blood?

WENDAL: No. What difference does it make how I got it?

REBA: You been lying to us. You been home here and you ain't said a word . . .

WENDAL: Every day I tried to tell you . . . I practiced this speech . . .

REBA: I don't want to hear no damn speech. I want to hear how the hell you got this? You're not one of them that why you got so mad at dinner?

WENDAL: Mama.

REBA: No. No. I know you're not. You've been living with Simone . . .

WENDAL: *(Carefully choosing his words.)* Mama, you know that I never was quite right like Daddy used to say . . . *(No response from REBA.)* Try to understand Mama. I have relationships with women and sometimes with men.

REBA: No you don't, un-un. No you don't. You're my son, just like Junior . . . you're a man. You're supposed to . . .

WENDAL: Supposed to what? Be like Daddy. His world don't stretch no farther than this couch . . .

REBA: Boy, who the hell are you to judge anybody?

WENDAL: Mama, it's not much different than you and Auntie May?

REBA: What you say?

WENDAL: It's not so different than how you feel about Auntie May . . .

REBA: How dare you? How dare you twist me and Maybelle's relationship into this sickness you talking. That woman is like a sister to me. You hear me? A sister!

WENDAL: A sister that might as well live here. You closer to her than you are to Daddy.

REBA: *(Enraged.)* You shut up. Shut your mouth. Shut your filthy mouth. Don't be trying to compare that shit . . . my life ain't the one on trial here.

WENDAL: I'm sorry. I just thought you might understand Mama.

REBA: UNDERSTAND! How can a mother understand that? How can I understand that you're one of them people, that I raised a liar for a son . . . I was so happy . . .

WENDAL: Mama, forgive me. I would've done anything to spare you . . .

REBA: Is that why you don't come home?

WENDAL: It's hard pretending.

REBA: You don't have to pretend with us. We're your parents . . .

WENDAL: Yeah, right. Dad can't stand to hear anything about my life and where does he get off having Dwayne call him Daddy?

REBA: *(His last words lost on her.)* Couldn't you have given us a chance? Maybe we would have . . .

WENDAL: *(Softly, tries to touch her.)* I am now Mama.

REBA: *(Shudders at his touch, sharply.)* Don't you tell your father. You hear me? I'll tell him. It'll kill him if it came from you. *(More to herself)* I should've never let you leave here. Bailey told me . . . said I kept you too close, wasn't no room left over for him . . . he told me no good would ever come to you . . . he told me . . . *(Yelling.)* You better get down on your knees right now boy and you better pray, beg God's forgiveness for your nasty wicked ways . . .

WENDAL: Pray! Mama, what in the hell you think I've been doing? I've prayed every night. I laid in that hospital bed thirty two days and thirty two nights and all I did was pray. You know how lonely it is Mama to lay in a bed that ain't even your own for thirty two days, nothing but tubes and your own shit to keep you company; what it is to bite into a pillow all night so people can't hear you screaming? No TV, I didn't even have a quarter to buy myself a paper. I tried to get right with your God, I asked him for some spare time, to keep me from pitching my guts every hour, to keep me from shitting all over myself, to give me the strength to wipe my ass good enough so I didn't have to smell myself all night. I prayed that they would stop experimenting on me, stop the rashes, the infections, the sores up my ass. I prayed Mama for some company. I prayed that somebody would get their room wrong and happen into mine so I could talk to somebody, maybe they would even put their arms around me 'cause I was so damn scared, maybe it would be somebody who would come back, somebody who would want to know me for who I really was and I prayed harder and I prayed to your God that if I could just hold on, if I could just get home . . . I'm not going to apologize Mama for loving who I loved, I ain't even gonna apologize for getting this shit, I've lived a lie and I'm gonna have to answer for that, but I'll be damn if I'm gon' keep lying, I ain't got the energy. I'm a deal with it just like you taught me to deal with everything else that came my way . . . but I could use a little help Mama . . .

REBA: No more. You hear me Wendal? No more. I never thought I'd see the day I'd be ashamed of you, that I wouldn't even want to know you. *(She exits.)*

WENDAL: *(Quietly to himself.)* Well, welcome home Wendal. *(Lights. The next morning.* WENDAL *is still asleep on the couch.* DWAYNE *enters from the kitchen.)*

DWAYNE: *(Nudging* WENDAL.*)* Daddy. Daddy. You woke?

WENDAL: Hmm.

DWAYNE: Daddy, you woke?

WENDAL: I am now.

DWAYNE: You want to watch videos?

WENDAL: It's a little early, isn't it? *(*DWAYNE *turns on the television.)*

BAILEY: *(Coming down the stairs.)* I don't see why we have to go to Church today, it ain't even Sunday.

WENDAL: Morning Dad.

BAILEY: Morning. You feeling better this morning?

WENDAL: Yeah.

REBA: Dwayne!!!!

BAILEY: I don't know what's gotten into that woman this morning.

WENDAL: Go see what your Grandma wants.

DWAYNE: Ok. Granddaddy, I made you some toast. I left it on the table.

BAILEY: Thanks, 'cause if it's up to your Grandma, I'm not getting nothing this morning. She in some kind of state. *(*DWAYNE *exits, a moment.)*

WENDAL: Sorry 'bout last night. You've done a good job with him.

BAILEY: I tried.

WENDAL: It shows. *(Neither speak for a minute.)* Dad.

BAILEY: *(Overlapping.)* Son. *(They laugh.)*

WENDAL: Age before beauty.

BAILEY: *(Playfully.)* All right boy, I can still take you out. Only reason I ain't is 'cause I don't wanna mess up my Sunday-go-to meetin' clothes.

WENDAL: Dad, you'll never change.

BAILEY: *(More than a hint of seriousness.)* Do you want me to?

WENDAL: *(A moment.)* I try not to want for things anymore, 'specially things I have no control over.

BAILEY: Yeah, I guess that's probably wise. *(Another pause.)*

REBA: *(Yelling from upstairs.)* Bailey!!!

BAILEY: *(Yelling back)* What? What Reba?

REBA: Are you ready?

BAILEY: Yes woman. Yes. I been ready. *(To* WENDAL.*)* Now where were we? What were we talking 'bout?

WENDAL: You were 'bout to tell me you glad I'm home.

BAILEY: *(Looks at him for a moment.)* Why you trying to pick around inside me boy?

WENDAL: I wasn't. I was just . . . forget it.

BAILEY: *(Pause.)* You know my offer still stands. If you ever want to come work for me . . . I got a lotta plans for the store. Did I tell you I'm thinking about expanding?

WENDAL: Yes.

BAILEY: Not interested, huh?

WENDAL: I didn't say that.

BAILEY: Yeah.

REBA: *(Coming down the stairs carrying an overnight bag, overlapping.)* Look how nasty this table-cloth is. *(Whisks the table-cloth off the table, looks around trying to figure out where to put it.)*

BAILEY: Reba, the tablecloth wasn't that dirty. Leave it on the chair, we can get it when we get back.

REBA: I said it was nasty. I want it out of my sight.

BAILEY: Sugar, I don't know why you so upset but . . .

DWAYNE: And I don't understand why I have to go to Aunt May's. I can stay here, clean out the basement. Dad and I can clean it out and get it done by the time you get back. Right Dad?

BAILEY: That basement is filthy. Reba, if he's not going to Church, then why can't he stay here?

REBA: FINE. WHATEVER YOU SAY IS FINE BAILEY. WHAT DO I HAVE TO SAY ABOUT ANYTHING AROUND HERE ANYWAY? WHAT HAVE I EVER HAD TO SAY ABOUT ANYTHING?

BAILEY: I didn't mean it like that Reba. I just thought the boy might wanna . . .

WENDAL: Dwayne, why don't you go start on the basement while your grandparents and I talk.

DWAYNE: But am I staying home?

WENDAL: Yes. Now go. (DWAYNE *exits.*)

BAILEY: What's going on here?

WENDAL: Dad . . .

REBA: *(Cutting him off.)* Nothing. Bailey, I wanna talk to Wendal. Alone. Please wait for me in the car. Please.

BAILEY: Somethin' I should know?

WENDAL: Yes.

REBA: *(Overlapping.)* No. Bailey please. Please honey. And take the suitcase with you.

BAILEY: *(Picks up the suitcase, mumbling to himself)* A suitcase to church . . . it ain't even Sunday . . . all morning 'bout to take my head off, now I gotta go wait in the car like some child. *(He exits.)*

WENDAL: Mama, I should tell . . .

REBA: Shut up. Just shut up. Don't say a word. I heard enough from you last night to last me a lifetime. I'm about to walk out that door and try and explain to that man out there why I don't have a home no more. I hate what you've done to my house Wendal. Spent my life here, inside these walls, trying to stay safe, keep my family safe . . . didn't know any better, maybe if I had, I could deal with what you done brought in here. See this slipcover, I made it. And that afghan, I made that too, these curtains . . . I made this tablecloth, see this lace. I made you. My son! And I took such pride . . . but last night you made me realize I hadn't made nothing, not a damn thing . . . been walking around fooling myself. . . . It's hard to look at something . . . I mean I look around here and it's like somebody came in and smeared shit all over my walls . . . I'm scared to touch anything . . . you hear me Wendal, scared to touch anything in my own house. . . . Nothing. Maybe if I could get outside these walls I could . . . I can't stay here and watch it fester, crumble down around me . . . right now I can't help you . . . I can hardly stand to even look at you . . . I can't help your father . . . what good am I? I don't know anymore. I just know this house is closing in on me and I got to get out of here.

WENDAL: But Mama I can go.

REBA: Wouldn't make any difference. This ain't a home no more.

WENDAL: Mama, can we at least talk? I need you . . . if you would just let me . . .

REBA: You need?! Hmph! You need?!! I don't give a damn about what you need Wendal. Did you give a damn about us?

WENDAL: You act like I got this just to hurt you. . . . Don't leave Mama . . . I . . .

REBA: I can't help you right now. You understand? Mama can't help you. *(Starting to exit.)*

WENDAL: But where are you going? (REBA *exits.* WENDAL *throws something, maybe hits the door behind her as his beeper goes off he retrieves his pill box, gets ready to take his medicine but instead throws the pills across the room, after a moment.)*

DWAYNE: *(Enters.)* Dad, you ok? (WENDAL *jumps.)*

WENDAL: *(Snaps.)* Man, don't come up behind me like that.

DWAYNE: I'm sorry. Can I ask you something? (WENDAL *nods yes.)* I only need 'bout forty more dollars. Schools almost out and I thought I could go back with you for the summer. Simone said it was ok.

WENDAL: You talked to Simone?

DWAYNE: Yeah we were gonna surprise you. She said she was fixing me up a room.

WENDAL: Dwayne, Simone and I ain't together no more. So you don't have to pack up, your Dad plans to be around here.

DWAYNE: *(Excited.)* Really? Wow, then we could go places, go to all the games . . . Daddy, I mean Granddaddy, he takes me to the games and he tries to play ball . . . don't tell him I said this, but he's kind of old . . .

WENDAL: You don't have to worry, I won't tell him that. *(Pause.)* There's so much I want to say to you, like be careful how you judge people, weigh a man carefully, you never know when you may get on the same scale . . .

DWAYNE: You don't want me to be like Granddad.

WENDAL: What I want is for you to think for yourself, make your own choices, you know the kind you can defend, not with your fists but in your heart.

DWAYNE: I got it. So what we gon' do today?

WENDAL: Why don't you go work in the basement for a while. I'll take a shower, then we'll go somewhere, maybe to the Center or take in a movie . . .

JUNIOR: *(Entering.)* How come nobody woke me up?

DWAYNE: 'Cause you were snoring. Granddaddy say you sound worse than Amtrak.

JUNIOR: Ok man. I don't want to have to bust no head today. Have to do you like I used to do your Dad.

WENDAL: Why you wanna lie to the boy? Wasn't a day in the week that somebody wasn't going upside your head. Your Uncle always had a lotta mouth Dwayne.

JUNIOR: Don't let him lie to you. Your Uncle spent all his time defending your Dad.

WENDAL: *(Obviously there's some truth in JUNIOR's statement.)* Dwayne, the basement's calling you.

DWAYNE: Ok. But I wanna hear . . .

JUNIOR: I'll tell you if you wanna hear some stories . . .

WENDAL: The basement Dwayne. You can listen to your Uncle's tales later.

DWAYNE: Ok. You gon' call me when you ready to go? *(WENDAL shakes his head yes; DWAYNE exits.)*

JUNIOR: Where's the folks?

WENDAL: Church.

JUNIOR: *(Looking for food in the kitchen.)* Wait a minute. It's not Sunday. Well, maybe it's some type of social. Mama didn't cook? *(Takes the milk carton out and drinks from it.)*

WENDAL: I don't think so. Why did you have to say that shit in front of him?

JUNIOR: What?

WENDAL: Defending me.

JUNIOR: What in the hell is wrong with you Wendal? I was just kidding. What happened to your sense of humor? And I did have to kick ass because of you. I know what it is. You must not be getting none? Is that your problem?

WENDAL: Drop it man.

JUNIOR: Hey, I was just trying to make conversation. I can take my black ass back upstairs.

WENDAL: Junior wait. I'm just a little uptight.

JUNIOR: I can see that.

WENDAL: Ok already. Next subject. Service seems to agree with you. You look good. Going back to school when you get out?

JUNIOR: Nan, I don't think so.

WENDAL: Don't they pay for it?

JUNIOR: Yep.

WENDAL: So what's stopping you?

JUNIOR: Correct me if I'm wrong, but I don't remember you going back to school.

WENDAL: I know I didn't, that's why I'm trying to talk to you knuckle-head. Man, look at you, you got a lot going for you . . .

JUNIOR: Guess who you starting to sound like? Reason you can't get along 'cause you two are too much alike. And I sure as hell wish you'd stop using me in ya'lls battles. . . .

WENDAL: Man, what you talking about?

JUNIOR: I'm not the favorite Wendal. Just your stand-in. God forbid you ever get your life together.

WENDAL: I'll look over that last comment and deal with your initial silly ass statement. Dad's been throwing you up to me ever since I can remember. If Junior did it, why didn't I figure out a way to do it better . . .

JUNIOR: Hit the nail on the head. Only time I count is when brother Wendal is fucking up . . .

WENDAL: I don't want to talk about him. I was just trying to tell you something for your own good. Junior you oughtta finish your education . . .

JUNIOR: My own good is just that, my own good.

WENDAL: Man, your problem is you don't listen.

JUNIOR: Look who's talking. Seem to me, I listened better than you.

WENDAL: Not from where I'm sittin.'

JUNIOR: Well, you need to go sit somewhere else then. Look, I ain't trying to be you. Ain't into making no big inroads. Call me Joe-Regular. Go to work, have a family, retire. Simple. I don't fault you for your life, so get up offa me 'bout mine.

WENDAL: I didn't mean no harm.

JUNIOR: Yeah right. As long as we straight.

WENDAL: Guess I was just playing big brother. Didn't mean no harm.

JUNIOR: *(Pause.)* Want you to be my best man.

WENDAL: Say what?

JUNIOR: Yeah. Yeah. When the right woman comes along . . . what can I say? She teaches school, one of them fine church-going woman. Her name is A-nita and she loves my dirty drawers and Lord knows I can smell hers all day long, you hear me?

WENDAL: Man you crazy. *(They both laugh, it's a needed tension release.)* Congratulations Junior. *(Goes to hug him.)*

JUNIOR: Go on Wendal, you still ain't learned 'bout hugging up on men . . .

WENDAL: I love you man, that's all.

JUNIOR: I know that . . . we brothers. Man you been smoking some funny shit this early . . . *(WENDAL starts coughing uncontrollably.)* What's wrong with you Wendal?

WENDAL: Junior . . .

DWAYNE: *(Enters.)* I need some garbage bags. Dad, I thought you were gon' take a shower? If we don't get to the Center early . . . *(BAILEY enters, it's obvious he's trying hard to control himself.)*

JUNIOR: *(To DWAYNE.)* I don't think your father feels too well . . .

DWAYNE: What's wrong?

BAILEY: Come here.

WENDAL: What?

BAILEY: I said come here. Bring your ass over here and look me in my face.

WENDAL: Dwayne, go finish what you were doing.

BAILEY: No, you don't. Stand right there. Don't you move.

WENDAL: Dad, please, not in front of him.

JUNIOR: Can somebody tell me what's going on here? Wendal come on . . . let me help you . . .

BAILEY: *(Overlapping.)* Little late to be ashamed. *(BAILEY roughly grabs and examines WENDAL's arms.)* Where's your marks? Where you hiding 'em?

WENDAL: What marks?

BAILEY: You know what I'm talking about. You been doing drugs.

WENDAL: Dwayne, get outta here.

BAILEY: No. It's time he know the truth. . . .

WENDAL: I don't know what you talking about. Dwayne . . .

BAILEY: You don't know what I'm talking about? You don't know what I'm talking about!!! I'm one step off your ass boy . . .

JUNIOR: Dad, please he's sick.

BAILEY: He's sick alright. Tell him. Let me hear you tell your brother, hear you tell your son, tell 'em you's a junkie. . . . Tell them why your mother was ashamed to stay in the same house with you. Tell 'em Mr. Junkie . . .

WENDAL: I'm not a junkie . . .

BAILEY: Then what the hell are you? *(The question hangs in the air, recognition, finally.)* I never laid a hand on you but you better get out my sight before I kick you straight to hell's door.

JUNIOR: Will somebody clue me in?

WENDAL: Dad, if you'd let me explain . . . I'm not sure how I got it. . . .

BAILEY: I don't wanna know how you got it. The sight of you breaks my heart. I oughtta kill you. *(Shoves him.)*

DWAYNE: Granddaddy, what's wrong?

WENDAL: It's ok Dwayne. Go on now. Your grandfather is just upset about something.

JUNIOR: *(Overlapping.)* Man stop it. Can't you see he's sick? I don't know what's going on here, but you gon' have to come through me 'cause I ain't gon' let you lay another hand on him . . .

BAILEY: Boy get out of my way. I'll go through you and anybody else. He won't need the AIDS when I get through. . . .

JUNIOR: What you say?

BAILEY: AIDS. That's what I said.

JUNIOR: Naw Wendal. It can't be. You ain't got that. Tell me you ain't got that.

DWAYNE: Dad?

WENDAL: Dwayne . . . I'm sorry. If you all would just let me explain . . . I didn't know if you'd understand. . . .

BAILEY: You right. I don't understand. You no son of mine. In my house. . . . Did you hear me? *(Violently throws* WENDAL *on the floor, who attempts to crawl away from him.)* Take your sissy fairy ass and get the hell out of my house.

JUNIOR: What the fuck you doing? He's sick. Look at him.

WENDAL: *(Reaches out for* DWAYNE.*)* Dwayne . . . (DWAYNE *backs off, exits.)*

JUNIOR: Wendal why? Naw, I can't deal with this. . . . Can't deal with this right now . . . I looked up to you . . . I looked up to him . . . I can't deal with this . . . I . . . I . . . can't . . .

BAILEY: *(To* JUNIOR.*)* Boy, stop that whining. (JUNIOR *is crying, turns his back, walks away to exit.)* Did you hear me? Stop all that whimpering. *(Just before* JUNIOR *is almost out the room.)* Where you think you goin'?

You just gon' turn your back? Raised you to turn your back on your
brother? *(JUNIOR stops, but doesn't turn around.)*

JUNIOR: Don't do it Dad . . .

BAILEY: I'm talking to you Junior. You a man or not? Are you a man or not?

JUNIOR: *(Pause, finally turns around, he's crying.)* It's not gon' work this
time. You hear me? It's not gon' work Dad. You got what you always
wanted. Right there. He's all yours. *(Turns around to exit.)*

BAILEY: Boy, don't you turn your back to me. Don't you ever turn your
back to me.

JUNIOR: Fuck you. Is that man enough for you? There's your son Dad.
There's the man you always wanted. *(He exits.)*

BAILEY: *(Pause.)* Get up. I said get up. Get up Wendal.

WENDAL: I can't Daddy.

BAILEY: *(A beat as the anger is replaced by grief.)* If you could've just told me.
Wendal, if you could've just told me. If you could've just told me . . . you my
son . . . what we gon' do? *(Eventually he drops to his knees, scoops up WEN-
DAL, maybe rocks him, cries.)* you my son . . . don't cry Wendal . . . don't cry,
we gon' get through this . . . we Bailey men don't give up, do we? . . . just
you and me now. Oh Wendal I been waitin' . . . waitin' so long for you to
grow into somethin' . . . you my son . . . God help me . . . what I got to wait
on now? *(Lights dim as attendants wheel hospital bed into the BAILEY living
room. WENDAL is placed in the bed, maybe BAILEY helps. IV is hooked up.
BAILEY exits. A passage of time—it's weeks later. BAILEY enters carrying
wood. He is a changed man: gone is the neat appearance, the sense of order
and control. He drops the wood, then opens WENDAL's saxophone case, crosses
to the kitchen, retrieves a towel, forgets why he has the towel . . . looks over at
WENDAL retrieves and puts on rubber gloves . . . cleans him up.)* You woke?

WENDAL: Where's Dwayne?

BAILEY: Maybelle's bringing him.

WENDAL: Mama?

BAILEY: *(An untruth)* She asked about you. *(Turning him to check the bed
pad.)*

WENDAL: Really?

BAILEY: Yeah.

WENDAL: She coming home?

BAILEY: Yeah. And she'll be sending your dinner after awhile . . .

WENDAL: I was gon' take him on the train with me. Remember when we
took the train.

BAILEY: Yeah. I remember. Look. I brought the wood in . . . member for the
cabinets? We can sand a little after you have your supper.

WENDAL: Look Wendal, you see it? That's red dirt . . . sweet Mississippi dirt. I see it Dad. Mama, you see it? Mama?

BAILEY: *(Helpless, but with forced cheerfulness.)* You hungry? Maybe a little something. It was something else I was 'bout to do. Now what was it. . . . Oh I know. I was gon' clean up your horn for you. Shine it up, so you'd be real slick when you start playing again. Got to get this place cleaned up before your Mama gets home. She'll have my head on a platter, letting this house go like this. *(Starts to pick up a little: maybe strewn newspapers, mail)* How 'bout a little soup? Couldn't get off to sleep last night, that couch ain't that comfortable, so I got up 'bout three with this bright idea. Thought I'd make you some soup . . . cut up a lot of vegetables in it. *(WENDAL moans.)* I know the sores hurt, *(Losing control.)* but how the hell you gon' get well if you don't eat somethin'? *(Recovers, less harsh, starts shining the saxophone.)* Yeah, I'll get this shined up for you. *(Blows a note or two on the horn.)* You wanna give it a try? *(Takes the horn to the bed, waits for WENDAL to take, no response.)* Well, maybe a little later. Later on maybe you'll feel like playing, a little something. *(Places the horn on the table.)* Yeah it's a beautiful day outside. I wish you could see it. *(Crosses to the window, to himself.)* Your Mama likes days like this, she'd be out there in that garden right now wearing that funny hat with the fruit on it . . . I got to figure out what I should put on to go over there. What you think? My blue suit or the black one? You wait a minute and I'm a go get 'em . . . then we can decide. *(Just then DWAYNE and MAYBELLE enter. MAYBELLE wears a hooded rain poncho, a wool scarf wrapped around her face and on her hands are oven mitts. DWAYNE has a large bruise on his face; gone is the innocence, the sweetness; he's an angry little boy who doesn't know what to do with his anger, with any of his feelings.)* Hi. I'm glad ya'll got here . . . just getting ready . . . Maybelle, what in the hell do you have on? It must be ninety degrees outside. If you don't look ridiculous . . .

MAYBELLE: I didn't want to take any chances. *(Looks around at all the things down in the house.)*

BAILEY: Maybelle, if it wasn't for ignorance, you wouldn't have no sense at all. And Dwayne what you hiding back there for? Come over here. *(Reluctantly DWAYNE crosses.)* Get over here! *(Notices the bruise.)* You been fighting? *(No response from DWAYNE who looks at him defiantly.)* Did you hear me ask you a question?

MAYBELLE: Them kids making that boy's life miserable.

DWAYNE: I can handle myself.

BAILEY: You try handling yourself some other kinda way. You speak to your Dad? *(No response from DWAYNE.)* Boy get over there before that ain't the only bruise you sportin'.

DWAYNE: *(Crosses to the bed, has a hard time looking at* WENDAL; *begrudgingly.)* Hi.

BAILEY: *(Takes* MAYBELLE *to the side.)* How's Reba today? *(Now that* BAILEY *isn't looking* DWAYNE *moves away from the bed.)*

MAYBELLE: The same. Driving me nuts. Bathing all day and when she ain't in the tub she's somewhere changing clothes. I swear she ain't never been a vain woman, but now she hangs in that mirror for hours . . . I don't know what she sees . . . I wish she'd cry or yell or do something . . . 'cause right now I can't reach her . . . everyday she slipping a little further away from me. *(Whispers.)* Spends half the night watching Dwayne sleep. That's right, I'm telling you the truth, she sits straight up in that chair and watches that boy sleep, and then she goes in the room and the rest of the night she's walking and talking, to who I don't know, to herself or God one. . . . She misses you.

BAILEY: Then she oughtta come home.

MAYBELLE: *(Pause.)* Today's menu: chicken and fried corn. I tried to get Reba to help . . .

BAILEY: *(Taking the tin foil off the plate.)* This looks good. Wendal likes fried corn. Look Wendal.

MAYBELLE: Bailey you know he can't eat that.

BAILEY: How you know what he can eat? How do any of y'all know what he can eat? I been in this house with this boy for weeks and has anybody come by? Has anyone bothered to come and see what he can eat?

MAYBELLE: I'm doing the best I can. I cook everyday for you . . . I don't know what else you expect . . . I'm taking care of Reba and that boy. Come on Dwayne let's go.

BAILEY: What you mean? Ya'll just got here. I was hoping you'd stay with him so I could go sit with Reba a while . . . *(*WENDAL *grunts, moans.)*

MAYBELLE: *(Timidly, waves.)* Hi Wendal. It's Maybelle, Auntie May. I can't stay . . .

BAILEY: What's wrong with you? Even if he wanted to, he ain't got the strength to bite your ass.

MAYBELLE: It ain't no cause for you to talk to me like that.

BAILEY: And it ain't no cause for you to be afraid of him like that. Why don't you touch him . . .

MAYBELLE: Have you gone nuts?

BAILEY: *(The cost of all the weeks of holding it together, he explodes; there's an edge of madness, grabs her, forces her to the bed.)* I said touch him. You used to rock him and sing to him, just like he was your own. . . . 'I want you to touch him . . . right now . . .

MAYBELLE: Bailey let go of me. You scaring me.

BAILEY: Good. Touch him. That's my son you treating like some leper. I said touch him.

MAYBELLE: *(Terrified, crying.)* Let me go Bailey. Let me go. I can't. Please.

BAILEY: What if it was one of your sons? Huh?

MAYBELLE: I wouldn't touch them either. I wouldn't have no AIDS in my house.

WENDAL: *(Overlapping.)* Dad, it hurts.

BAILEY: *(Quickly letting go of* MAYBELLE, *who retreats.)* I'm right here Wendal.

WENDAL: I wanna go. Help me. It hurts. I gotta go see Simone . . .

BAILEY: Now hold on Wendal. Dwayne's here. *(To* DWAYNE.*)* Say something to him.

DWAYNE: *(Still defiant.)* What?

BAILEY: Tell him you love him. *(No response from* DWAYNE, *pleading.)* Please Dwayne. Tell him something. Anything. He's still your father. You may not get another chance. . . . He's still . . . (DWAYNE *doesn't move.)*

WENDAL: *(Overlapping.)* You see that plot of land, that's where your man started kicking . . .

BAILEY: *(Panicking.)* Fight Wendal. Remember what I told you 'bout fighting. Don't let him take you out. Stay on the ropes son. . . . You can't give up. Come on. Don't give up. I'm in there with you. Ain't gon' let you go yet. . . . Come on son, fight now.

MAYBELLE: I got to get out of here. I'll send Reba. Come on Dwayne. (DWAYNE *doesn't move).* Wendal, Auntie May love you. I'm so sorry. *(She exits.)*

WENDAL: *(Overlapping)* I'm riding Dad. I'm on the train. I see you . . . Junior. I see Dwayne . . . Mama . . . (SIMONE *enters in profile on the other side of the stage, a special light.)* Simone . . . *(Gasping for breath.)* She's pregnant. Oh my God no . . . I'm so sorry Simone . . . I'm sorry . . .

BAILEY: I'm right here Wendal, but don't die on me. Please, don't leave me. . . . (BAILEY *screams.)* NO. . . . *(Sobbing.)* Don't take him. Don't take him. God, give me some more time with him . . . just one more day, please don't take him. *(Lights on* SIMONE. SIMONE *takes off her earrings, then her wig and then the robe and transforms into* ANGEL PETERSON *from Act One.)*

SIMONE: *(Fully transformed.)* God don't have nothing to do with it. Time to get on board Wendal Bailey. Welcome to the family . . . *(As lights go down,* ANGEL *sings the same song* WENDAL *was singing in the first scene in the reception area).*

The End